High-Yield™

Comprehensive USMLE STEP 1 REVIEW

High-Yield™
Comprehensive USMLE STEP 1 REVIEW

Barbara Fadem, PhD
Professor
Department of Psychiatry
University of Medicine and Dentistry
of New Jersey
New Jersey Medical School
Newark, New Jersey

Ronald W. Dudek, PhD
Professor of Anatomy
East Carolina University
Brody School of Medicine
Greenville, North Carolina

Pamela C. Champe, PhD
Professor Emeritus
Department of Biochemistry
University of Medicine and Dentistry
Robert Wood Johnson Medical School
Piscataway, New Jersey

Richard A. Harvey, PhD
Professor Emeritus
Department of Biochemistry
University of Medicine and Dentistry
Robert Wood Johnson Medical School
Piscataway, New Jersey

Ivan Damjanov, MD, PhD
Professor of Pathology
University of Kansas Medical School
Kansas City, Kansas

Arthur G. Johnson, PhD
Professor Emeritus
Department of Medical Microbiology
and Immunology
University of Minnesota
Duluth School of Medicine
Duluth, Minnesota

Charles R. Craig, PhD
Professor of Neurobiology and Anatomy
School of Medicine, West Virginia University
Director of the West Virginia University Office
of Research Compliance
Morgantown, West Virginia

Todd Nelson, MD
Resident Physician
Department of Anesthesia
University of Iowa Hospitals and Clinics
Iowa City, Iowa

Edward A. Monaco III, PhD
College of Physicians & Surgeons
Columbia University
New York, New York

⊞ Lippincott Williams & Wilkins
a Wolters Kluwer business
Philadelphia · Baltimore · New York · London
Buenos Aires · Hong Kong · Sydney · Tokyo

Acquisitions Editor: Donna Balado
Developmental Editor: Kathleen H. Scogna
Marketing Manager: Emilie Linkins
Production Editor: Christina Remsberg
Designer: Doug Smock
Compositor: Circle Graphics
Printer: Courier

Printed in the United States of America

Library of Congress Cataloging-in-Publication Data

High-yield comprehensive USMLE step 1 review / Barbara Fadem ... [et al.].
     p. ; cm.
 ISBN-13: 978-0-7817-7427-7
 ISBN-10: 0-7817-7427-6
1. Medicine—Examinations, questions, etc. 2. Physicians—Licenses—United States—Examinations—Study guides.
 [DNLM: 1. Clinical Medicine—Examination Questions. WB 18.2 H638 2007]
I. Fadem, Barbara.
R834.5.H54 2007
610.76—dc22

                     2005027313

To purchase additional copies of this book, call our customer service department at **(800) 638-3030** or fax orders to **(301) 824-7390**. International customers should call **(301) 714-2324**.

Visit Lippincott Williams & Wilkins on the Internet: *http://www.LWW.com.* Lippincott Williams & Wilkins customer service representatives are available from 8:30 am to 6:00 pm, EST.

06 07 08 09 10
1 2 3 4 5 6 7 8 9 10

Dedication

TO OUR EXTRAORDINARY MEDICAL STUDENTS—*as teachers and authors, we greatly appreciate the opportunity to again help you successfully complete the requirements for licensure and practice.*

Preface

High-Yield Comprehensive USMLE Step 1 Review is designed to be used to study for the first of the three steps of the United States Medical Licensing Examination (USMLE). The aim of the authors is to provide an inclusive yet manageable tool containing only the highest yield information for the USMLE Step 1. The book covers all of the major topics tested on the exam in a tabular format designed to make the best use of the limited study time available to medical students.

The book is divided into seven major sections: Behavioral Science; Gross Anatomy, Embryology, and Histology/Cell Biology; Physiology; Pathology; Microbiology/Immunology; Biochemistry; and Pharmacology. The authors of each section are experts in their fields; most have authored review books, and all have expert knowledge of the material required for the USMLE Step 1. Most sections of the book were also edited by Dr. Edward Monaco and Dr. Todd Nelson, who, as senior medical students/residents were recently highly successful in their personal encounters with USMLE Steps 1 and 2.

Each major section of the book begins with a TEN TOP TIPS table. These tables contain the highest yield USMLE topics in that discipline, including for each tip a representative Step 1 focus clinical example. These identified high-yield topics are then discussed in detail in each section using only the most USMLE relevant material.

The **Behavioral Science** section is written by **Barbara Fadem**, PhD, professor of psychiatry, New Jersey Medical School in Newark, New Jersey. Dr. Fadem's popular review books include *BRS Behavioral Science, High -Yield Behavioral Science, High-Yield Psychiatry*, and *Psychiatry Recall*. Her recently published text book, *Behavioral Science in Medicine*, has been adopted as a course text by a number of medical schools and related programs.

The **Gross Anatomy, Embryology, Histology/Cell Biology** section is written by **Ronald Dudek**, PhD, professor, East Carolina University, Brody School of Medicine in Greenville, North Carolina. Dr. Dudek is the author of the well-received review books *BRS Embryology, High-Yield Embryology, High-Yield Histology, High-Yield Cell and Molecular Biology*, and *High-Yield Gross Anatomy*. He is currently preparing a series of high-yield books with a systems approach, the first of which, *High-Yield Lung,* has recently been published.

Edward A. Monaco III, who wrote the **Physiology** section, holds a Ph.D. in Neuroscience from SUNY Upstate Medical University and is currently completing his medical studies at Columbia University College of Physicians and Surgeons in New York City. Dr. Monaco also helped to design and edit both the Anatomy and Microbiology sections of the book. **Todd Nelson**, MD, a medical resident at the University of Iowa, was closely involved in creative and editorial work involving the Biochemistry, Pharmacology, and Pathology sections of the book.

The **Pathology** section is written by **Ivan Damjanov**, MD, PhD, professor of pathology, University of Kansas Medical School in Kansas City, Kansas. Dr. Damjanov is the author of *High-Yield Pathology, Histopathology Atlas,* and *Pathology Secrets.*

The **Microbiology/Immunology** section is written by **Arthur G. Johnson**, PhD, professor emeritus, University of Minnesota—Duluth School of Medicine in Duluth, Minnesota. Dr. Johnson is the author of *High-Yield Immunology.*

Pamela Champe, PhD, and **Richard Harvey**, PhD, professors emeriti of Biochemistry, University of Medicine and Dentistry—Robert Wood Johnson Medical School in Piscataway, New Jersey, are the authors of the **Biochemistry** section. Drs. Champe and Harvey have written many books for medical students, including the popular *Lippincott Illustrated Reviews: Pharmacology, Lippincott Illustrated Reviews: Biochemistry,* and *Lippincott Illustrated Reviews: Microbiology.*

The **Pharmacology** section is written by **Charles R. Craig**, PhD, professor of neurobiology and anatomy in the School of Medicine, West Virginia University, and Director of the West Virginia University Office of Research Compliance in Morgantown, West Virginia. Dr. Craig is also the author of *Modern Pharmacology with Clinical Applications* (with Dr. Bob Stitzel), which is currently in the sixth edition.

Acknowledgments

The authors acknowledge with great thanks Kathleen Scogna and the staff at Lippincott, Williams & Wilkins for their able, helpful, and available assistance.

Figure Credits

I-1   Adapted from Wedding D. *Behavior and Medicine.* St. Louis: Mosby-Year Book, 1995:416.

I-2   From Fadem B. *High-Yield Behavioral Science,* 2nd ed. Baltimore: Lippincott Williams & Wilkins, 2003:114.

II-1   From Dudek RW. *High-Yield Embryology,* 2nd ed. Baltimore: Lippincott Williams & Wilkins, 2001:20.

II-2   From Dudek RW, Fix JD. BRS *Embryology,* 3rd ed. Baltimore: Lippincott Williams & Wilkins, 2005:65.

II-3   From Dudek RW. *High-Yield Embryology,* 2nd ed. Baltimore: Lippincott Williams & Wilkins, 2001:61.

II-4   From Dudek RW, Fix JD. *BRS Embryology,* 3rd ed. Baltimore: Lippincott Williams & Wilkins, 2005:54.

II-5   From Moore KL, Dalley AF. *Clinically Oriented Anatomy,* 5th ed. Baltimore: Lippincott Williams & Wilkins, 2005:527.

II-6   From Dudek RW. *High-Yield Gross Anatomy,* 2nd ed. Baltimore: Lippincott Williams & Wilkins, 2002:17.

II-8   Adapted from Moore KL. *Clinically Oriented Anatomy,* 3rd ed. Baltimore: Lippincott Williams & Wilkins, 1992:210.

II-7   From Dudek RW. *High-Yield Systems: Heart.* Baltimore: Lippincott Williams & Wilkins, 2006: Fig. 2-4.

II-9   From Dudek RW. *High-Yield Gross Anatomy,* 2nd ed. Baltimore: Lippincott Williams & Wilkins, 2002:59.

II-10   Adapted from Ernest WA. *NMS Anatomy,* 2nd ed. Media, PA: Harwal, 1990:225.

II-11   From Dudek RW. *High-Yield Gross Anatomy,* 2nd ed. Baltimore: Lippincott Williams & Wilkins, 2002:158.

II-12   From Fix JD. *High-Yield Neuroanatomy,* 3rd ed. Baltimore: Lippincott Williams & Wilkins, 2005:29.

II-13   From Fix JD. *High-Yield Neuroanatomy,* 3rd ed. Baltimore: Lippincott Williams & Wilkins, 2005:132.

II-14   From Fix JD. *High-Yield Neuroanatomy,* 3rd ed. Baltimore: Lippincott Williams & Wilkins, 2005:117.

II-15   From Fix JD. *High-Yield Neuroanatomy,* 3rd ed. Baltimore: Lippincott Williams & Wilkins, 2005:146.

II-16   From Fix JD. *High-Yield Neuroanatomy,* 3rd ed. Baltimore: Lippincott Williams & Wilkins, 2005:139.

II-17   From Fix JD. *High-Yield Neuroanatomy,* 3rd ed. Baltimore: Lippincott Williams & Wilkins, 2005:62.

II-18   Adapted from April EW. *NMS Clinical Anatomy,* 3rd ed. Baltimore: Williams & Wilkins, 1997.

II-19   From Dudek RW. *High-Yield Gross Anatomy,* 2nd ed. Baltimore: Lippincott Williams & Wilkins, 2002:152.

II-20   From Fix JD. *High-Yield Neuroanatomy,* 3rd ed. Baltimore: Lippincott Williams & Wilkins, 2005: 119.

II-21   From Fix JD. *High-Yield Neuroanatomy,* 3rd ed. Baltimore: Lippincott Williams & Wilkins, 2005:70.

II-22   From Dudek RW. *High-Yield Histology,* 3rd ed. Baltimore: Lippincott Williams & Wilkins, 2004:179.

II-23   From Dudek RW. *High-Yield Histology,* 3rd ed. Baltimore: Lippincott Williams & Wilkins, 2004:210.

II-24   From Dudek RW. *High-Yield Histology,* 3rd ed. Baltimore: Lippincott Williams & Wilkins, 2004:133.

II-25   From Dudek RW. *High-Yield Histology,* 3rd ed. Baltimore: Lippincott Williams & Wilkins, 2004:128.

III-1   Adapted from Cohen JJ, Kassirer JP. *Acid/Base.* Boston: Little, Brown, 1982.

IV-1   From Damjanov I. *High-Yield Pathology,* 2nd ed. Baltimore: Lippincott Williams & Wilkins, 2005:3.

IV-2   From Damjanov I. *High-Yield Pathology,* 2nd ed. Baltimore: Lippincott Williams & Wilkins, 2005:3.

IV-3   From Damjanov I. *High-Yield Pathology,* 2nd ed. Baltimore: Lippincott Williams & Wilkins, 2005:44.

IV-4   From Damjanov I. *High-Yield Pathology,* 2nd ed. Baltimore: Lippincott Williams & Wilkins, 2005:53.

IV-5   From Damjanov I. *High-Yield Pathology,* 2nd ed. Baltimore: Lippincott Williams & Wilkins, 2005:71.

IV-6   From Damjanov I. *High-Yield Pathology,* 2nd ed. Baltimore: Lippincott Williams & Wilkins, 2005:77.

IV-7   From Damjanov I. *High-Yield Pathology,* 2nd ed. Baltimore: Lippincott Williams & Wilkins, 2005:86.

IV-8   From Damjanov I. *High-Yield Pathology,* 2nd ed. Baltimore: Lippincott Williams & Wilkins, 2005:87.

IV-9   From Damjanov I. *High-Yield Pathology,* 2nd ed. Baltimore: Lippincott Williams & Wilkins, 2005:140.

V-1   Adapted from Atlas RM. *Microbiology: Fundamentals and Application,* 2nd ed. New York: Macmillan, 1988:215.

V-2   Adapted from Benjamini E. *Immunology: A Short Course,* 3rd ed. New York: Wiley-Liss, Inc., a subsidiary of John Wiley & Sons, 1996:98.

V-3   Johnson AG, Clarke BL. *High-Yield Immunology,* 2nd ed. Baltimore: Lippincott Williams & Wilkins, 2006:30.

V-4   Adapted from Kuby J. *Immunology,* 3rd ed. New York: WH Freeman, 1997.

V-5   Johnson AG, Clarke BL. *High-Yield Immunology,* 2nd ed. Baltimore: Lippincott Williams & Wilkins, 2006:69.

VII-1   From Craig CR, Stitzel RE. *Modern Pharmacology with Clinical Applications,* 6th ed. Baltimore: Lippincott Williams & Wilkins, 2004:84.

VII-3   From Christ D. *High-Yield Pharmacology,* 2nd ed. Baltimore: Lippincott Williams & Wilkins, 2004:80.

VII-2   Adapted from Mycek MJ, Gertner SB, Perper MM [Harvey RA, Champe PC, ed]. *Lippincott's Illustrated Reviews: Pharmacology,* 2nd ed. Philadelphia: Lippincott-Raven, 1997:224.

VII-4   From Christ D. *High-Yield Pharmacology,* 2nd ed. Baltimore: Lippincott Williams & Wilkins, 2004:57.

VII-5   From Christ D. *High-Yield Pharmacology,* 2nd ed. Baltimore: Lippincott Williams & Wilkins, 2004:101.

VII-6   From Craig CR, Stitzel RE. *Modern Pharmacology with Clinical Applications,* 6th ed. Baltimore: Lippincott Williams & Wilkins, 2004:568.

VII-7   From Ramachandran A. *Pharmacology Recall.* Philadelphia: Lippincott Williams & Wilkins, 2000:278.

Contents

I Behavioral Science 1

Barbara Fadem, PhD

II Gross Anatomy, Embryology, and Histology/Cell Biology 41

Ronald Dudek, PhD

III Physiology 89

Edward A. Monaco III, PhD

IV Pathology 151

Ivan Damjanov, MD, PhD

V Microbiology/Immunology 219

Arthur G. Johnson, PhD

VI Biochemistry 259

Pamela C. Champe, PhD and Richard A. Harvey, PhD

Behavioral Science

10 Top Tips

Behavioral Science

Topic	Main Focus	USMLE Example
1 The Life Cycle	Physical, social, and cognitive development in children	• A normal 3-year-old child can ride a tricycle, speak in complete sentences, and show parallel play. She is toilet trained, has no conception that death is final, and willingly goes to nursery school for four hours each day.
2 Biological Bases of Behavior	Neurological changes in psychiatric illness	• A functional magnetic resonance image of the brain of a 45-year-old man with schizophrenia shows increased size of the cerebral ventricles, decreased frontal lobe activity, and decreased limbic system activity.
3 Psychological Bases of Behavior	Defense mechanisms and related issues	• A 35-year-old man who was very sloppy as a child grows up to become a famous abstract painter. This is an example of use of the mature defense mechanism of sublimation.
4 Psychopathology	Emotional illness that presents as physical illness	• A 32-year-old woman who, in the absence of physical findings, has been tired, has headaches, and has lost interest in her usual activities over the past 3 months should be evaluated for major depressive disorder.
5 Sleep and Sleep Disorders	Sleep stages and brain changes in aging and in depression	• The sleep pattern of an 85-year-old man is characterized by decreased delta and rapid eye movement (REM) sleep and poor sleep efficiency.

(Continued)

10 Top Tips

Behavioral Science *(Continued)*

Topic	Main Focus	USMLE Example
6 Sexuality and Aggression	Action by the physician in suspected child, elder, and domestic partner abuse	• A 1-year-old child has an unexplained head injury and a fractured radius. This should be reported to state health authorities; neither parental notification nor permission to treat is required.
7 The Doctor–Patient Relationship	Physicians' responses to difficult situations involving patients	• A 27-year-old patient asks his physician for a date. The physician should refuse. It is not appropriate for a physician to have a romantic relationship with a patient, former patient, patient's relative, or patient's friend.
8 Psychoactive Substance Abuse	Substance abuse presenting as psychiatric illness	• A 23-year-old man in the ER shows paranoia and anxiety. A toxicology screen should be done. The patient is more likely to have abused a substance than to have a psychotic illness such as schizophrenia.
9 Legal and Ethical Issues in Medicine	Making health care decisions	• An 18-year-old Jehovah's witness refuses to have a life-saving blood transfusion. Respect her wishes but note that she cannot refuse necessary treatment for her child or spouse.
10 Epidemiology and Biostatistics	How sensitivity, specificity, and predictive values are calculated and how they are related to the prevalence of disease	• If the prevalence of a disease is higher in one population than another (e.g. prostate cancer is more prevalent in old men than in young men), the sensitivity and specificity of screening tests for the illness will be the same in both populations but positive predictive value will be higher and negative predictive value will be lower in the group where prevalence is higher (e.g. old men).

Topic **1**

The Life Cycle

Must
Knows

- Motor, social, and cognitive skills of children ages 4 months, 8 months, 18 months, 3 years, 8 years, and 15 years (Table I-1)

- The definitions of developmental milestones such as the social smile, stranger anxiety, separation anxiety, object permanence, and conscience/empathy (the superego)

- The distinction between a normal grief reaction (bereavement) and an abnormal grief reaction (depression)

CHILDBIRTH AND THE POSTPARTUM PERIOD

Infant mortality in the United States
- Rates are higher than in other developed countries
- Rates are at least twice as high among African American infants as white American infants

TABLE I-1	MOTOR, SOCIAL, AND VERBAL AND COGNITIVE DEVELOPMENT OF NORMAL CHILDREN		
	Skill Area		
Age	**Motor**	**Social**	**Verbal and Cognitive**
4 months	• Supports own head	• Shows the social smile	• Coos and babbles
8 months	• Turns over, sits alone	• Shows stranger anxiety	• Imitates sounds
18 months	• Walks alone • Climbs stairs using one foot • Scribbles on paper	• Shows separation anxiety • Shows object permanence	• Uses 10 words in one- or two-word sentences
3 years	• Rides a tricycle • Climbs stairs using alternate feet • Copies a circle and cross	• Shows parallel play • Develops gender identity • Is toilet trained	• Uses 900 words in complete and understandable sentences
8 years	• Rides a bicycle • Competes in games	• Has only same sex friends • Develops morality and empathy	• Reads, calculates, thinks logically
15 years	• Skills near adult levels	• Behavior influenced most strongly by peers	• Thinks abstractly

The Apgar score	• Quantifies physical condition of newborns at 1 and 5 (or 10) minutes after birth using five measures
	• Each measure can have a score of 0, 1, or 2 (highest score = 10)
	• Measures are heart rate (slow to fast), respiratory effort (slow to good), muscle tone (limp to active), color of body and extremities (blue to pink), and reflex irritability (low to high)
	• Score > 7 = no imminent survival threat; score < 4 = imminent survival threat
Maternal reactions to childbirth	• The "baby blues" (emotionality, crying) is common and normal
	• Baby blues starts within a few days and can last 1 to 2 weeks after childbirth
	• Management of baby blues involves support and practical help
	• More serious and less common, major depression, with or without psychotic features or brief (lasting less than 4 weeks) psychotic disorder can also occur
	• If psychotic, the mother may harm the infant
	• Management of mothers with these more serious conditions involves appropriate psychopharmacology and hospitalization if necessary

INFANTS (AGE 0 TO 1 YEAR) AND TODDLERS (AGE 1.0 TO 2.5 YEARS): TASKS AND MILESTONES

Major task	• To form an intimate attachment to the primary caregiver, usually the mother (infants)
	• To learn to separate from the primary caregiver (toddlers)
Developmental milestones (see Table I-1)	• The social smile: Smiling in response to a human face (1–2 months)
	• Stranger anxiety: Showing fear when confronted with an unfamiliar person (7–8 months)
	• Object permanence: Maintaining the mental image of an object or person without seeing it (12 months)
	• Normal separation anxiety (fearfulness when the mother leaves) (1–3 years)
	• Parallel play: Playing alongside but not cooperatively with other children (2–4 years)
	• First words and first steps occur on or about the first birthday
	• At age 2 years, "no" is the favorite word
Fears, illness, and death	• With extended absence (or lack of responsiveness) of the mother, infants are at risk for depression, developmental delay, and poor health and growth (formerly called failure to thrive; now called reactive attachment disorder of infancy or early childhood)
	• Greatest fear when ill is separation from caregiver
	• Has no conception of death

PRESCHOOL CHILDREN (AGE 2.5 TO 6 YEARS): TASKS AND MILESTONES

Major task	• To learn to function and interact with other people
Developmental milestones	• Can spend a few hours away from the mother in the care of others (e.g., in day care). If not able to do this by age 3 years, the child is experiencing separation anxiety disorder • Is toilet trained (3 years) • Plays cooperatively with other children (4 years) • Has imaginary friends (4 years) • Begins to develops a conscience (the superego) and feelings of empathy (see below) and morality (6 years)
Fears, illness, and death	• Life stress (e.g., moving, gaining a new sibling) may result in regression, a defense mechanism in which the child temporarily behaves in a "baby-like" way (e.g., bedwetting) • Has transient irrational fears (i.e., phobias) • Greatest fear when ill is bodily injury or disfigurement • Does not yet understand that death is permanent and typically expects that a dead pet or relative will come back to life

SCHOOL AGE CHILDREN (AGE 6 TO 12 YEARS)

Major task	• To develop a sense of competence and self-esteem
Developmental milestones	• Identifies with the parent of the same gender • Psychosexual issues are dormant (Freud's "latency" stage) • After age 6 years, the child can put her- or himself in another person's place (i.e., show empathy) • Develops the capacity for logical thought (e.g., an object can be both red and metal at the same time) and can follow rules • Understands the concept of conservation (e.g., no matter how many pieces you cut a hot dog in, it is still only one hot dog). • Involvement with people outside of the family (e.g., teachers; group leaders; and friends, especially same-sex friends) increases
Fears, illness, and death	• Copes well with separation from parents • Best age for elective surgery • Gains an understanding that death is final (about age 6 years) • Understands that he or she can also die (about age 9 years)

TEENAGERS (AGE 13 TO 18 YEARS)

Major task	• To develop a personal identity
Developmental milestones	• Puberty (11–12 years in girls; 13–14 years in boys) • Preoccupation with gender roles, body image, and popularity

- Hetero- and homosexual practicing are normal
- Concern with humanitarian issues and world problems (17–18 years)
- Development of the ability for abstract reasoning (e.g., calculus)

Fears, illness, and death	• Feelings of omnipotence (e.g., "Nothing bad can possibly happen to me") • May challenge the authority of doctors • Compliance with medical advice gained mainly by concerns about appearance (e.g., "I will not smoke because smoking will discolor my teeth") or peer pressure (e.g., "I do not smoke because none of my friends smoke")

AGING

Life expectancy in the United States	• Average, 75 years; about 7 years longer for women • Asian Americans are the longest lived American group • African Americans are the shortest lived American group
Brain changes	• Decreased brain weight and blood flow • Enlarged ventricles and sulci • Intelligence remains the same (if there is no dementia)
Psychological changes	• Depression is common and may mimic dementia (pseudodementia) because it is associated with cognitive problems • Poor sleep quality (e.g., decreased delta and REM sleep and poor sleep efficiency; see Topic 5)

DYING AND DEATH

Stages of dying	• Denial ("It's not my lab report.") • Anger ("It's all the doctor's fault.") • Bargaining ("I will never smoke again.") • Depression ("I just want to be left alone.") • Acceptance ("I am ready to get my affairs in order.") • "DANG BAD ACT"
Normal grief (bereavement)	• Example: A 64-year-old woman whose husband died 6 months ago reports that on one occasion, she briefly followed a man down the street who resembled her late husband. The patient also relates that she enjoys visits and outings with her friends and family but that she often starts crying when she thinks about her husband. • Mild insomnia and minor weight loss • Illusions (misperceiving that someone unrelated is the lost loved one) • Sadness and intermittent crying

Abnormal grief (depression; and see Topic 4)	• Example: A 64-year-old man whose wife died 6 months ago feels very guilty, is poorly groomed, and has lost 20 pounds.
	• Significant weight loss (e.g., > 5% of body weight)
	• Intense guilt
	• Suicidal ideation and attempts
	• Psychotic features (e.g., hallucinations, delusions)
	• Anhedonia (inability to experience pleasure)
Physician's role in normal grief	• Provide personal support with regular visits
	• Encourage socialization
	• Provide information about grief support groups
Physician's role in abnormal grief	• Provide personal support with regular visits
	• Treat with antidepressants or electroconvulsive therapy
	• Hospitalize if the patient is suicidal

Topic **2**

Biologic Bases of Behavior

Must Knows

- Concordance rates for relatives of patients with schizophrenia and bipolar disorder
- Effects of brain lesions on neuropsychological function
- Effects of alterations in neurotransmitters on behavior

BEHAVIORAL GENETICS

Schizophrenia	• Occurs cross-culturally in 1% of the population
	• Equal occurrence in males and females
	• 50% concordance rate in monozygotic (MZ) twins
	• 12% concordance rate in first-degree relatives (sibling, child, or dizygotic (DZ) twin)
Bipolar disorder	• Occurs cross-culturally in 1% of the population
	• Equal occurrence in males and females
	• 70% concordance rate in MZ twins
	• 20% concordance rate in first-degree relatives

Major depressive disorder	• Occurs cross-culturally in 10% to 20% of the population • Twice as common in women • Lower concordance rates than schizophrenia or bipolar disorder
Alzheimer's disease	• Family history and increasing age increase risk • Chromosome 21 is implicated because individuals with Down syndrome ultimately develop Alzheimer's disease • Chromosomes 1, 14, and 19 (site of the apolipoprotein E_4 gene) are also implicated
Alcoholism	• Four times more prevalent in the biological children of alcoholics even if they are raised by nondrinking adoptive parents • 60% concordance rate in MZ and 30% in DZ twins • Male children of alcoholics are at greater risk than female children

BEHAVIORAL NEUROANATOMY

Hemispheric dominance	• The right (nondominant) hemisphere is associated with perception, spatial relations, and musical and artistic abilities • The left (dominant) hemisphere is associated with language function in almost all right-handed and most left-handed persons
Frontal lobe lesions	• Dorsolateral convexity: Difficulty with motivation, concentration, attention, orientation, and problem solving • Orbitofrontal: Difficulty with judgment and inhibitions; emotional and personality changes • Left-sided: Inability to speak fluently (i.e., Broca's aphasia), depressed mood
Temporal lobe lesions	• Impaired memory • Psychomotor seizures • Changes in aggressive behavior • Left-sided: Inability to understand language (i.e., Wernicke's aphasia)
Limbic lobe lesions	• Hippocampus: Poor new learning • Amygdala: Kluver-Bucy syndrome (decreased aggression and fear, increased sex drive)
Parietal lobe lesions	• Right sided: Impaired processing of visual-spatial information • Left sided: Gerstmann's syndrome: Impaired processing of verbal information (e.g., cannot tell left from right, do simple math, name fingers, or write)
Occipital lobe lesions	• Visual hallucinations and illusions • Inability to identify camouflaged objects • Blindness

Reticular system lesions	• Changes in sleep–wake mechanisms (e.g., decreased REM sleep)
	• Loss of consciousness
Basal ganglia lesions	• Disorders of movement: Parkinson disease (substantia nigra), Huntington disease (caudate and putamen) and Tourette syndrome (caudate)
Hypothalamus lesions	• Ventromedial nucleus: Hunger leading to obesity
	• Lateral nucleus: Loss of appetite leading to weight loss
	• Effects on sexual activity and body temperature regulation

NEUROTRANSMITTERS (NTS)

Classification	• The three major classes of NTs are biogenic amines (monoamines), amino acids, and neuropeptides (e.g., endorphins)
Regulation of synaptic NT concentrations	• Reuptake by the presynaptic neuron
	• Degradation by enzymes such as monoamine oxidase (MAO)
Monoamine theory of mood disorders	• Lowered monoamine activity results in depression
Monoamines: Dopamine	• Major metabolite: Homovanillic acid (HVA)
	• HVA is increased in schizophrenia and mania
	• HVA is decreased in depression and Parkinson's disease
Monoamines: Norepinephrine	• Most neurons are located in the locus ceruleus
	• Major metabolites are vanillylmandelic acid (VMA) and 3-methoxy-4-hydroxyphenylglycol (MHPG)
	• VMA is high in pheochromocytoma (adrenal medulla tumor)
	• MHPG is low in depression and anxiety
Monoamines: Serotonin	• Most neurons located in the dorsal raphe nuclei
	• Major metabolite: 5-hydroxyindoleacetic acid (5-HIAA)
	• 5-HIAA is low in depression, impulsiveness, fire setting, Tourette syndrome, alcohol abuse, and bulimia
Amino acids: GABA (γ-aminobutyric acid)	• Inhibitory neurotransmitter
	• Decreased in anxiety and Huntington disease
Amino acids: Glutamate	• Excitatory neurotransmitter
	• Increased in Alzheimer disease (excitotoxic action)
	• Dysregulated in schizophrenia

Topic **3**

Psychologic Bases of Behavior

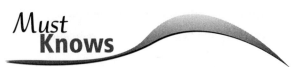

Must
Knows

● Clinical examples of patients' uses of defense mechanisms
● Definitions and clinical examples of transference and countertransference

DEFENSE MECHANISMS

Acting out	"I never had sex with a boy before but had sexual relationships with many different boys after my parents got divorced."
Denial	"I do not have a problem with alcohol. I can stop drinking whenever I want to."
Displacement	"Every time I have a fight with my wife, the female residents say that I get very nasty toward them."
Dissociation	"I cannot remember anything about the accident in which I was driving and my younger sister was killed."
Intellectualization	"My illness is terminal in 20% of patients, remits in 20%, and causes lasting impairment in the other 60%."
Rationalization	"Since I lost my vision, my hearing has become much better."
Reaction formation	"I used to hate my ex-wife, but now every time I see her, I want to kiss her."
Regression	"Since I have been sick, I crave ice cream and chocolate."
Splitting	"All of the doctors in the group practice are wonderful, but all of the office workers in the practice are terrible."
Sublimation	"When my child was killed by a drunk driver, I joined an organization called Mothers Against Drunk Driving."
Suppression	"I do not want to talk about my illness now. Let's just have a good time at the party."
Undoing	"I will give all my money to charity if I can get rid of this illness."

TRANSFERENCE AND COUNTERTRANSFERENCE

Definitions	Transference and countertransference are unconscious mental attitudes based on important past personal relationships (e.g., with parents) that can influence physician–patient interactions
Transference	Example: A male patient becomes angry at a middle-aged female doctor when the doctor asks him if he has been taking his medication. The doctor reminds the patient of his overbearing mother.
Countertransference	Example: A female doctor becomes angry at a young male patient when the patient fails to take his medication. The patient has a strong physical resemblance to the doctor's own difficult son.

Topic **4**

Psychopathology

Must Knows

- Rule out physical illness and drug abuse before diagnosing psychopathology
- The time requirements for distinguishing schizophrenia from other psychotic disorders (e.g., persistence of symptoms for at least 6 months in schizophrenia)
- Distinction between obsessive-compulsive disorder (OCD) and obsessive-compulsive personality disorder (e.g., personal distress about the symptoms in OCD)
- Features that distinguish cognitive disorders from dissociative disorders (e.g., presence of an identifiable psychological stressor in dissociative disorders)
- Features that distinguish bulimia nervosa from anorexia nervosa (e.g., abnormal body image in anorexia nervosa)
- Features that distinguish oppositional defiant disorder from conduct disorder in children (e.g., child with conduct disorder breaks societal rules)

SCHIZOPHRENIA

Patient example	• A 28-year-old man living in a group home tells the doctor that his roommates have been spying on him for the past year by listening to his thoughts through the television set (a delusion). He is unkempt and seems preoccupied by what he describes as "people giving him instructions in his head (auditory hallucination)."

Epidemiology	• 1% of the population cross-culturally
	• No ethnic or gender differences
	• "Downward drift" of patients with schizophrenia into poverty because they cannot earn a living
Neurological abnormalities	• Enlargement of the lateral and third ventricles
	• Cortical atrophy
	• Decreased activity in the frontal lobes
	• Decreased activity in the limbic system
Positive and negative symptoms	• Positive symptoms: Hallucinations (i.e., false perceptions; mainly auditory) and delusions (false beliefs)
	• Negative symptoms: Flat affect, social withdrawal
Characteristics	• Positive and negative symptoms for at least 6 months
	• Normal level of consciousness
	• Chronic social and occupational impairment
Prognosis	• Generally poor, but better for women
	• Suicide is common, especially just after a psychotic episode
First-line treatment	• Atypical antipsychotic agents (e.g., risperidone, olanzapine)
Second-line treatment	• Typical antipsychotic agents (e.g., haloperidol)
Third-line treatment	• Clozapine (an atypical antipsychotic agent) is most effective against negative symptoms, but side effects (e.g., agranulocytosis and seizures) limit its usefulness

OTHER DISORDERS WITH PSYCHOTIC SYMPTOMS

Brief psychotic disorder	• Example: A 22-year-old man who was fired from his job 2 weeks ago is brought to the emergency room (ER) by his girlfriend. She reports that since he lost his job, he has begun to show bizarre behavior and claims that his old boss is trying to kill him.
	• Psychotic symptoms lasting more than 1 day, but less than 1 month not better accounted for by a mood disorder with psychotic features
	• Precipitating psychosocial factors (e.g., life stressor)
Schizophreniform disorder	• Psychotic symptoms lasting 1 to 6 months
Delusional disorder	• Example: A 65-year-old woman states that her neighbor has been trying to get her evicted from her apartment for years by telling lies about her to the landlord. The patient is married and is retired from her job as a secretary.
	• Fixed, nonbizarre delusional system; few, if any, other thought disorders
	• Typically begins in middle age
	• Relatively normal social and occupational functioning

Delirium (and see Cognitive Disorders below)	• Psychotic symptoms: Visual hallucinations and illusions (misperceptions of reality) occurring as a consequence of physical illness or substance abuse • Clouding of consciousness

MOOD DISORDERS

Epidemiology	• No ethnic differences • Major depressive disorder and dysthymic disorder are more common in women • No gender difference in bipolar disorder and cyclothymic disorder
Major depressive disorder patient	• Example: A 40-year-old man states that he has little interest in activities he used to enjoy. He has lost 11 pounds, reports that he wakes up 2 hours before his alarm goes off, and admits to thoughts of suicide. He says that although he feels tired most of the time, he seems to feel somewhat better in the evening than in the morning (i.e., diurnal improvement in symptoms).
Definition of major depressive disorder	• At least one episode of depression lasting at least 2 weeks
Signs and symptoms of depression	• Decreased pleasure and interest in activities • Reduced energy and appetite • Insomnia and early morning awakening • Feelings of intense guilt • Suicidality • When severe, may have psychotic features (e.g., erroneous belief that one has a fatal illness or is already dead)
First-line treatment of major depressive disorder	• Selective serotonin reuptake inhibitors (SSRIs) because they have few adverse effects
Other treatments for major depressive disorder	• Cyclic antidepressants, monoamine oxidase inhibitors, and other antidepressants • Electroconvulsive therapy is used for patients with severe depression who are nonresponsive or intolerant to antidepressants or who are suicidal or psychotic • Psychological treatment in conjunction with pharmacologic treatment is more effective than either form of treatment alone
Bipolar I disorder patient	• A 28-year-old accountant is brought to the ER by police because he tried to enter a federal building to "talk to the president" about conducting a worldwide telethon to cure AIDS (grandiosity). When stopped from entering the building, he attacks a guard.
Definition of bipolar I disorder	• At least one manic episode with or without episodes of depression

Signs and symptoms of mania	• Greatly elevated mood that negatively affects judgment and social or occupational functioning • Grandiosity, expansiveness, irritability • Behavioral disinhibition (e.g., lack of modesty) • Pressured speech (feels compelled to speak quickly) • Flight of ideas (ideas follow each other rapidly)
Definition of bipolar II disorder	• At least one hypomanic episode (elevated mood that does not negatively affect function) plus at least one episode of depression
Treatment of bipolar disorder	• Lithium for classic bipolar disorder • Anticonvulsants (e.g., divalproex) for rapid cycling bipolar disorder (> 4 episodes/year) • Sedatives or antipsychotics (e.g. risperidone) for agitation
Dysthymic disorder patient	• Example: A 26-year-old woman has been feeling "low" since graduating from college 4 years ago. Her family members say that she never seems really happy, even at family occasions, and that she resists their suggestions to seek psychotherapy.
Definition of dysthymic disorder	• Chronic mild depression lasting at least 2 years in adults or at least 1 year in children
Cyclothymic disorder patient	• Example: A 30-year-old man has seemed full of energy and optimism for no obvious reason (an "up" or hypomanic period) for the past 4 months. Previously, he had been described by friends and family as being "down in the dumps."
Definition of cyclothymic disorder	• Chronic alternating mild depression and hypomania lasting at least 2 years in adults or at least 1 year in children
Differential diagnosis of the mood disorders	• Medical illness (e.g., decreased thyroid function can lead to depressive symptoms) • Substance use or withdrawal (e.g., use of stimulants causes elevated mood; withdrawal causes depression) • Cognitive or neurological disorder (e.g., dementia in elderly patients can present with depression)
Prognosis of the mood disorders	• Episodes are self-limiting (1 year for depression; 3 months for mania) • Episodes typically recur

COGNITIVE DISORDERS

Delirium	• Example: An 84-year-old woman is brought to the emergency room (ER) by her son when she is found wandering down the street in her nightclothes. The patient seems confused and mistakes the ER physician for her nephew. Physical examination reveals evidence of pneumonia. The son notes that before today, the patient was oriented and alert.

- Hallmark: Impaired consciousness
- Etiology: Physical illness, drug abuse, drug withdrawal
- Treatment: Find the cause and remove or treat it

Dementia
- Example: An 84-year-old woman is brought to the ER by her son when she is found wandering down the street in her night-clothes. The patient is alert but cannot state her name or identify her son. Physical examination is unremarkable. The son notes that for the past few months, the patient has seemed "different" and has sometimes not seemed to recognize him.
- Hallmark: Loss of memory and intellectual abilities with normal level of consciousness
- Etiology: Alzheimer's disease (65% of cases); vascular dementia (15% of cases)
- Major differential diagnosis: Delirium, depression or effects of sensory loss or disease in normal aging

Management of Alzheimer's patient
- Emotional support for patient and family
- Provide orienting cues, e.g., put an identifying label on the door of the bathroom
- Acetylcholinesterase inhibitors (e.g., donepezil, rivastigmine, galantamine), and N-methyl-D-aspartate (NMDA) receptor blockers (e.g., memantine) may slow progression but do not restore function already lost

ANXIETY DISORDERS

Generalized anxiety disorder (GAD)
- Example: A 35-year-old woman says that since she was a teenager, she has frequently felt "nervous" and often has an "upset stomach" and "palpitations."
- Chronic (> 6 months) fearfulness without adequate cause
- Symptoms include agitation, tremor, tachycardia, dizziness, tingling in the extremities, perioral loss of sensation, diarrhea, and urinary urgency
- Treatment: Antidepressants (e.g., venlafaxine), buspirone

Panic disorder (with or without agoraphobia)
- Example: A 22-year-old medical student experiences a sudden onset of shortness of breath and racing pulse and is convinced that she is having an asthma attack and will suffocate.
- Episodic (about twice weekly) periods of intense fearfulness that have a sudden onset, include feelings of impending doom, and last approximately 30 minutes
- May be associated with agoraphobia (i.e., fear of open places)
- ER treatment: Benzodiazepines (e.g., alprazolam)
- Maintenance treatment: antidepressants (e.g., paroxetine)

Phobias
- Specific phobia: Irrational fear of specific objects or environmental situations (e.g., dogs, heights)

	• Social phobia: Irrational fear of embarrassing oneself in public (e.g., public speaking, eating in a restaurant, using a public restroom) • Psychological treatment: Desensitization using gradual (e.g., systematic desensitization) or overwhelming (e.g., flooding) exposure to the feared stimulus • Physiological treatment: β-adrenergic antagonists (e.g., propranolol) to decrease autonomic arousal; antidepressants
Obsessive-compulsive disorder (OCD)	• Example: A 40-year-old man gets out of bed repeatedly during the night to recheck the locks on the doors and to be sure the gas jets on the stove are turned off. • Recurrent thoughts, feelings, and images (i.e., obsessions) that cause anxiety and repetitive actions (i.e., compulsions such as hand washing) that relieve the anxiety • Treatment: Serotonergic antidepressants (e.g., fluvoxamine or other SSRI, clomipramine)
Acute stress disorder (ASD-lasting between 2 days and 4 weeks) and posttraumatic stress disorder (PTSD- lasting more than 4 weeks)	• Emotional symptoms of four types: 1) re-experiencing (e.g., daytime intrusive memories, nightmares), 2) hyperarousal (e.g., anxiety), 3) emotional numbing (e.g. inability to feel love) and 4) avoidance of associated places or feelings, after a physical or psychological event that was potentially life threatening (e.g., earthquake, fire, rape, serious accident) • Treatment: Psychotherapy, support groups, group therapy, psychoactive medication
Adjustment disorder	• Example: Three months after moving, a teenager who was formerly outgoing and a good student seems sad and begins to do poor work in school. • Emotional symptoms (e.g., depression, anxiety, conduct disturbances) causing social or work impairment that occur within 3 months and last less than 6 months after a serious (but usually not life threatening) event (e.g., divorce, changing residency, bankruptcy) • Treatment: Psychotherapy, group therapy, medication for associated symptoms (e.g., depression, anxiety)

SOMATOFORM DISORDERS, FACTITIOUS DISORDER AND MALINGERING

Overview of somatoform disorders	• Physical symptoms that cause emotional distress but do not have an organic cause • Patients truly believe that they are ill • Management includes reassurance from and regularly scheduled appointments with the physician
Somatization disorder	• Example: A 45-year-old woman has a 20-year history of vague physical complaints including nausea, painful menses, and loss of feeling in her legs.

- Multiple (at least eight) physical symptoms (e.g., nausea, dyspnea, menstrual problems) over years

Conversion disorder	• Example: A 29-year-old man experiences sudden weakness of his right arm and leg but appears unconcerned. He reports that just before the onset of hemiparesis, he saw his girlfriend with another man. • Sudden loss of sensory (e.g., blindness) or motor function • Stressful life event in the recent past • Patient is relatively unconcerned: "La belle indifference"
Hypochondriasis	• Example: A 50-year-old man, convinced that he has prostate cancer, insists on having a prostate specific antigen test every month. • Exaggerated concern with health and illness • Concern persists despite reassurance from the physician • Goes "doctor shopping" to seek other opinions
Body dysmorphic disorder	• Example: Despite the fact that his nose is of normal size for his face, a 25-year-old man repeatedly seeks plastic surgery to make his "huge" nose smaller. • Normal-appearing person believe he or she is physically abnormal
Factitious disorder	• Example: A 24-year-old nurse is admitted to the hospital with a diagnosis of "pain of unknown origin." After 4 days in the hospital, the nurse shows little evidence of pain and seems "remarkably content." • Healthy person (often a health care worker) feigns or induces illness in self or child (factitious disorder by proxy) because of a need to get attention from physicians • Becomes angry when confronted with the truth
Malingering	• Example: A 24-year-old man complains of severe back pain after a car accident. His pain remits after he receives a cash settlement from the other driver. • Healthy person feigns physical or emotional illness for actual gain (e.g., money in a lawsuit, getting out of prison) • Becomes angry when confronted with the truth

PERSONALITY DISORDERS (PDs)

Characteristics	• Long-standing, rigid, unsuitable patterns of relating to others that cause significant problems in social or occupational functioning
DSM-IV-TR Clusters	• Cluster A: Paranoid, schizoid, schizotypal • Cluster B: Histrionic, narcissistic, antisocial, borderline • Cluster C: Avoidant, obsessive-compulsive, dependent

Paranoid pd: Suspicious, mistrustful, litigious	• A 45-year-old hospital aide relates that she has been laid off because by working too hard she made her supervisor look lazy. She reports that when the same thing happened in a previous job, she filed a lawsuit against that hospital
Schizoid PD : Lifelong pattern of voluntary social withdrawal	• The parents of a 26-year-old man state that they are concerned about him because he has no friends and spends most of his time hiking in the woods. He states that he is content with his solitary life, and there is no evidence of a formal thought disorder.
Schizotypal PD: Peculiar person	• An oddly dressed 32-year-old woman tells the doctor that she likes to walk in the woods because the birds seem to communicate with her. She says she never goes out on Thursdays, however, because they are "dangerous days."
Histrionic PD: Dramatic, emotional, sexually provocative	• A 28-year-old male patient is dressed in a cape lined with red satin. He reports that his mild sore throat feels like "a hot poker" when he swallows and says that he feels so warm that he "must have a fever of at least 106°."
Narcissistic PD: Grandiosity, envy, and a sense of entitlement	• A 38-year-old male patient asks for a referral to a physician who graduated from a top medical school. He says that he is "better" than most other people.
Antisocial PD: Criminality, absence of conscience or empathy	• A 35-year-old man brags that he has been sexually assaulting women since high school but has never been caught. He has also been arrested for passing bad checks.
Borderline PD: Unstable, impulsive, suicide attempts, boredom, emptiness, cutting one's skin, eating disorders	• A 20-year-old student relates that, because she was afraid to be alone again, she tried to commit suicide after a man with whom she had had two dates failed to call her again. She states that her current doctor is wonderful but no other doctor has ever understood her problems (use of "splitting" as a defense mechanism).
Avoidant PD: Socially withdrawn, shy, sensitive	• A 35-year-old woman who works as a laboratory assistant lives with her elderly mother and rarely socializes. She reports that when coworkers ask her to join them for lunch, she refuses because she is afraid that they will not like her.
Obsessive-compulsive PD: Orderly, stubborn, indecisive, perfectionistic	• A 33-year-old man reports that each night, he makes up a written schedule for his behavior and for all of the food that he will eat for the next day. He tells the doctor that his wife recently moved out because she could not conform to his demands that she follow the same schedule.
Dependent PD: Lacks self-confidence; lets others assume responsibility	• A 32-year-old female patient states that her husband is very angry at her because she calls him at the office many times a day to ask him to make trivial, everyday decisions for her.

DISSOCIATIVE DISORDERS

Characteristics	• Psychologically based loss of memory; problems with personal identity or feelings of detachment
	• Often related to a stressful psychological event in the recent or remote past
	• Normal level of conciousness
Dissociative amnesia	• Inability to remember important personal information
Dissociative fugue	• Amnesia combined with sudden wandering from home
Dissociative identity disorder	• At least two separate personalities within an individual
	• Formerly known as multiple personality disorder
Depersonalization disorder	• Feelings of detachment from the patient's own body or the social situation; feeling of being in a dream
Derealization disorder	• Feeling that objects and people within the environment are unreal or changed

EATING DISORDERS

Characteristics	• More common in adolescent and young adult women
	• Menstrual irregularities (at least 3 months of amenorrhea in anorexia nervosa)
	• Binge eating followed by vomiting or other compensatory mechanism (most people with bulimia and 50% of people with anorexia)
	• Compensatory mechanisms include laxatives, diuretics, enemas, and excessive exercising
	• If vomiting, there are esophageal varices, calluses on the backs of the hands (from inducing vomiting), dental caries, parotid gland swelling or abscess, electrolyte disturbances (e.g., hypokalemia leading to cardiac arrhythmias)
Anorexia nervosa	• A 16-year-old gymnast who is 5 ft., 6 inches tall and weighs 85 pounds tells the doctor that she needs to lose another 15 pounds for her dancing career. Radiographic examination reveals evidence of early osteoporosis, and fine body hair (lanugo) is seen during the physical examination.
Bulimia nervosa	• A 17-year-old dancer who is 5 ft., 4 inches tall and weighs 118 pounds has been eating an entire cheesecake every night. Then, to avoid gaining weight, she has been putting her fingers down her throat to force herself to vomit.
Major distinction between anorexia nervosa and bulimia nervosa	• Anorexia: Disturbance of body image (feels fat when thin), denies problem, body weight at least 15% below normal
	• Bulimia: Depression, insight that eating behavior is abnormal, normal body weight

NEUROPSYCHIATRIC DISORDERS IN CHILDHOOD

Autistic spectrum disorders	• Rare; more common in boys: Diagnosed in the first 3 years of life • Diminished ability to form social relationships • Deficits in language skills • Often mentally retarded in the more severe form • Repetitive behavior (e.g., spinning) • Unusual abilities in some (i.e., savants) • Management includes behavioral training and emotional support for care givers • Most remain severely socially impaired throughout life
Child with autistic disorder	• Concerned parents report that their 3-year-old boy cries whenever he is changed or bathed. When given paper and crayons, the child sits on the floor folding and unfolding a piece of the paper and does not make eye contact when spoken to.
Attention deficit hyperactivity disorder (ADHD)	• Occurs in 3% to 5% of children; more common in boys • Hyperactivity or limited attention span • Impulsive; prone to accidents • Emotional lability and irritability • Most have normal intelligence • Management includes central nervous system stimulants (e.g., methylphenidate) • Persists into adulthood in 20% of patients • Example: A 10-year-old boy interrupts the teacher, disturbs the other students, and cannot seem to sit still in class or at home. However, the child works well and productively when he is alone with his math tutor.
Oppositional defiant disorder	• Persistent defiant, noncompliant behavior that does not violate social norms (e.g., "talking back" to parents and teachers) • Management includes family therapy • Example: A 10-year-old boy talks back to the teacher and his parents but is kind to his younger siblings and pets.
Conduct disorder	• Persistent behavior that grossly violates social norms (e.g., abusing animals, setting fires, stealing) • Management includes family therapy • Cannot be diagnosed as antisocial personality disorder before age 18 years • Example: A 10-year-old boy is brought to the principal when he sets a fire in the coat closet. The child has a history of stealing lunch money from the children in his class and of pinching the class pet hamster when no one is watching.

Topic **5**

Sleep and Sleep Disorders

Must **Knows**

● Characteristics of rapid eye movement (REM) and non-REM sleep

● Meaning of the terms *sleep latency, REM latency,* and *sleep efficiency*

● Changes in sleep architecture with depression, in aging, or with the use of sedative agents

● Three major symptoms of narcolepsy

● The most appropriate treatments for insomnia, narcolepsy, and sleep apnea

● The difference between sleep terror disorder and nightmare disorder

SLEEP ARCHITECTURE (FIG. I-1)

Stages: Rapid eye movement (REM) sleep	• "Sawtooth," beta, alpha, and theta waves • 25% of the night • Dreaming • Penile and clitoral erection • Increased pulse, respiration, and blood pressure (BP) • Absence of skeletal muscle movement
REM latency	• Time from falling asleep until the first REM period • Is typically 90 minutes long • REM periods (10–40 minutes each) occur every 90 minutes throughout the night
REM rebound	• Increased REM resulting from previous deprivation of REM
Stages: Non-REM sleep and stages 1, 2, 3, and 4	• Stage 1: Theta waves: 5%: Lightest stage of sleep characterized by peacefulness, slowed pulse and respiration, decreased BP, and episodic body movements • Stage 2 sleep spindles and K-complexes: 45%: Largest percentage of total sleep time; tooth grinding • Stages 3 and 4: Delta waves (slow-wave sleep): 25%; deepest, most relaxed part of sleep

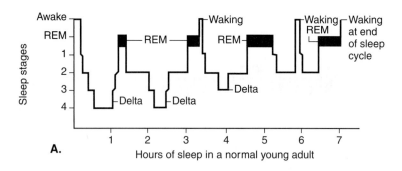

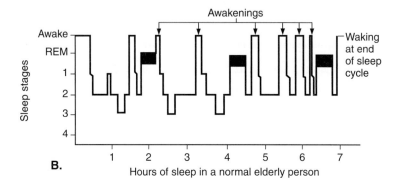

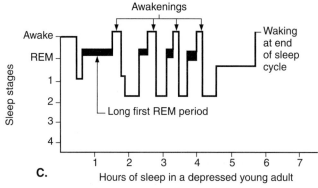

● **Figure I-1** Sleep architecture in a normal young adult (**A**), a normal elderly person (**B**), and a depressed young adult (**C**). (adapted from Wedding D. *Behavior & Medicine*, St.Louis: Mosby Year Book, 1995:416)

Changes with aging	
	• Increased sleep latency (time from closing the eyes to falling asleep)
	• Normal REM latency (time from falling asleep to the first REM period)
	• Poor sleep efficiency (time sleeping per time spent in bed)
	• Repeated nighttime awakenings
	• Waking too early in the morning
	• Reduced % slow-wave sleep
	• Decreased % REM sleep

Changes with depression	• Shortened sleep latency
	• Shortened REM latency
	• Poor sleep efficiency
	• Repeated nighttime awakenings
	• Waking too early in the morning
	• Reduced % slow wave sleep
	• Increased % REM sleep

SLEEP DISORDERS

Insomnia	• Problems falling asleep or staying asleep that occur 3 times per week for at least 1 month and lead to sleepiness during the day or result in problems fulfilling social or occupational obligations
	• Management: Eliminate caffeine from the diet, set up a regular sleep–wake schedule, limited use of non-benzodiazepine sleep agent (e.g., zolpidem) or sedating antidepressants (e.g., trazodone)
Narcolepsy	• Hypnagogic and hypnopompic hallucinations, which occur, respectively, while falling asleep or waking up
	• Cataplexy, which is when an individual suddenly collapses because of loss of all muscle tone with a cough, sneeze, or when startled; occurs in about 50% of individuals with narcolepsy
	• Sleep paralysis (brief inability to move after waking)
	• Management: Planned daytime naps, stimulant agent (e.g., modafinil)
Sleep apnea	• Condition characterized by multiple brief periods of apnea during sleep; seen more frequently in elderly and obese individuals
	• In obstructive sleep apnea, the most common type of sleep apnea, respiratory effort and snoring are present, but an airway obstruction prevents air from reaching the lungs
	• Management: Weight loss (if appropriate), continuous positive airway pressure (CPAP) during sleep
Sleep terror disorder	• An extreme form of fright in which a person, usually a child, awakens in great fear
	• Occurs during slow-wave sleep; there is no memory of arousal or dreaming
	• May be an early sign of temporal lobe epilepsy
	• Management: Temporary use of benzodiazepines to decrease slow-wave sleep

Topic **6**

Sexuality and Aggression

Must Knows

- The distinction between gender identity, gender role, and sexual orientation
- Similarities and differences between males and females in events occurring during the stages of the sexual response cycle
- Identifying and reporting child and elder abuse

SEXUALITY DEFINITIONS

Gender identity	• An individual's sense of being male or female • Is present and fixed by age 3 years
Gender role	• The expression of one's gender identity in society (e.g., clothes preference)
Sexual orientation	• Preference for members of one's own gender (homosexuality) or the opposite gender (heterosexuality) for sex and love
Homosexuality, heterosexuality, bisexuality	• Forms of normal sexual expression • More closely related to genetic and perinatal hormonal influences than to life experiences

STAGES OF THE SEXUAL RESPONSE CYCLE

Excitement	• Penile and clitoral erection • Vaginal lubrication • Tenting effect (uterus rises in the pelvic cavity) • Nipple erection in both sexes • Increased heart rate, blood pressure, and respiration
Plateau	• Testes move upward • Skin flushing occurs just before orgasm on abdomen, chest, neck, and face in both genders
Orgasm	• Seminal fluid is forcibly expelled • Uterine contractions • Contractions of the anal sphincter in both genders • Skeletal muscle contractions in both genders

| **Resolution** | • Return of sexual organs and cardiovascular system to prestimulation state |
| | • Rapid restimulation possible in women but not in men |

SEXUAL DYSFUNCTION

Male erectile disorder	• Inability to maintain erection until completion of the sexual act
	• Most common male sexual disorder
	• Often first caused by alcohol abuse
	• Presence of early-morning or REM erections suggests a psychogenic cause
	• Management: Relaxation techniques or phosphodiesterase inhibitors (e.g., sildenafil, tadalafil), which work as vasodilators in the penis, causing the erection to persist
Premature ejaculation	• Ejaculation occurs before the man wishes
	• No plateau phase
	• Anxiety is present
	• Management: Behavioral strategies (e.g., the "squeeze" technique) and selective serotonin reuptake inhibitors (SSRIs)
Functional pain disorders	• Dyspareunia: Persistent pain associated with sexual intercourse without physical pathology
	• Vaginismus: Spasm of the outer one third of the vagina, causing difficulty during intercourse and gynecologic examination; associated with a history of rape or incest
	• Management: Relaxation techniques, vaginal dilators for vaginismus
In aging	• Decreased sexual performance despite continued sexual interest
	• In men: Need for more direct genital stimulation, slower time to erection, diminished intensity of ejaculation, and increased length of the resolution stage
	• In women: Vaginal thinning and vaginal dryness
Management	• Primary care physicians make recommendations for specific behavioral techniques and pharmacotherapy

DRUGS AND SEXUALITY

Antihypertensives (e.g., propranolol)	• Neurotransmitter action: Decrease norepinephrine β
	• Sexual effect: Erectile dysfunction
Antidepressants	• Neurotransmitter action: Increase serotonin
	• Sexual effect: Prolong time to orgasm and ejaculation
	• Trazodone can cause persistent erection (i.e., priapism)
Antipsychotics	• Neurotransmitter action: Decrease dopamine; increase prolactin
	• Sexual effect: Erectile dysfunction

Abused drugs	• Alcohol use leads to erectile dysfunction
	• Cocaine and amphetamines increase sexual interest
	• Opioids decrease sexual interest

CHILD ABUSE

Evidence of physical abuse	• Old, healed fractures
	• Cigarette burns, belt marks
	• Bruises on buttocks or lower back
	• Subdural hematomas and retinal hemorrhage or detachment in infants ("shaken baby syndrome")
Evidence of sexual abuse	• Genital or anal trauma
	• Sexually transmitted disease
	• Child's report of inappropriate adult behavior
	• Urinary tract infection
Emotional neglect	• Withholding of love and attention
	• Harsh criticism
The child abuser	• Socially isolated
	• Substance abuser
	• Physically or sexually abused as a child
Role of the physician when abuse is suspected	• Report the case to the appropriate social service agency
	• Admit the child to the hospital to ensure his or her safety
	• Neither parental notification nor permission to treat is required

ABUSE OF ADULTS

Sexual assault (e.g., rape)	• The victim knows the assaulter
	• Most instances are not reported
	• The emotional results often last for 1 year or longer (i.e., post-traumatic stress disorder)
	• The victim (not the physician) must report the assault to law enforcement
Domestic partner abuse	• Common
	• Never blame the victim
	• The doctor should offer suggestions to ensure future safety
	• The victim must report the abuse to law enforcement authorities
Elder abuse (victim is age 65 or older)	• The abuser is most often the caretaker (e.g., spouse or adult child)
	• The victim is often mildly demented or incontinent
	• The doctor must protect the victim by reporting the case to the appropriate state social service agency

Topic **7**

The Doctor–Patient Relationship

Must Knows

- Appropriate responses by physicians to questions asked or statements made by patients
- Rules for giving patients bad news
- Factors associated with compliance with medical advice

PATIENTS' STATEMENTS AND DOCTORS' RESPONSES: THE "QUOTE" QUESTIONS

The mother of a 15-year-old girl states: "Please give my daughter a prescription for birth control pills."	"Please wait in the outer office. I would like to speak to your daughter alone." Speak to teenagers alone particularly when the issue involves sex or abused substances
The mother of a 15-year-old girl asks: "Does my daughter have gonorrhea?"	"I cannot tell you your daughter's diagnosis. Please ask your daughter." (see page 34 "Confidentiality")
An anxious patient says: "Do not tell me the results of the biopsy."	"Please tell me when you feel ready to hear the report." (see page 28 "Giving Patients Bad News")
A terminally ill 9-year-old patient asks: "Am I going to die?"	"What have your parents told you about your illness?" It is up to the parents to decide if how and when information will be given to their ill child
A diabetic man states: "My wife and I are having problems in bed."	"Please tell me what you mean by 'problems in bed.'" Do not assume that you know what the patient means. Get more information.
A male patient asks: "What are the side effects of the fluoxetine I have been taking for the past 4 months?"	"Please tell me what side effects you have been experiencing." Patients are often reticent to report sexual side effects of drugs. Ask more questions.
A patient states: "My wife says that my drinking is ruining the family."	"What do you think the impact of your drinking is on your family?" Be nonjudgmental; elicit the patient's perspective and address it.

A patient on chemotherapy states: "I want to stop this treatment. It is making me feel too sick."	"I will work on (or "I will consult with an oncologist about") adjusting the medication to make the treatment more acceptable to you." While patients can refuse needed treatment (autonomy) finding a more acceptable treatment is a better path.
A heavy smoker states: "I know it is bad for me, but I just cannot give up smoking."	"Many people have difficulty when they try to stop smoking. Why do you think it is difficult for you?" Express understanding and get more information
An abused wife states: "My husband beat me up because I was drunk when he came home from work."	"Do you think it is safe for you to return home?" Be nonjudgmental; ensure the patient's safety
A cancer patient who is being released from the hospital states: "Doctor, I have a gun in my house."	"I think it would be best if you stayed in the hospital for a few more days." Statements like this when made to a physician can indicate suicidal intent. Ensure the patient's safety
A married mastectomy patient states "After the surgery I began to feel so ugly."	"Please tell me how the surgery has affected your relationship with your husband." Avoid the tendency to immediately reassure the patient; get more information
An angry patient asks: "Why is your office always so disorganized?"	"I apologize. How do you think we can improve things in the office in the future?" Do not be defensive when you are criticized by a patient; address the patient's concerns

GIVING PATIENTS BAD NEWS

When to tell the patient bad news	• The doctor can delay telling the patient the diagnosis until the patient is ready to receive it • Ask the patient if he or she wants to have someone with them when you give them the news
How to tell the patient	• Speak to competent adult patients directly, not through relatives or anyone else • Sit at eye level and avoid putting a desk or table between you and the patient • Wait for the patient to adjust to a negative diagnosis • When a patient cries, offer a tissue and remain attentive but silent
What to tell the patient	• Tell patients the complete truth about their illness and prognosis • Check the patient's understanding regularly • Do not cover up the errors of colleagues
If the patient refuses a test or treatment	• Find out why the patient has refused • Suggest a more acceptable option • Do not try to frighten a patient into consenting to a medical test or treatment

PATIENT COMPLIANCE/ADHERENCE WITH MEDICAL ADVICE

Increased by	• Good physician–patient relationship • Patient feels ill • Disruption of patient's usual activities by the illness • Written instructions for taking medication
Decreased by	• Lack of rapport with the doctor • Few symptoms • Little disruption in usual activities • Verbal instructions for taking medication
Not related to	• Gender or race • Religion or socioeconomic status • Intelligence or education

Topic **8**

Psychoactive Substance Abuse

Must Knows

● Difference between substance abuse and substance dependence

● Four major classes of abused agents

● Effects of use and withdrawal of abused agents

DEFINITIONS

Substance abuse	• A pattern of abnormal substance use that leads to impairment of occupational, physical, or social functioning
Substance dependence	• Substance abuse plus withdrawal symptoms, tolerance, or a pattern of repetitive use
Tolerance	• Need for increased amounts of the substance to achieve the same positive physical and psychological effects
Major classes of abused agents	• Stimulants • Sedatives • Opioids • Hallucinogens and related agents

STIMULANTS

Agents	• Cocaine and amphetamines • Nicotine and caffeine are minor stimulants
Major neurotransmitter (NT) action	• Increase dopamine (DA)
Labs	• Benzoylecgonine (cocaine metabolite) • Cotinine (nicotine metabolite)
Effects of use	• A 19-year-old man is brought to the ER claiming that he is "on top of the world" because he is communicating mentally with the governor (a delusion). Physical examination reveals dilated pupils, erythema of the nose (from "snorting" cocaine), hypertension, and tachycardia.
Effects of withdrawal	• A 24-year-old woman who has been taking amphetamines during exam week complains of a low mood, tiredness, headache, and intense hunger the day after the exams are over.
Acute treatment (detoxification)	• Benzodiazepines to decrease agitation • Antipsychotics for psychotic symptoms
Maintenance treatment	• Education for maintenance of abstinence

SEDATIVES

Agents	• Alcohol • Benzodiazepines • Barbiturates
Major NT action	• Increase γ-aminobutyric acid (GABA)
Effects of use	• A 35-year-old woman who has taken a large dose of alprazolam (a benzodiazepine) appears relaxed and has slurred speech. Her gait is unsteady, and she laughs inappropriately.
Effects of withdrawal	• A 65-year-old woman who has been drinking large amounts of alcohol for the past 10 years is hospitalized for a fractured hip. Two days later, the woman begins to show an intense hand tremor and tachycardia. She states that there are insects crawling on her arms and on the walls (hallucinations). Later that day, she has a seizure.
Acute treatment	• Hospitalization • Substitution of long-acting sedative agents (e.g., benzodiazepines) in decreasing doses
Maintenance treatment for alcohol abuse	• Alcoholics Anonymous (AA) or other peer support groups (12-step programs)

- Disulfiram (Antabuse), which causes a toxic reaction when alcohol is ingested
- Naltrexone
- Acamprosate (Campral)

OPIOIDS

Agents	• Heroin and methadone • Medically used opioids (e.g., morphine)
Major NT action	• Increase DA
Effects of use	• A 17-year-old woman is brought to the hospital by her father. She is very relaxed, her breathing is shallow, her pupils are constricted and she keeps falling asleep as the doctor tries to interview her.
Effects of withdrawal	• A 28-year-old man in the emergency room (ER) is complaining of stomach cramps, muscle aches, and diarrhea. He is sweating, has a runny nose, and has goose bumps on his skin (piloerection). His pupils are dilated, and he appears agitated. Both his pulse rate and blood pressure are elevated.
Acute treatment	• For overdose: Naloxone (blocks opioid receptors) • For withdrawal symptoms: Clonidine for autonomic instability • Substitution of long-acting opioid (e.g., methadone) in decreasing doses
Maintenance treatment	• Methadone or l-α-acetylmethadol acetate (LAMM) maintenance program • Naloxone, naltrexone, or buprenorphine (a partial opioid agonist) used prophylactically to block the positive effects of abused opioids)

HALLUCINOGENS AND RELATED AGENTS

Agents	• Lysergic acid diethylamide (LSD) • Phencyclidine (PCP) • Marijuana • Mescaline, peyote • Ketamine • Inhalants
Major NT action	• LSD increases serotonin • PCP increases glutamate
Effects of use	• A 29-year-old man is hospitalized after jumping from the roof of one apartment building to another after taking PCP. His friends relate that before the jump, the man angrily threatened them because they would not follow suit. Physical examination reveals an agitated man with vertical nystagmus.

- While lying on the examining table in the ER, a 22-year-old woman who previously ingested LSD states that she feels as if she is floating and the sun is big and glaring above her.

Effects of withdrawal	• None
Acute treatment	• Calming or "talking down" the patient to decrease agitation while the agent wears off
	• Benzodiazepines to decrease agitation
	• Antipsychotics to treat psychotic symptoms
Maintenance treatment	• Abstinence and education

Topic **9**

Legal and Ethical Issues in Medicine

Must Knows

- The standards for emancipation of minors
- The components of informed consent
- The rights of the mother versus those of the fetus
- Instances in which the confidentiality of teenagers can be maintained
- Types of advance directives
- Criteria for the legal standard of death

ETHICAL AND LEGAL ISSUES

Overview	• Ethical behavior is a standard based on moral issues
	• Legal conduct conforms to written law
	• Ethical standards typically exceed legal standards

PROFESSIONAL BEHAVIOR

Impaired physicians	• If a physician knows that another doctor is impaired by alcohol, drugs, illness, or old age, he or she must prevent the impaired doctor from treating patients
	• The impaired doctor should be reported to his or her supervisor (e.g., residency training director, department chairperson)

Inappropriate relationships	• Doctors should not have romantic relationships with patients, patient's relatives, or former patients
	• Doctors should not accept valuable gifts from patients
Medical malpractice	• Occurs when harm comes to a patient by the actions or inactions of a physician
	• The 4 Ds of malpractice are <u>d</u>ereliction (failure to follow the normal standards of care) of a <u>d</u>uty (there is an established doctor-patient relationship) leading to <u>d</u>amages (injury) <u>d</u>irectly to the patient
	• Malpractice suits have increased because of increased awards to successful plaintiffs and breakdowns in doctor–patient relationships

LEGAL COMPETENCE

Minors	• Everyone 18 years of age and older is assumed to be legally competent to make health care decisions for themselves, even if they are mentally retarded or demented
	• Emancipated minors are younger than age 18 years but can make their own health care decisions
Criteria for the status of emancipated minor (only one criterion needed)	• Is self-supporting
	• Is in the military
	• Is married
	• Has children whom he or she cares for
Parents request genetic testing for their child	• If the disorder starts in childhood and there is no treatment (e.g., Tay-Sachs disease), test the child
	• If the disorder starts in adulthood and there is no treatment (e.g., Huntington's disease), do not test the child
	• If the disorder starts in childhood or adulthood and can be treated, test the child
Questions of competence	• A judge (not the patient's family or physician) makes the determination of competence

INFORMED CONSENT

Components of informed consent	• Patients must understand the diagnosis, risks, benefits, alternatives, and likely outcome of treatment in order to give informed consent
Pregnant women	• Pregnant women can refuse diagnostic, medical, or surgical intervention needed to protect the health or life of the fetus
Obtaining informed consent	• Only the physician can obtain informed consent

Unexpected findings during surgery	• If the finding does not require emergency intervention, wake the patient and obtain consent before taking action
	• If the finding requires emergency intervention, perform the procedure immediately without obtaining consent

CONFIDENTIALITY

Expectations of the physician	• Maintain the confidentiality of adult patients unless the patient is suspected of child or elder abuse, is at significant risk for suicide, or poses a serious threat to another person
Confidentiality of teenagers	• Maintain their confidentiality and treat teenagers when the issue relates to sexuality (e.g., sexually transmitted diseases) or substance abuse
Reportable illnesses	• Illnesses that must be reported vary by state but typically include childhood infectious illnesses (e.g., varicella); hepatitis A, B, and C; tuberculosis; and most sexually transmitted diseases
	• HIV infection is not reportable in all states, but AIDS is reportable in all states

ADVANCE DIRECTIVES

Durable power of attorney or health care proxy	• A document in which the patient designates another person to be his or her legal representative when the patient is incompetent
Living will	• A document in which a person gives directions for his or her future health care
Surrogates	• Surrogates are persons who make decisions for patients if there is no health care proxy or living will

DEATH AND EUTHANASIA

Legal standard of death	• Brain death (irreversible cessation of all functions of the entire brain) is the legal standard of death and commonly includes absence of: responses to external events or pain; spontaneous respiration; cephalic reflexes; electrical potentials of cerebral origin; and cerebral blood flow
	• Physicians can remove life support from brain-dead patients
Organ donation	• Organs usually cannot be harvested after death unless the patient has signed a document or informed surrogates of his or her wish to donate
Euthanasia	• Euthanasia (mercy killing or physician-assisted suicide) is illegal and unethical
	• Withholding and withdrawing life-sustaining treatment (e.g., food, water, ventilator support) at a competent patient's request are both legal and ethical
	• Pain relief can be provided to a terminally ill patient even if it may coincidentally shorten his or her life. This is not euthanasia.

Topic **10**

Epidemiology and Biostatistics

Must Knows

- The relationship between incidence and prevalence
- Calculate sensitivity, specificity, positive predictive value, and negative predictive value
- What happens to these measures when prevalence increases or when cutoff values change
- The difference between cohort and case-control studies
- Calculate relative risk and odds ratio
- Measures of central tendency: Mean, median, mode, standard deviation, and standard error
- Calculate confidence intervals

INCIDENCE AND PREVALENCE

Incidence rate	• Number of new cases per population at risk
Prevalence rate	• Number of existing cases at a point in time (e.g., on March 4, 2006) or during a specific period (e.g., during 2006) per population at risk
Relationship between incidence and prevalence	• Prevalence is greater than incidence if the disease is long lasting (e.g., AIDS)

SCREENING TESTS

To calculate sensitivity	• Of the truly sick people, what percentage are correctly identified as sick by the screening test TP/TP + FN
	• Only include sick people (true positives and false negatives), whether they are identified by the test or not
To calculate specificity	• Of the truly well people, what percentage are correctly identified as well by the screening test TN/TN + FP
	• Only include well people (true negatives and false positives), whether they are identified by the test or not
To calculate positive predictive value	• Of the people with a positive test result, what percentage are truly sick (TP/TP + FP)
	• Only include people with a positive test result, whether they are really sick or not

To calculate negative predictive value	• Of the people with a negative test result, what percentage are truly well (TN/TN + FN) • Only include people with a negative test result, whether they are really well or not
Effect of increased prevalence	• No change in sensitivity or specificity • Increased positive predictive value • Decreased negative predictive value
Effect of making it easier to declare a test result positive (e.g., for a prostate specific antigen [PSA] test result to be considered positive, a patient only needs to score 3 ng/mL rather than 4 ng/mL, the former cutoff value)	• Increase sensitivity • Increase negative predictive value • Decrease specificity • Decrease positive predictive value
Effect of making it harder to declare a test result positive (e.g., for a PSA test result to be considered positive, a patient must score at least 5 ng/mL)	• Decrease sensitivity • Decrease negative predictive value • Increase specificity • Increase positive predictive value
Precision, accuracy, reliability, and validity	• Example: A patient's true blood pressure (BP) is 120/80 mm Hg. However, on four weekly visits, the doctor has obtained readings of 140/90, 140/85, 142/87, and 140/85 mm Hg. This result is precise and reliable (i.e., the readings are similar to each other) but is not accurate or valid (the mean BP obtained by the doctor is different from the patient's real BP)

RESEARCH STUDY DESIGN

Case-control study example	• Compare the smoking histories of hospitalized women with and without lung cancer to determine the increased chances (odds ratio) of having lung cancer if one had been a smoker
Odds ratio for this case-control study	• Of 200 women in a hospital, 50 have lung cancer. Of these patients, 45 are smokers. Of the remaining 150 women, 60 are smokers. The odds ratio of 13.5 means that in this group of women, a woman with lung cancer was 13.5 times more likely to have smoked than a woman without lung cancer
Cohort study example	• Follow healthy adults from age 20 to age 50 years to compare the incidence rate of lung cancer in those who smoke versus those who do not smoke (relative risk)

Relative risk for this cohort study	• If the incidence rate of lung cancer among the smoking group is 50:1000 and the incidence rate of lung cancer among the nonsmoking group is 2:1000, the relative risk is 50:2, or 25 (i.e., the risk of lung cancer is 25 times higher for smokers than for nonsmokers)
Attributable risk for this cohort study	• Given the above data, the risk of lung cancer attributable to smoking (the attributable risk) is 50:1000–2:1000, or 48:1000 (i.e., 48:1000 cases of lung cancer can be attributed to smoking)
Cross-sectional study example	• Conduct a large telephone survey to determine if people who smoke are more likely to cough during daytime hours than those who do not smoke
Cross-over study	• Subjects in group 1 first receive the drug, and subjects in group 2 first receive the placebo. Later in the study, the groups switch (i.e., those in group 1 receive the placebo and those in group 2 receive the drug)
Power analysis	• Determination in advance how large a sample size to use in a study in order to detect a statistically significant difference between groups
Meta-analysis	• Combination of the results of many studies to determine if the null hypothesis (see below) should be rejected

THE NULL HYPOTHESIS AND STATISTICAL TESTS

Hypothesis	• A statement or expectation based on observations, literature, or preliminary studies • The statement postulates that a difference exists between two groups • The possibility that the observed difference occurred by chance is tested with statistical procedures
The null hypothesis	• The null hypothesis postulates that there is no difference between the two groups • This hypothesis is either rejected or not rejected after statistical analysis
Type I α and type II β error	• A type I error occurs when the null hypothesis is rejected even though it is true • A type II error occurs when the null hypothesis is not rejected even though it is false
Statistical probability	• The P (probability) value is the chance that a type I error has been made ◦ If a P value is equal to or less than 0.05, it is unlikely that a type I error has been made (i.e., a type I error is made five or fewer times out of one hundred attempts) • A P value equal to or less than 0.05 is generally considered statistically significant

STATISTICS

Descriptive statistics: Measures of central tendency	• The mean is the average score • The median is the middle value when the scores are ordered sequentially • The mode is the value that appears most often
Normal (i.e., Gaussian, bell-shaped) distribution	• Mean = median = mode (Fig. I-2)
Measures of dispersion	• Standard deviation (S): The average distance of observations from their mean • Standard error (SE) is the standard deviation divided by the square root of the number of scores (n) in the set • A z score is the difference between an individual variable and the population mean in units of standard deviation: 2 is used for the 95% confidence interval; 3 is used for the 99.7% confidence interval
Confidence intervals	• Calculated by the mean ± z score (SE)
t Tests and analyses of variance (ANOVA)	• Used when means and standard deviations can be obtained • Independent (nonpaired) test. Two different groups of people are sampled on one occasion: E.g., tests the difference between the mean body weights of people in group A and people in group B at time 1.

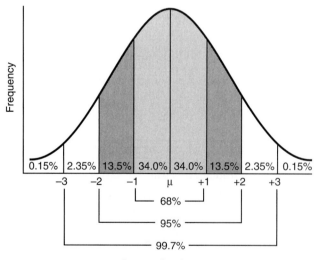

Area under the curve

● **Figure I-2** The normal (Gaussian) distribution. The number of standard deviations (–3 to +3) from the mean is shown on the *x* axis. The percentage of the population that falls under the curve within each standard deviation is shown.

- Dependent (paired) test. The same people are sampled on two occasions: E.g., tests the difference between mean body weights of people in group A at time 1 and time 2.
- ANOVA tests the differences between the means of more than two samples.

Chi-square test	• Tests the differences between frequencies in a sample
	• Used when the distribution of scores in a population is not normal or the sample is small
	• Example: Tests the difference between the percentage of subjects who lose weight is those who fail to lose weight in groups A and B
Correlation	• Tests the mutual relation between two continuous variables
	• Correlation coefficients are negative to −1 (i.e., if one variable increases as the other decreases)
	• Correlation coefficients are positive to +1 if both variables change in the same direction
	• Example: Tests the relationship between number of calories consumed and body weight in each group

Gross Anatomy, Embryology, and Histology/Cell Biology

10 Top Tips

Anatomy

Topic	Main Focus	USMLE Example
1 Pregnancy and Early Life	Events during pregnancy affect embryological development and maternal health.	• A 24-year-old pregnant woman at 13 weeks' gestation with her first pregnancy is diagnosed with a molar pregnancy. The pathological appearance of this tissue resembles a "cluster of grapes."
2 Embryology of Body Systems	Embryological processes establish the organization of the adult.	• A 35-year-old woman with trigeminal neuralgia has intermittent severe pain in areas near her nose and mouth. These areas are innervated by cranial nerve (CN) V and are the product of the first pharyngeal arch.
3 Embryological Anomalies	Abnormalities of development have distinct underlying mechanisms and sequelae after birth.	• A 3-day-old girl spits up, coughs, and chokes while feeding. A radiographic study demonstrates the presence of a tracheoesophageal fistula.
4 Teratology	Perinatal infection and toxic exposure result in dysgenesis of the developing fetus.	• A 30-year-old pregnant woman regularly consumes alcohol during pregnancy. Her child is later observed to have intellectual defects, microcephaly, growth deficiency, and facial dysmorphisms.
5 Gross Anatomy	Normal anatomy	• A 60-year-old man is admitted to the hospital with episodes of severe chest pain unrelieved by rest or sublingual nitroglycerin. A thallium stress test shows decreased perfusion to the anterior wall of the left ventricle caused by occlusion of the left anterior descending coronary artery.

(Continued)

10 Top Tips

Anatomy *(Continued)*

Topic	Main Focus	USMLE Example
6 Anatomic Pathology	Injury to or abnormalities of anatomical structures present with distinct signs and symptoms.	• A 57-year-old man who has been abusing alcohol for 30 years is brought to the emergency room because he has been vomiting large amounts of blood. Physical examination and laboratory studies reveal ruptured esophageal varices secondary to portal hypertension and liver cirrhosis.
7 Neuroanatomy	Normal neuroanatomy	• After carotid endarterectomy, a 68-year-old woman shows denervation atrophy of the muscles of the left side of her tongue and protrusion of her tongue toward the affected side. These signs indicate that the woman's left hypoglossal nerve was injured during surgery.
8 Neuropathology	Characteristic neurologic deficits result from specific nervous system lesions.	• A 38-year-old man sustains an anterior shoulder dislocation and subsequent axillary nerve injury in an accident. Subsequently, it is observed that the sensation of the skin overlying the lower portion of the deltoid muscle is impaired.
9 Cytology	Cellular differentiation allows for diverse functions.	• Shortly after birth, a premature infant begins to show signs of respiratory distress. This condition is a result of deficient surfactant production by type II pneumocytes.
10 Microscopic Anatomy	Characteristic features of tissues and organs provide insight into function.	• A newborn girl shows significant clitoral enlargement. Laboratory studies reveal a defect in adrenal cortical synthesis of steroid hormones (congenital adrenal hyperplasia).

Topic **1**

Pregnancy and Early Life

Must
Knows

- Features of normal pregnancy and its detection
- Identification of important abnormalities of pregnancy
- Pathology of prematurity

FEATURES OF FERTILIZATION AND PREGNANCY

Oocyte maturation	• Primary oocytes arrest in prophase I until puberty
	• Secondary oocytes progress to metaphase II with ovulation
	• Secondary oocyte remains arrested until fertilization
Male gametogenesis	• At puberty, primordial germ cells differentiate into type A spermatogonia. These cells undergo mitosis to yield stem cells for future gamete formation, as well as differentiation to type B spermatogonia
	• Type B spermatogonia enter meiosis I and undergo DNA replication to form primary spermatocytes
	• Primary spermatocytes complete meiosis I to form two secondary spermatocytes
	• Secondary spermatocytes undergo meiosis II to form spermatids
	• Spermatids undergo spermiogenesis (e.g., formation of acrosome, neck, tail) to form sperm
Human chorionic gonadotropin (hCG)	• Glycoprotein produced by syncytiotrophoblasts
	• α and β subunits: The α subunit is identical to luteinizing hormone, follicle-stimulating hormone, and thyroid-stimulating hormone
	• Maintains the corpus luteum until the eighth week of pregnancy
	• Presence in blood or urine is the basis of pregnancy tests
	• Low levels may signal spontaneous abortion or ectopic pregnancy
	• High levels may signal multiple gestations, hydatidiform mole, or trophoblast neoplasm

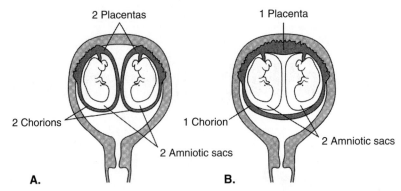

● Figure II-1 Arrangement of the placenta, chorion, and amniotic sac of (**A**) dizygotic twins and 35% of monozygotic twins and (**B**) 65% of monozygotic twins. In general, dizygotic twins can be distinguished from monozygotic twins by an inspection of the afterbirth. However, please note that in approximately 35%, the determination will be in error.

Twinning (Fig. II-1)	• Monozygotic: Fertilization of a secondary oocyte by one sperm, resulting blastocyst splits in two = genetically identical twins
	• Dizygotic: Fertilization of two secondary oocytes by two distinct sperm = as identical as non-twin siblings
	• All dizygotic and 35% of monozygotic twins are diamniotic–dichorionic
	• 65% of monozygotic twins are diamniotic–monochorionic

ABNORMALITIES OF PREGNANCY

Ectopic pregnancy	• Occurs when blastocyst implants outside the uterus
	• Approximately 99% occur in the fallopian tube
	• Results from damage to the fallopian tubes (e.g., pelvic inflammatory disease, endometriosis)
	• Diagnosis is based on patient history (abdominal/pelvic pain, vaginal bleeding), physical examination (adnexal mass, cervical bleeding), and laboratory results (low hCG)
	• Rupture is a surgical emergency (i.e., salpingectomy)
Hydatidiform moles	• Complete mole: Fertilization of enucleate ovum by normal sperm; sperm duplicates chromosomes to give 46,XX karyotype, which is composed of only trophoblastic elements. Has greater malignant potential. Tissue appears as "cluster of grapes".
	• Incomplete or partial mole: Ovum is fertilized by two sperm, commonly 69,XXY karyotype, which is composed of both trophoblastic and fetal elements. Has less malignant potential.
Amniotic fluid abnormalities	• Polyhydramnios: > 1.5 to 2 L of fluid; associated with gastrointestinal abnormalities (esophageal or duodenal atresia) or anencephaly
	• Oligohydramnios: < 0.5 L; associated with renal abnormalities (renal agenesis, Potter's syndrome, maternal diabetes mellitus)

Complications of prematurity	• Respiratory distress syndrome (RDS)
	   ○ Caused by a deficiency of surfactant
	   ○ Signs and symptoms: dyspnea, tachypnea, and cyanosis
	   ○ Antenatal maternal steroids reduce risk
	• Intraventricular hemorrhage
	   ○ Germinal matrix bleeding second to asphyxia or hypertensive injury
	   ○ Can cause neurological sequelae, including cerebral palsy or mental retardation
	   ○ Antenatal maternal steroids reduce risk
	• Necrotizing enterocolitis
	   ○ A syndrome of intestinal infarction and necrosis of complex etiology (e.g., vascular instability, infection, impaired mucosal defense)
	   ○ Antenatal maternal steroids may reduce risk

Topic **2**

Embryology of Body Systems

Must Knows

● Early embryological features

● Pharyngeal arch derivatives

● Differences between fetal and adult circulation

EARLY LIFE

Early hematopoiesis	• Yolk sac: 3 to 8 weeks' gestation • Liver: 6 to 30 weeks' gestation • Spleen: 9 to 28 weeks' gestation • Bone marrow: From 28 weeks' gestation on

Embryologic derivatives	• Ectoderm
	   ○ Surface ectoderm: Anterior pituitary (Rathke's pouch), eye lens, epithelial linings, epidermis
	   ○ Neuroectoderm: Posterior pituitary, central nervous system neurons, oligodendrocytes, astrocytes, pineal gland

○ Neural crest: Autonomic nervous system (ANS), dorsal root ganglia (DRG), melanocytes, chromaffin cells of adrenal medulla, pia, Schwann cells, C cells of thyroid

- Mesoderm: Dura, muscle, bone, cardiovascular system, lymphatics, blood, urogenital structures, serous linings, spleen, adrenal cortex
- Endoderm: Gut tube epithelium and derivatives (lungs, liver, pancreas, thymus, thyroid, parathyroid)

Neural tube vesicle development (Fig. II-2)

- Prosencephalon (forebrain) Gives rise to telencephalon and diencephalon

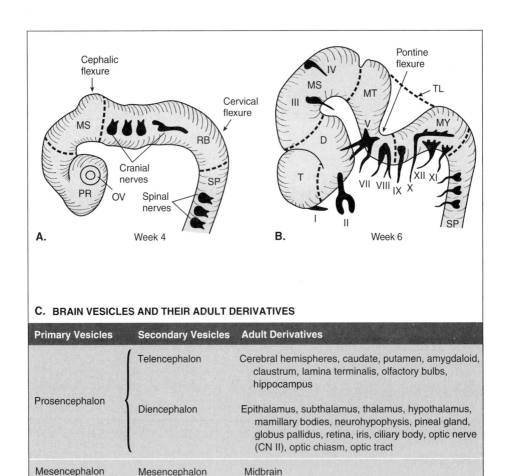

C. BRAIN VESICLES AND THEIR ADULT DERIVATIVES

Primary Vesicles	Secondary Vesicles	Adult Derivatives
Prosencephalon	Telencephalon	Cerebral hemispheres, caudate, putamen, amygdaloid, claustrum, lamina terminalis, olfactory bulbs, hippocampus
	Diencephalon	Epithalamus, subthalamus, thalamus, hypothalamus, mamillary bodies, neurohypophysis, pineal gland, globus pallidus, retina, iris, ciliary body, optic nerve (CN II), optic chiasm, optic tract
Mesencephalon	Mesencephalon	Midbrain
Rhombencephalon	Metencephalon	Pons, cerebellum
	Mylencephalon	Medulla

● **Figure II-2** The developing brain vesicles. (**A**) Three-vesicle stage of the brain in a 4-week-old embryo. Divisions are indicated by *dotted lines*. (**B**) Five-vesicle stage of the brain in a 6-week-old embryo. Divisions are indicated by *dotted lines*. Cranial nerves (CNs) are indicated by *Roman numerals*. CN VI is not shown because it exits the brain stem from the ventral surface (**C**) Table indicating the brain vesicles and their adult derivatives. D = diencephalon; MS = mesencephalon; MT = metencephalon; MY = myelencephalon; OV = optic vessel; PR = prosencephalon; RB = rhombencephalon; SP = spinal cord; T = telencephalon; TL = tela choroidea.

- Mesencephalon (midbrain) Remains the mesencephalon
- Rhombencephalon (hindbrain): Metencephalon and myelencephalon
- Cephalic flexure (midbrain flexure): Between the prosencephalon and rhombencephalon
- Cervical flexure: Between the rhombencephalon and future spinal cord

Primitive heart tube dilations	• Truncus arteriosis: Give rise to the ascending aorta and pulmonary trunk • Bulbus cordis: Smooth portions of the left and right ventricles • Primitive ventricle: Trabeculated portions of the left and right ventricles • Primitive atria: Trabeculated portions of the left and right atria • Sinus venosus: Coronary sinus and smooth portion of the right atrium
Pharyngeal apparatus (Fig. II-3)	• Contains five arches (1 to 4 and 6), four pouches (1 to 4), and four clefts (1 to 4) • Arch 5 is rudimentary in humans and disappears early • Clefts are derived from ectoderm, arches from mesoderm, and neural crest and pouches from endoderm • In general, mesoderm differentiates into muscle and arteries and neural crest differentiates into bones • Derangements in development can manifest as first-arch syndromes, Di George syndrome, or pharyngeal cysts
Pharyngeal arch 1 derivatives	• Meckel's cartilage: Mandible, malleus, incus, sphenomandibular ligament • Muscles: Muscles of mastication, tensor tympani, tensor veli palatini, mylohyoid, anterior belly of digastric • Nerve: Cranial nerve (CN) V_3
Pharyngeal arch 2 derivatives	• Reichert's cartilage: Stapes, styloid process, lesser horn of hyoid, stylohyoid ligament • Muscles: Muscles of facial expression, stapedius, stylohyoid, posterior belly of digastric • Nerve: CN VII
Pharyngeal arch 3 derivatives	• Cartilage: Greater horn of hyoid • Muscle: Stylopharyngeus • Nerve: CN IX
Pharyngeal arches 4 to 6 derivatives	• Cartilages: laryngeal cartilages • Muscles: Fourth (pharyngeal and laryngeal constrictors); sixth (intrinsic laryngeals) • Nerves: Fourth (CN X); sixth (recurrent laryngeal, or CN X)

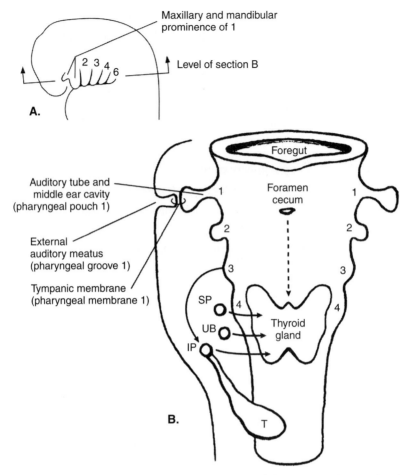

● **Figure II-3** (**A**) Lateral view of an embryo in week 4 of development, showing the pharyngeal arches. Note that pharyngeal arch 1 consists of a maxillary and mandibular prominence, which may cause some confusion in numbering of the arches. (**B**) Migration of the superior (SP) and inferior (IP) parathyroid glands, thymus (T), ultimobranchial body (UB), and thyroid gland. Note that the parathyroid tissue derived from pouch 3 is carried further caudally by the descent of the thymus than parathyroid tissue from pouch 4. The foramen cecum evaginates to form the thyroid diverticulum, which migrates caudally along the midline (*dotted arrow*). In addition, pharyngeal pouch 1, pharyngeal membrane 1, and pharyngeal groove 1 are shown to give rise to structures of the adult ear. 2 = pharyngeal pouch 2; 3 = pharyngeal pouch 3; 4 = pharyngeal pouch 4.

Pharyngeal cleft derivatives	• First cleft: External auditory meatus, external surface of the tympanic membrane
	• Second to fourth clefts: Temporary cervical sinuses that are obliterated during development
Pharyngeal pouch derivatives	• First pouch: Middle ear cavity, eustachian tube, mastoid air cells
	• Second pouch: Epithelial lining of palatine tonsil
	• Third pouch dorsal wings: Inferior parathyroids
	• Third pouch ventral wings: Thymus
	• Fourth pouch: Superior parathyroids

Tongue development

- Anterior two thirds: Formed from one median and two distal tongue buds associated with pharyngeal arch 1; therefore, general sensation is provided by CN V_3 and taste from CN VII
- Posterior third: Formed from the copula and hypobranchial eminence, associated with pharyngeal arches 2, 3, and 4; therefore, general sensation and taste are largely via CN IX

SYSTEMS EMBRYOLOGY

Fetal circulation (Fig. II-4)

- Before birth, the lungs do not function; oxygenated blood is shunted away via the foramen ovale and ductus arteriosus

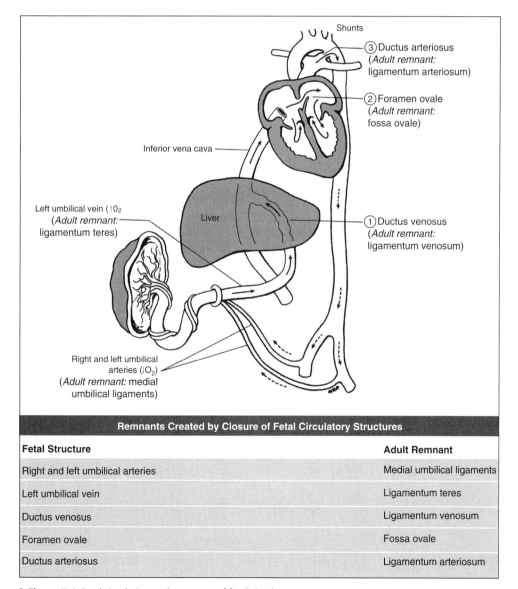

Shunts

③ Ductus arteriosus
(*Adult remnant:*
ligamentum arteriosum)

② Foramen ovale
(*Adult remnant:*
fossa ovale)

Inferior vena cava

Left umbilical vein ($\uparrow O_2$
(*Adult remnant:*
ligamentum teres)

Liver

① Ductus venosus
(*Adult remnant:*
ligamentum venosum)

Right and left umbilical
arteries ($\downarrow O_2$)
(*Adult remnant:* medial
umbilical ligaments)

Remnants Created by Closure of Fetal Circulatory Structures

Fetal Structure	Adult Remnant
Right and left umbilical arteries	Medial umbilical ligaments
Left umbilical vein	Ligamentum teres
Ductus venosus	Ligamentum venosum
Foramen ovale	Fossa ovale
Ductus arteriosus	Ligamentum arteriosum

● **Figure II-4** Fetal circulation and remnants of fetal circulatory structures.

- After birth, with the infant's first breath, decreased pulmonary vascular resistance occurs. Left atrial pressure increases above right atrial pressure, the foramen ovale closes, and increased oxygen triggers closure of ductus arteriosus (DA).
- Indomethacin closes the DA by blocking prostaglandin synthesis

Fetal circulation derivatives	• Umbilical vein: Ligamentum teres hepatic
	• Umbilical arteries: Medial umbilical ligaments
	• Ductus arteriosus: Ligamentum arteriosum
	• Ductus venosus: Ligamentum venosum
	• Foramen ovale: Fossa ovalis
Male/female genital homologues	• Corpus spongiosum = Vestibular bulbs
	• Bulbourethral glands (Cowper's) = Greater vestibular glands (Bartholin's)
	• Prostate gland = Glans clitoris
	• Ventral penile shaft = Labia minora
	• Scrotum = Labia majora

Topic **3**

Embryologic Anomalies

Must Knows

- Nervous system abnormalities
- Gastrointestinal (GI) abnormalities
- Genitourinary abnormalities

NERVOUS SYSTEM

Neural tube defects	• Spina bifida: Lumbosacral region; bony vertebral arches fail to close
	○ Occulta: Mildest form; evidence by tuft of hair
	○ Spina bifida with rachischisis: Most severe, secondary to failure of posterior neuropore closure; paralysis from the level of the defect downward
	• Anencephaly: Failure of the anterior neuropore to close; results in failure of the brain and cranium to develop; incompatible with extrauterine life

- Diagnosed prenatally by elevated maternal serum α-fetoprotein level and ultrasonography
- Approximately 75% can be prevented by use of preconceptual folic acid

Arnold-Chiari malformation	• Caudal vermis, cerebellar tonsils, and medulla through the foramen magnum; can be associated with obstructive hydrocephalus • Signs and symptoms from compression of medulla and stretching of CN 9, 10, and 12
Neuroblastoma	• Most common solid extracranial neoplasm; *N-myc* oncogene, chromosome 1p deletion • Primitive neuroblasts derived from neural crest, arranged in Homer-Wright pseudorosettes • 60% along sympathetic chain, 40% in adrenal medulla • Urine markers: Increased vanillylmandelic acid (VMA) and metanephrine levels • Treatment: Surgery, chemotherapy
Pheochromocytoma	• Secrete norepinephrine and epinephrine • Associated with multiple endocrine neoplasia (MEN) IIA and IIB • Classic symptom triad: Episodic headache, sweating, and tachycardia in the setting of hypertension • Rule of 10's: 10% malignant, 10% bilateral, 10% extraadrenal, 10% calcify, 10% in children, 10% are familial • Treatment: Surgery and α-antagonist phenoxybenzamine before β-blocker therapy

GASTROINTESTINAL

Cleft lip and palate	• Cleft lip: Occurs when maxillary prominence fails to fuse with the medial nasal prominence
	• Cleft palate
	  ◦ Anterior: When the palatine shelves fail to fuse with the primary palate
	  ◦ Posterior: When the palatine shelves fail to fuse with each other and with the nasal septum

Pyloric stenosis	• Hypertrophy of muscularis externa with narrowing of pyloric lumen • Signs and symptoms: Nonbilious projectile vomiting; palpable "olive-like" mass
Abdominal wall herniation	• Omphalocele: Persistent herniation of abdominal contents into umbilical and supraumbilical portions of abdominal wall; possesses a membranous sac • Gastroschisis: Full-thickness paraumbilical wall defect associated with evisceration of abdominal contents; attributable to vascular accident disruption of normal abdominal wall development; no sac

Meckel's diverticulum	• When remnant of the vitelline duct persists, forming an out-pouching on the antimesenteric border of the ileum • Most common congenital GI abnormality • Rule of 2's: 2 inches long; 2 feet from ileocecal valve; 2% of population presents during first 2 years of life, can possess 2 types of epithelium • Signs and symptoms: GI bleeding, obstruction
Hirschsprung's disease	• Caused by the arrest of neural crest caudal migration • Absence of ganglion cells in myenteric and submucosal plexuses • Massive colonic dilation precedes aganglionic portions • 50% familial and 15% sporadic cases are associated with *RET* proto-oncogene mutations • Signs and symptoms: Inability to pass meconium, abdominal distension
Tracheoesophageal fistulas (TEs)	• Abnormal connection between the esophagus and trachea; most common is complete esophageal atresia with a connection between the distal esophagus and trachea • Caused by improper division of the foregut by TE septum • Associated with polyhydramnios • Signs and symptoms: coughing or cyanosis on feeding, recurrent aspiration pneumonia • Diagnosis: Inability to pass a nasogastric tube into the stomach

GENITOURINARY

Urinary system abnormalities	• Renal ectopia: One or both kidneys fails to ascend (i.e., pelvic kidney) • Renal fusion (horseshoe kidney): Inferior poles of both kidneys fuse; ascent is then arrested secondary to the presence of IMA • Urachal cyst or fistula: persistent remnants of the allantois
Congenital penile abnormalities	• Hypospadias: Urethral folds fail to fuse completely, resulting in a ventral external urethral orifice • Epispadias: External urethral orifice opens on the dorsal surface
Female pseudointersexuality	• 46,XX; ovarian tissue present and masculinization of the female external genitalia • Caused most commonly by congenital adrenal hyperplasia (i.e., 21β- or 11β-hydroxylase deficiency) • "Salt-wasting" form: Aldosterone synthesis does not occur, producing hyponatremia and hyperkalemia
Male pseudointersexuality	• 46,XY; testes present but with female or ambiguous external genitalia • Caused most commonly by androgen insensitivity secondary to a mutation in the androgen receptor gene; X-linked recessive • Appear to be girls but with no internal female organs (secondary to Müllerian inhibiting factor) and a blind-pouch vagina

Topic **4**

Teratology

Must Knows

● TORCH organisms

● Teratogenic drugs

TORCH organisms

- *Toxoplasma gondii,* a protozoan parasite
  - Transmitted through ingestion of oocyst in water or food, cyst-containing undercooked meat
  - Transmitted transplacentally
  - Results in miscarriage, perinatal death, chorioretinitis, microcephaly, hydrocephalus, and encephalomyelitis with cerebral calcification
- Others, including *Treponema pallidum,* a spirochete
  - Transmitted via sexual contact
  - Transmitted transplacentally
  - Results in miscarriage, perinatal death, hepatosplenomegaly, focal erosions of the proximal medial tibia (Wimberger sign), saw-toothed appearance of the metaphysis of long bones, Hutchinson teeth
- Rubella virus: Togaviridae, enveloped, ss-RNA
  - Transmitted transplacentally; risk greatest during the first trimester
  - Results in cardiac triad (patent ductus arteriosus, pulmonary artery stenosis, atrioventricular septal defects)
  - Results in intrauterine growth retardation, eye involvement, bluish-purple lesions on yellow jaundiced skin ("blueberry muffin spots"), sensorineural deafness
- Cytomegalovirus (CMV): Herpesviridae, enveloped, ds-DNA
  - Transmitted transplacentally; more severe during the first trimester
  - Results in sensorineural deafness, intrauterine growth retardation, microcephaly, chorioretinitis, hepatosplenomegaly, osteitis

- Herpes simplex virus (HSV-1 and 2): Herpesviridae, enveloped, ds-DNA
  - Transmitted by direct contact via passage through an infected birth canal, most commonly by HSV-2
  - CNS involvement includes lethargy, bulging fontanelles, focal or generalized seizures, opisthotonus, decerebrate posturing, and coma
  - Hematogenous spread causes multiorgan disease

Drugs
- Angiotensin-converting enzyme inhibitors: Renal damage
- Ethanol: Fetal alcohol syndrome
- Diethylstilbestrol: Vaginal clear-cell carcinoma
- Iodide: Congenital goiter or hypothyroidism
- Retinoic acid: High risk of multiple birth defects
- Phenytoin: Fetal hydantoin syndrome
- Thalidomide: Fetal limb reduction (e.g., meromelia, amelia)
- Valproic acid: Neural tube defects
- Warfarin: Bone and cartilage abnormalities

Topic **5**

Gross Anatomy

Must Knows

- Spinal cord segmentation and key dermatomal anatomy
- Coronary artery anatomy
- Abdominal anatomy

SEGMENTAL ANATOMY

Lumbar puncture
- Procedure to withdraw cerebrospinal fluid from the subarachnoid space
- Needle is inserted between L4 and L5 at level of iliac crests
- Structures pierced (Fig. II-5):
  - Skin → Superficial fascia → supraspinous ligament → interspinous ligament → ligamentum flavum → epidural space → duramater → arachnoid → subarachnoid space

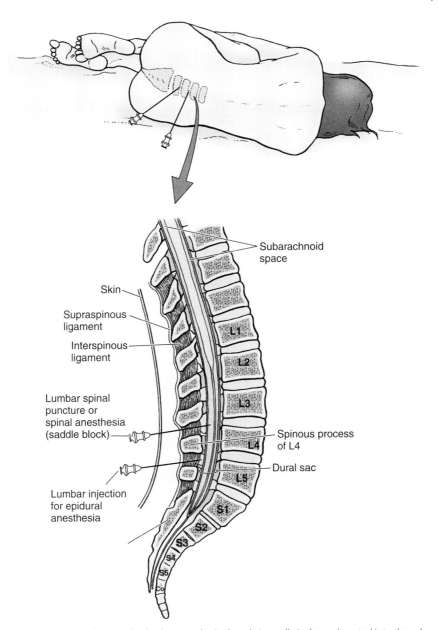

● **Figure II-5** Lumbar vertebral column and spinal cord. A needle is shown inserted into the subarachnoid space above the spinous process of L4 (L3–4 interspace) to withdraw cerebrospinal fluid or administer spinal anesthesia. A second needle is shown inserted into the epidural space to administer lumbar epidural anesthesia. Note the sequence of layers (superficial to deep) that the needle must penetrate.

| **Spinal cord** | • 31 spinal nerves: Eight cervical, 12 thoracic, five lumbar, five sacral, one coccygeal |
| | • Cord extends to level of L1–L2, below which lies the cauda equina; subarachnoid space extends to S2 |

Dermatomes (Fig. II-6)

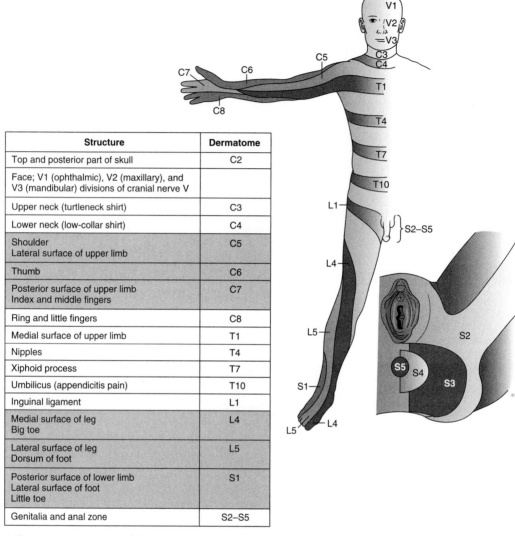

Structure	Dermatome
Top and posterior part of skull	C2
Face; V1 (ophthalmic), V2 (maxillary), and V3 (mandibular) divisions of cranial nerve V	
Upper neck (turtleneck shirt)	C3
Lower neck (low-collar shirt)	C4
Shoulder Lateral surface of upper limb	C5
Thumb	C6
Posterior surface of upper limb Index and middle fingers	C7
Ring and little fingers	C8
Medial surface of upper limb	T1
Nipples	T4
Xiphoid process	T7
Umbilicus (appendicitis pain)	T10
Inguinal ligament	L1
Medial surface of leg Big toe	L4
Lateral surface of leg Dorsum of foot	L5
Posterior surface of lower limb Lateral surface of foot Little toe	S1
Genitalia and anal zone	S2–S5

● **Figure II-6** Anterior view of dermatomes. Although dermatomes are shown as distinct segments, some overlap occurs between any two adjacent dermatomes. *Shaded areas* in the table indicate dermatomes that are affected by a herniated disk. (The sensory innervation of the face does not involve dermatomes. It is provided by cranial nerve V [CN V]: V1 [ophthalmic division], V2 [maxillary division], and V3 [mandibular division].) Knowledge of dermatomes is important because clinical vignette questions include a description of sensory loss at a specific dermatome level.

Diaphragm structures

- Inferior vena cava (IVC): Perforates at level of T8
- Esophagus and vagus: Perforate at level of T10
- Aorta, thoracic duct, azygous vein: perforate at level of T12

THE HEART

Heart surfaces

- The posterior surface (base) consists of the left atrium
- The apex consists of the left ventricle at intercostal space 5 along the midclavicular line

- The sternal surface consists of the right ventricle
- The diaphragmatic surface consists of the left ventricle

Heart borders	• Right border: Right atrium and superior vena cava (SVC) • Left border: Left ventricle and atrium, pulmonary trunk, and aortic arch • Inferior border: Right ventricle • Superior border: SVC, aorta, and pulmonary trunk

Coronary arterial anatomy (Fig. II-7)	• The right coronary artery (RCA) arises from the right aortic sinus
	
	  ○ Courses in the coronary sulcus
	
	  ○ Right-side dominant (approximately 80%): Posterior inter-ventricular artery arises from the RCA
	
	  ○ Supplies the sinoatrial and atrioventricular nodes
	
	• The left main coronary artery (LMCA) arises from the left aortic sinus
	
	  ○ Left-side dominant (approximately 20%): Posterior inter-ventricular artery arises from the LMCA
	
	  ○ Important branches: Circumflex artery, left anterior descending (LAD) coronary artery
	
	  ○ LAD: Most commonly occluded

Valves and auscultation sites	• Tricuspid valve: Between the right atrium and ventricle; three leaflets
	
	  ○ Auscultation site = Over the sternum at the fifth intercostal space
	
	• Pulmonary semilunar valve: At outflow of right ventricle, three cusps
	
	  ○ Orifice is directed to the left shoulder
	
	  ○ Auscultation site: Lateral to the sternum at the left second intercostal space
	
	• Mitral valve: Between the left atrium and ventricle; two leaflets
	
	  ○ Auscultation site: At cardiac apex, left fifth intercostal space
	
	• Aortic semilunar valve: At the outflow of the left ventricle; three cusps
	
	  ○ Orifice is directed to the right shoulder
	
	  ○ Auscultation site: Lateral to sternum at the right second intercostal space

THE ABDOMEN

Intra- and extraperitoneal structures	• Intraperitoneal: Stomach, first portion of duodenum, jejunum, ileum, cecum, appendix, transverse colon, sigmoid colon, liver, gallbladder, tail of pancreas, spleen

Arterial Supply

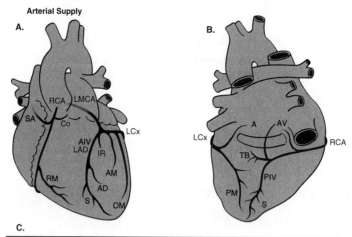

C.

	Branches	Structures Supplied
Right coronary artery	SA nodal artery Conus branch Right marginal artery AV nodal artery Terminal branches Posterior interventricular artery Septal branches	SA node Right atrium Right ventricle Diaphragmatic surface of the left ventricle AV node Posterior third of the interventricular septum

Left main coronary artery	**Left circumflex artery**
	    Anterior marginal artery
	    Obtuse marginal artery
	    Atrial branches
	    Posterior marginal artery
	Intermediate ramus
	Anterior interventricular artery
	(left anterior descending)
	    Anterior diagonal artery
	    Septal branches
		Left atrium
		Majority of the left ventricle
		Right and left bundle branches of the
		  bundle of His
		Anterior two-thirds of the interventricular
		  septum

Venous Drainage

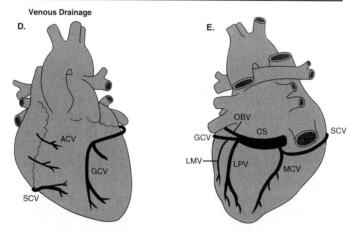

● **Figure II-7** Arterial supply of the heart. (**A**) Anterior (sternocostal) surface of the heart. (**B**) Inferior (diaphragmatic) surface of the heart. (**C**) The branches of the right and left coronary arteries and the structures supplied by each. Venous drainage of the heart. (**D**) Anterior (sternocostal) surface of the heart. (**E**) Inferior (diaphragmatic) surface of the heart. A = atrial branches; ACV = anterior cardiac veins; AD = anterior diagonal artery; AIV = anterior interventricular artery; AV = atrioventricular nodal artery; Co = conus branch; CS = coronary sinus; GCV = great cardiac vein; IR = intermediate ramus; LAD = left anterior descending artery; LCx = left circumflex artery; LMCA = left main coronary artery; LMV = left marginal vein; LPV = left posterior vein; MCV = middle cardiac vein; OBV = oblique vein of the left atrium; OM = obtuse marginal artery; PIV = posterior interventricular artery; PM = posterior marginal artery; RCA = right coronary artery; RM = right marginal artery; S = septal branches; SA = sinoatrial nodal artery; SCV = small cardiac vein; TB = terminal branch.

- Retroperitoneal: Second to fourth portion of duodenum, ascending colon, descending colon, rectum, pancreatic head/neck/body, kidneys, ureters, adrenal glands, abdominal aorta, IVC

Gastrointestinal blood supply	• Celiac artery: Supplies the foregut
	   ○ Stomach to duodenum; liver, gallbladder, pancreas
	• Superior mesenteric artery: Supplies the midgut
	   ○ Duodenum to proximal two thirds of the transverse colon
	• Inferior mesenteric artery: Supplies the hindgut
	   ○ Distal third of the transverse colon to the upper rectum

THE EXTREMITIES

Muscles of the rotator cuff	• Supraspinatus, infraspinatus, teres minor, subscapularis

Topic **6**

Anatomic Pathology

Must Knows

- Distinguish between the mechanisms of pneumothorax
- Biliary tree obstruction: Jaundice versus non-jaundice
- Portosystemic anastomoses
- Abdominal wall hernias
- Common injuries to the extremities

THORAX

Postductal aortic coarctation	• Congenital anomaly that causes upper extremity hypertension and poor lower extremity pulses • Collateral circulation: Internal thoracic • Intercostals: Superior epigastrics • Inferior epigastrics: External iliacs • "Rib notching" occurs secondary to erosion of ribs by intercostal arteries

Cardiac tamponade	• Accumulation of fluid in the pericardial cavity
	• Compresses the heart because the fibrous pericardium is inelastic
	• Beck's triad: Classical presentation of the three D's: decreased blood pressure, distended neck veins, and decreased heart sounds
Pneumothorax	• Spontaneous: Air enters pleura via ruptured bleb, causes lung collapse
	• Signs and symptoms: Chest pain, cough, dyspnea
	• Open: Pleural cavity opened to outside atmosphere; collapses lung; commonly caused by trauma
	• Tension: Ball-valve injury; air enters pleura but cannot escape; causes tracheal shift away from injury, jugular venous distention, and absent breath sounds; may cause sudden death

ABDOMEN AND PELVIS

Biliary tree obstruction	• Biliary colic: Intermittent epigastric pain secondary to stone transiently lodge in cystic duct; no jaundice present
	• Acute cholecystitis: Inflammation of the gallbladder; causes pain secondary to entrapped stone in the cystic duct; no jaundice, but Murphy's sign is present
	• Choledocholithiasis: Gallstone becomes lodged in the common bile duct, blocking biliary flow from the gallbladder and liver; causes jaundice
Portosystemic anastomoses (Fig. II-8)	• Left gastric-azygous: Esophageal varices
	• Superior-middle or inferior rectal: Hemorrhoids
	• Paraumbilical-inferior epigastric: Caput medusae
	• Retroperitoneal: Renal and paravertebral
Abdominal hernias (Fig. II-9)	• Diaphragmatic: Defect through which abdominal organs may pass into thorax; can be congenital; hiatal, in which the stomach herniates through esophageal hiatus, is the most common form
	• Direct inguinal: Protrudes through Hesselbach's triangle, bulges medial to inferior epigastric artery, and passes through external inguinal ring only; common in older men
	• Indirect inguinal: Protrudes though the internal and external inguinal rings, passes into the scrotum, protrudes lateral to the inferior epigastric artery; common in infants; attributable to failure of processus vaginalis closure
	• Femoral: Protrudes below the inguinal ligament into the femoral canal, protrudes medial to femoral vein; common in women; prone to early strangulation
Anal canal and hemorrhoids (Fig. II-10)	• Anal canal has upper and lower parts, divided by the pectinate line. It is surrounded by the internal anal sphincter under involuntary control via autonomic innervation and the external anal sphincter with striated muscle under voluntary control via the pudendal nerve.

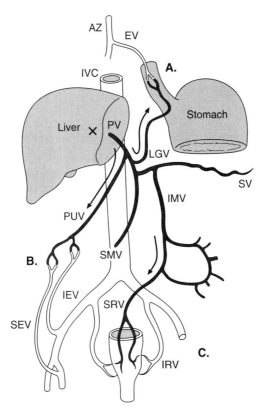

● **Figure II-8** The azygous venous system and the inferior vena cava (IVC). Note that the left gonadal vein (LGV) drains into the left renal vein (LRV). This pathway has clinical implications in males (e.g., left testicular varicocele). The azygous vein provides a route of collateral venous returns (*arrows*) if the IVC is blocked (X). AZ = azygous vein; EV = esophageal vein; IEV = inferior epigastric vein; IMV = inferior mesenteric vein; IRV = inferior rectal vein; PUV = paraumbilical vein; PV = portal vein; SEV = superior epigastric vein; SMV = superior mesenteric vein; SRV = superior rectal vein; SV = splenic vein.

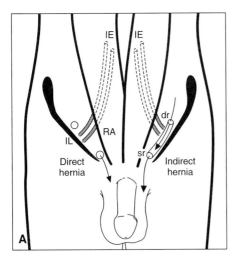 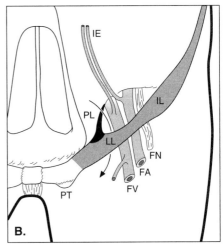

● **Figure II-9** (**A**) Anatomy associated with direct and indirect inguinal hernias. (**B**) Anatomy associated with a femoral hernia. dr = deep inguinal ring; FA = femoral artery; FN = femoral nerve; FV = femoral vein; IE = inferior epigastric artery and vein; IL = inguinal ligament; LL = lacunar ligament; PL = pectineal (Cooper) ligament; PT = pubic tubercle; RA = rectus abdominis muscle; sr = superficial inguinal ring.

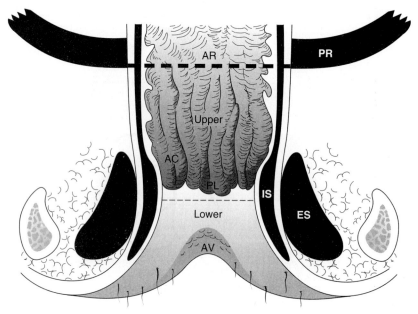

● **Figure II-10** The anal canal. Note the following structures: ampulla of the rectum (AR), puborectalis muscle (PR), anal columns (AC), anal verge (AV), pectinate line (PL; *thin dotted line*), internal anal sphincter (IS), and external anal sphincter (ES). The *thick dotted line* marks the anorectal junction. (Adapted with permission from Ernest WA: *NMS Anatomy,* 2nd ed. Media, PA: Harwal, 2000: 225.)

- Internal hemorrhoids: Varicosities of superior rectal veins, located above the pectinate line
  - Signs and symptoms: Bleeding, mucus discharge, prolapse, pruritus, painless
- External hemorrhoids: Varicosities of inferior rectal veins; located below pectinate line
  - Signs and symptoms: Bleeding, swelling, and pain

EXTREMITIES

Fracture of the scaphoid	- Most commonly fracture carpal bone; associated with osteonecrosis - Signs and symptoms: Tenderness of the "anatomical snuff box" (formed by the tendons of the extensor pollicis longus, extensor pollicis brevis, and abductor pollicis longus); radiographs may not show the fracture
Colles' fracture	- Fracture of the distal radius in which the distal fragment is displaced posteriorly ("dinner fork deformity") - Occurs during a fall on an outstretched hand with the wrist extended - Commonly accompanied by a fracture of the ulnar styloid process
Boxer's fracture	- Fracture at the head of the fifth metacarpal when a closed fist is used to hit something hard

- Signs and symptoms: Pain on the ulnar side of hand; depression of the head of the fifth metacarpal; flexing the fifth digit elicits pain

Femoral neck fracture	- Common in elderly women with osteoporosis - The lower limb is externally rotated and shorter than the normal limb - Avascular necrosis of the femoral head may occur
Posterior hip dislocation	- The hip is commonly dislocated in a posterior direction (e.g., car accident in which the flexed knee hits the dashboard); the lower limb is internally rotated, adducted, and shorter than the normal limb - Avascular necrosis of the femoral head may occur; the sciatic nerve may be damaged
The terrible triad of O'Donahue	- Result of fixation of a semi-flexed leg receiving a violent lateral blow (e.g., clipping in football); causes abduction and lateral rotation (Fig. II-11)

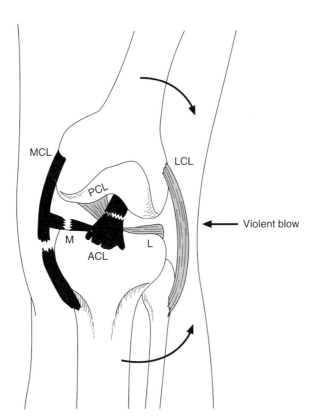

● **Figure II-11** The "terrible triad of O'Donoghue." Injury to the left knee caused by a violent blow to the lateral side of the knee (e.g., football "clipping"). The *curved arrows* indicate the direction of movement at the knee joint (abduction and lateral rotation). The anterior cruciate ligament (ACL), medial meniscus (M), and medial collateral ligament (MCL) are torn. Other structures of the knee are uninjured. LCL = lateral collateral ligament; PCL = posterior cruciate ligament; L = lateral meniscus.

- The anterior cruciate ligament (ACL) is torn; the medial meniscus is torn as a result of its attachment to the medial collateral ligament; and the medial collateral ligament is torn because of excessive abduction of the knee joint
- Anterior draw sign = Torn ACL

Topic **7**

Neuroanatomy

Must Knows

- Cranial nerve function and anatomy
- Vascular anatomy of the brain
- Synaptic anatomy of the basal ganglia
- Spinal cord pathways
- Brachial plexus components

THE BRAIN

Blood–brain barrier (BBB)
- An anatomic and physiologic separation of blood from the extracellular fluid in the central nervous system (CNS)
- Consists of the zonula occludens (tight junctions) between nonfenestrated intracerebral capillary endothelial cells; the surrounding basal lamina; and astrocytic foot processes, which promote the formation of tight junctions
- Water, gases, and small lipid-soluble molecules freely diffuse across the BBB; glucose and amino acids cross via carrier protein-mediated transport; the BBB excludes many drugs from the CNS
- Dopamine does not cross the BBB, but L-DOPA (used to treat Parkinson's disease) does

Cranial nerves
- The butcher's plea: Oh, oh, oh, to try and find very good veal and ham
  - I. Olfactory: Smell
  - II. Optic: Vision
  - III. Oculomotor: Eye movement (all eye muscles except for LR and SO; remember the chemical formula LR_6SO_4), pupil constriction, accommodation, eyelid opening

IV. Trochlear: Eye movement; innervates superior oblique muscle

V. Trigeminal: Mastication, facial sensation

VI. Abducens: Eye movement; innervates lateral rectus

VII. Facial: Muscles of facial expression, taste on the anterior two thirds of the tongue, salivation, lacrimation

VIII. Vestibulocochlear: Mediates equilibrium and balance (vestibular) and hearing (cochlear)

IX. Glossopharyngeal: Taste on posterior third of the tongue, salivation, swallowing, input from the carotid body and sinus

X. Vagus: Taste, swallowing; innervates the viscera of the thorax and abdomen

XI. Accessory: Innervates the sternocleidomastoid and trapezius muscles

XII. Hypoglossal: Innervates the intrinsic and extrinsic tongue muscles

Cranial nerve passageways	• Cribriform plate: I • Optic canal: II • Superior orbital fissure: III, IV, V$_1$, VI • Foramen rotundum: V$_2$ • Foramen ovale: V$_3$ • Internal auditory meatus: VII, VIII • Jugular foramen: IX, X, XI • Hypoglossal canal: XII
Extraocular muscles	• Superior rectus (cranial nerve [CN] III): The patient is asked to look to the side and then upward • Medial rectus (CN III): The patient is asked to look toward the nose • Inferior rectus (CN III): The patient is asked to look to the side and then downward • Inferior oblique (CN III): The patient is asked to look at the nose and then upward ("up and in") • Superior oblique (CN IV): The patient is asked to look at the nose and then downward ("down and in") • Lateral rectus (CN VI): The patient is asked to look to the side
Circle of Willis (Fig. II-12)	• Anterior cerebral artery: Supplies motor and sensory cortex for legs; occlusion results in contralateral paralysis and anesthesia of the leg • Middle cerebral artery: Supplies lateral aspects of the brain; occlusion of the main stem results in contralateral hemiplegia and hemianesthesia, homonymous hemianopia, and aphasia (dominant hemisphere only)

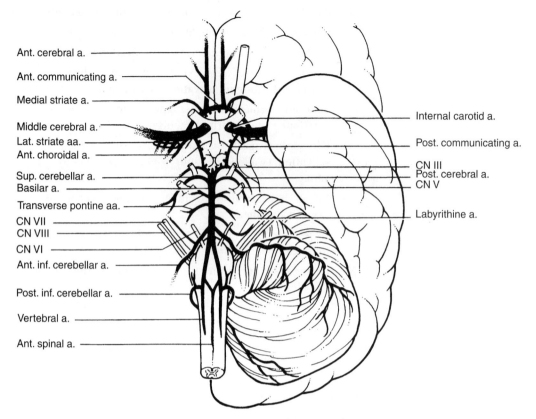

Ant. cerebral a.

Ant. communicating a.

Medial striate a.

Middle cerebral a.

Lat. striate aa.

Ant. choroidal a.

Sup. cerebellar a.

Basilar a.

Transverse pontine aa.

CN VII

CN VIII

CN VI

Ant. inf. cerebellar a.

Post. inf. cerebellar a.

Vertebral a.

Ant. spinal a.

Internal carotid a.

Post. communicating a.

CN III

Post. cerebral a.

CN V

Labyrithine a.

● **Figure II-12** Arteries of the base of the brain and brain stem, including the arterial circle of Willis. CN = cranial nerve.

- Lenticulostriate arteries (deep branches or lateral striate): Supply the basal ganglia and internal capsule; occlusion causes the classic "paralytic stroke" with contralateral hemiplegia and hemianesthesia. These arteries are prone to hemorrhagic infarction attributable to hypertension or atherosclerotic occlusion.
- Anterior communicating artery: Connects the anterior cerebral arteries; most common site of an aneurysm (e.g., Berry aneurysm)
- Posterior communicating artery: Connects the anterior and posterior circulations; second most common site of an aneurysm; can cause oculomotor nerve (CN III) paralysis

Hypothalamus (Fig. II-13)

Thalamic nuclei (Fig. II-14)

- The thalamus functions to integrate the sensory and motor systems
- Lateral geniculate: Vision
- Medial geniculate: Hearing
- Ventral posterior, lateral part: Body senses (proprioception, light touch, pain, vibration, pressure)
- Ventral posterior, medial part: Facial sensation
- Ventral anterior and lateral: Motor function

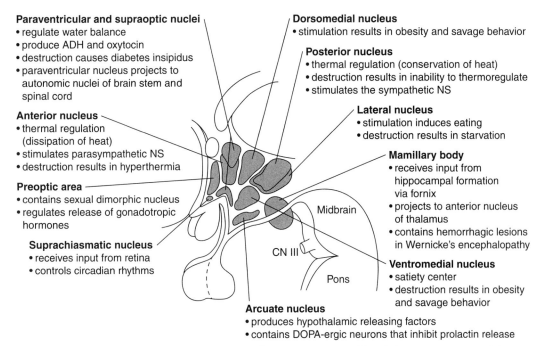

Paraventricular and supraoptic nuclei
- regulate water balance
- produce ADH and oxytocin
- destruction causes diabetes insipidus
- paraventricular nucleus projects to autonomic nuclei of brain stem and spinal cord

Anterior nucleus
- thermal regulation (dissipation of heat)
- stimulates parasympathetic NS
- destruction results in hyperthermia

Preoptic area
- contains sexual dimorphic nucleus
- regulates release of gonadotropic hormones

Suprachiasmatic nucleus
- receives input from retina
- controls circadian rhythms

Dorsomedial nucleus
- stimulation results in obesity and savage behavior

Posterior nucleus
- thermal regulation (conservation of heat)
- destruction results in inability to thermoregulate
- stimulates the sympathetic NS

Lateral nucleus
- stimulation induces eating
- destruction results in starvation

Mamillary body
- receives input from hippocampal formation via fornix
- projects to anterior nucleus of thalamus
- contains hemorrhagic lesions in Wernicke's encephalopathy

Ventromedial nucleus
- satiety center
- destruction results in obesity and savage behavior

Arcuate nucleus
- produces hypothalamic releasing factors
- contains DOPA-ergic neurons that inhibit prolactin release

Midbrain

CN III

Pons

● **Figure II-13** Major hypothalamic nuclei and their functions. ADH = antidiuretic hormone; CN = cranial nerve; DOPA = dopamine; NS = nervous system.

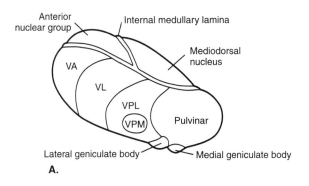

Anterior nuclear group

Internal medullary lamina

Mediodorsal nucleus

VA

VL

VPL

VPM

Pulvinar

Lateral geniculate body

Medial geniculate body

A.

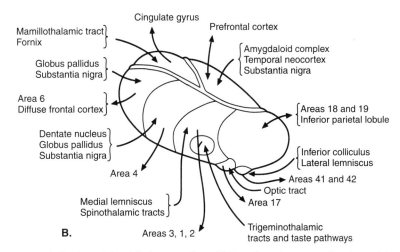

Mamillothalamic tract
Fornix

Cingulate gyrus

Prefrontal cortex

Amygdaloid complex
Temporal neocortex
Substantia nigra

Globus pallidus
Substantia nigra

Area 6
Diffuse frontal cortex

Areas 18 and 19
Inferior parietal lobule

Dentate nucleus
Globus pallidus
Substantia nigra

Inferior colliculus
Lateral lemniscus

Area 4

Areas 41 and 42
Optic tract
Area 17

Medial lemniscus
Spinothalamic tracts

B.

Areas 3, 1, 2

Trigeminothalamic tracts and taste pathways

● **Figure II-14** Major thalamic nuclei and their connections. (**A**) Dorsolateral aspect and major nuclei. (**B**) Major afferent and efferent connections. VA = ventral anterior nucleus; VL = ventral lateral nucleus; VPL = ventral posterior lateral nucleus; VPM = ventral posterior medial nucleus.

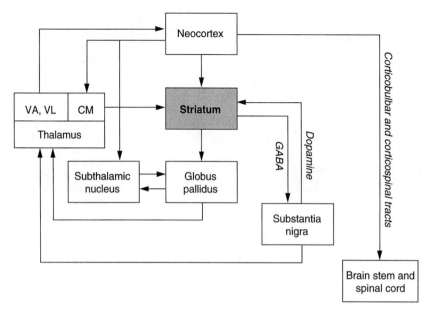

● **Figure II-15** Major afferent and efferent connections of the striatal system. The striatum receives major input from three sources: the thalamus, neocortex, and substantia nigra. The striatum projects to the globus pallidus and substantia nigra. The globus pallidus is the effector nucleus of the striatal system; it projects to the thalamus and subthalamic nucleus. The substantia nigra also projects to the thalamus. The striatal motor system is expressed through the corticobulbar and corticospinal tracts. CM = centromedian nucleus; GABA = γ-aminobutyric acid; VA = ventral anterior nucleus; VL = ventral lateral nucleus.

Basal ganglia (Fig. II-15)	• Striatum: Caudate and putamen
	• Lentiform nucleus: Globus pallidus and putamen
	• Corpus striatum: Lentiform nucleus and caudate
	• Has a role in the initiation and execution of somatic motor activity (especially willed movement); also involved in postural and reflex motor activity
Limbic system (Fig. II-16)	• Serves as the anatomic basis for behavioral and emotional expression (e.g., feeding, sexual behavior, fear, anger)
Cerebellum	• Maintenance of posture and balance; maintenance of muscle tone; coordination of voluntary motor activity
	• Major cerebellar pathway: Purkinje cells of cortex project to cerebellar nuclei; dentate nucleus (major nucleus) projects through the superior cerebellar peduncle via the dentatothalamic tract to the contralateral ventral lateral thalamic nucleus; VL nucleus projects to primary motor cortex of the precentral gyrus; motor cortex projects as the corticopontine tract to the pontine nuclei; pontine nuclei project as the pontocerebellar tract to the contralateral cerebellar cortex, terminating on mossy fibers

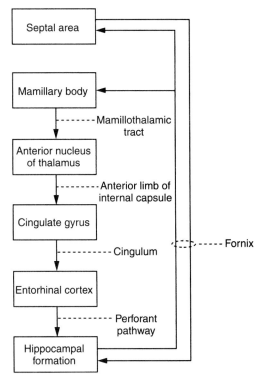

● **Figure II-16** Major afferent and efferent limbic connections of the hippocampal formation. This formation has three components: the hippocampus (cornu Ammonis), subiculum, and dentate gyrus. The hippocampus projects to the septal area, the subiculum projects to the mamillary nuclei, and the dentate gyrus does not project beyond the hippocampal formation. The circuit of Papez follows this route: hippocampal formation to mamillary nucleus to anterior thalamic nucleus to cingulate gyrus to entorhinal cortex to hippocampal formation.

THE SPINAL CORD AND PERIPHERAL NERVOUS SYSTEM

Tracts of the spinal cord (Fig. II-17)

- Dorsal column-medial lemniscal tract: Mediates proprioception, vibration, pressure, two-point discrimination

  ○ Pathway: First-order neurons in the dorsal root ganglia (DRG) → fasciculi gracilis and cuneatus → second-order neurons in the gracile and cuneate nuclei → decussating axons (medial lemniscus) to the ventroposterolateral (VPL) of the thalamus → third-order neurons from the VPL to the postcentral gyrus (posterior limb of the internal capsule)

  ○ Transection above decussation leads to a contralateral deficit; transection below leads to an ipsilateral deficit

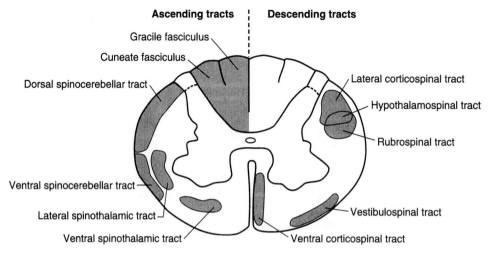

● **Figure II-17** The major ascending and descending pathways of the spinal cord. The ascending sensory tracts are shown on the *left,* and the descending motor tracts are shown on the *right.*

- Spinothalamic tract: Relays pain, temperature, nondiscriminatory touch
  - Pathway: First-order neurons in the DRG → project to cord via the tract of Lissauer → second-order neurons in the dorsal horn → decussating axons to the contralateral lateral funiculus (spinothalamic tract) → third-order neurons from the VPL of the thalamus → postcentral gyrus (posterior limb of the internal capsule)
  - Transection: Contralateral loss of modalities below the lesion
- Corticospinal tract: Volitional control of the limbs and trunk
  - Pathway: Neurons in the precentral gyrus, premotor cortex, and postcentral gyrus → (85%) decussate in the ventral medulla → descend as the lateral corticospinal tract (LCT) → terminate on the ventral horn motor neurons or (15%) do not decussate → descend in the spinal cord as the ventral corticospinal tract
  - Transection above decussation leads to contralateral loss of motor function, spastic paresis, a positive Babinski sign; transection below leads to ipsilateral loss of motor function, spastic paresis, a positive Babinski sign

Brachial plexus (Fig. II-18)

Lumbosacral plexus (Fig. II-19)

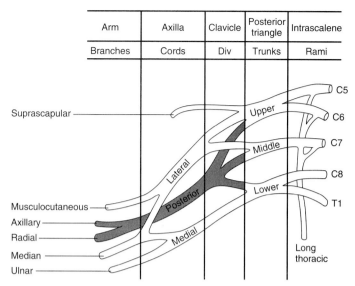

Arm	Axilla	Clavicle	Posterior triangle	Intrascalene
Branches	Cords	Div	Trunks	Rami

● Figure II-18 The rami, trunks, divisions (Div), cords, and five major terminal branches of the brachial plexus, along with their anatomic positions. Erb-Duchenne and Klumpke injuries to the brachial plexus. (Part A Adapted with permission from April EW: *NMS Clinical Anatomy,* 3rd ed. Baltimore: Williams & Wilkins, 1997.)

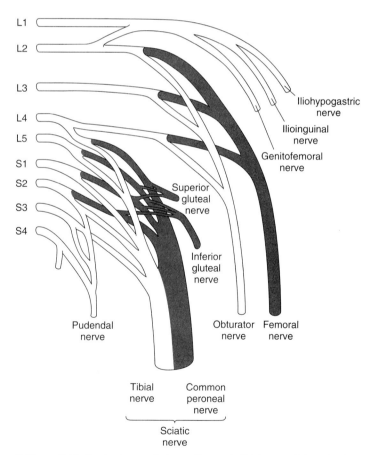

● Figure II-19 The lumbosacral plexus. The rami, divisions, and six major terminal branches are shown. The posterior divisions and branches are shown in *black*. The pudendal nerve is also shown.

Topic **8**

Neuropathology

Must
Knows

- Anatomy of visual system defects
- Brain lesions and their sequelae
- Intervertebral disc herniation
- Lesions of the spinal cord
- Peripheral nerve injury

CNS AND CRANIAL NERVE PATHOLOGY

Visual system defects (Fig. II-20)	The visual pathway from the retina to the visual cortex is shown. The location of various visual system defects is indicated by the numbers 1–7 along with the attendant anopia.
Brain lesions	• Broca's area: Damage to the inferior frontal gyrus of the dominant hemisphere; causes expressive aphasia; effortful, nonfluent speech; poor repetition
	• Wernicke's area: Dominant posterior temporal lobe damage; causes receptive aphasia with poor comprehension; speech is fluent with no meaning; paraphasic errors
	• Arcuate fasciculus: Conduction aphasia; repetition is poor, comprehension is good, and speech is fluent
	• Amygdala: Bilateral damage causes Klüver-Bucy syndrome (hyperorality, hypersexuality, disinhibition)
	• Frontal lobe: Personality changes, concentration difficulties, problems with orientation and judgment
	• Right parietal lobe: Spatial neglect syndrome; agnosia for the contralateral side
	• Reticular activating system: Coma
	• Mamillary bodies: Bilateral damage causes Wernicke-Korsakoff's encephalopathy; occurs in chronic alcoholics; causes confabulation and anterograde amnesia
Intracranial hemorrhage	• Epidural: Caused by skull fracture and associated tearing of the middle meningeal artery; classic history of loss of consciousness with lucid interval

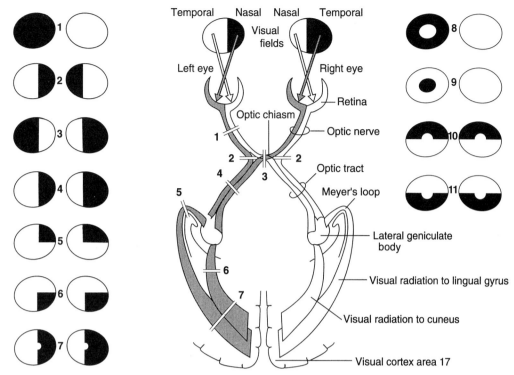

● Figure II-20 The visual pathway from the retina to the visual cortex showing visual field defects. (**1**) Ipsilateral blindness. (**2**) Binasal hemianopia. (**3**) Bitemporal hemianopia. (**4**) Right hemianopia. (**5**) Right upper quadrantanopia. (**6**) Right lower quadrantanopia. (**7**) Right hemianopia with macular sparing. (**8**) Left constricted field as a result of end-stage glaucoma. Bilateral constricted field may be seen in hysteria. (**9**) Left central scotoma as seen in optic (retrobulbar) neuritis in multiple sclerosis. (**10**) Upper altitudinal hemianopia as a result of bilateral destruction of the lingual gyri. (**11**) Lower altitudinal hemianopia as a result of bilateral destruction of the cunei.

- Computed tomography (CT) shows biconcave (lens-shaped) density near the skull; blood is located between the skull and dura
- Signs and symptoms: Ipsilateral blown pupil; contralateral hemiparesis
- Subdural: Caused by tearing of the bridging veins between the cortical surface and the dural venous sinuses
  - CT shows crescent shaped density that hugs brain contours; blood is located between dura and arachnoid
  - Can be acute, subacute, or chronic
- Subarachnoid: Caused by a contusion or laceration injury to the brain; cerebral or communicating arteries can be damaged
  - CT shows density in basal cistern, fissures, sulci, thickening of falx, and blood within the subarachnoid space
  - Signs and symptoms: "Worst headache of my life," meningismus, decreased mental status

Facial nerve lesions

- Central lesion: Upper motor neuron injury; causes contralateral lower facial paralysis

- Bell's palsy: Lower motor neuron injury; causes ipsilateral paralysis of facial expression of upper and lower face, loss of corneal reflex (efferent limb), loss of taste from the anterior two thirds of the tongue, and hyperacusis
  - Signs and symptoms: Inability to raise the eyebrow or blink; inability to seal the lips or smile properly on the affected side
  - Causes: AIDS, Lyme disease, sarcoidosis, tumors, diabetes

Recurrent laryngeal nerve	• Supplies intrinsic muscles of the larynx except for the cricothyroid; the left nerve wraps around the aortic arch; the right nerve around the right subclavian artery; nerves can be injured as a complication of thyroid surgery • Unilateral damage: Hoarse voice, shift of ipsilateral vocal fold to midline • Bilateral damage: Results in dyspnea with both vocal folds paralyzed at the midline

SPINAL CORD INJURY

Upper motor neuron (UMN) vs. lower motor neuron (LMN) signs	• UMN: Spastic paralysis or paresis; no significant atrophy; hyperreflexia (clonus); Babinski sign present; fibrillation and fasciculation absent • LMN: Flaccid paralysis or paresis; pronounced atrophy; hyporeflexia or areflexia; Babinski sign absent; fibrillation and fasciculation
Herniated disk (Table II-1)	• Disk consists of the annulus fibrosus and nucleus pulposus; the nucleus pulposus generally herniates in a posterior-lateral direction and compresses a nerve root

Spinal cord lesions (Fig. II-21)	• Poliomyelitis and Werdnig-Hoffman disease: LMN only
	
	• Amyotrophic lateral sclerosis (ALS): UMN and LMN; no sensory loss
	
	• Tabes dorsalis: Loss of tactile discrimination, position sense, vibration sensation; pain, paresthesia, and Romberg sign
	
	• Brown-Séquard syndrome: Combined motor and sensory loss
	  ○ Ipsilateral spastic paresis with pyramidal signs below the lesion
	  ○ Ipsilateral flaccid paralysis
	  ○ Ipsilateral loss of tactile discrimination as well as position and vibration sense
	  ○ Contralateral loss of pain and temperature sensation one segment below
	  ○ Ipsilateral Horner syndrome if the lesion is above T1
	
	• Ventral spinal artery occlusion: Combined motor and sensory loss
	  ○ Bilateral spastic paresis with pyramidal signs below the lesion

VERTEBRAL LEVELS OF HERNIATED DISK*

TABLE II-1

Herniated Disk Between	Compressed Nerve Root	Dermatome Affected	Muscles Affected	Movement Weakness	Nerve and Reflex Involved
C4–C5	C5	C5 Shoulder Lateral surface of upper limb	Deltoid	Abduction of arm	Axillary nerve ↓ biceps jerk
C5–C6	C6	C6 Thumb	Biceps brachialis Brachioradialis	Flexion of forearm Supination or pronation	Musculocutaneous nerve ↓ biceps jerk ↓ brachioradialis jerk
C6–C7	C7 Posterior surface of upper limb Middle and index fingers	Triceps Wrist extensors	Extension of forearm Extension of wrist	Radial nerve	↓ triceps jerk
L3–L4	L4	L4 Medial surface of leg Big toe	Quadriceps	Extension of knee	Femoral nerve ↓ knee jerk
L4–L5	L5	L5 Lateral surface of leg Dorsum of foot	Tibialis anterior Extensor hallucis longus Extensor digitorum longus	Dorsiflexion of ankle (cannot stand on heels) Extension of toes	Common peroneal nerve Absent or ↓ knee jerk
L5–S1 (most common)	S1	S1 Posterior surface of lower limb Little toe	Gastrocnemius Soleus	Plantar flexion (cannot stand on toes) Flexion of toes	Tibial nerve ↓ ankle jerk

*Note the correspondence between the dermatome affected and the compressed nerve root (shaded)

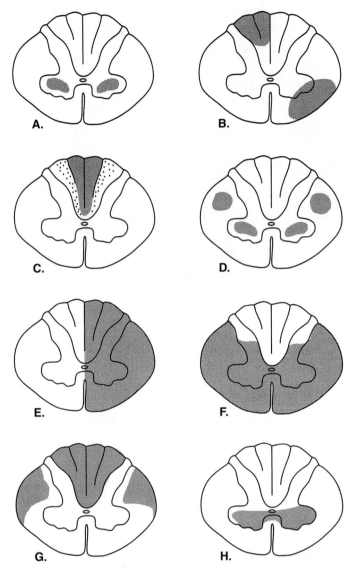

● **Figure II-21** Classic lesions of the spinal cord. (**A**) Poliomyelitis and progressive infantile muscular atrophy (Werdnig-Hoffmann disease). (**B**) Multiple sclerosis. (**C**) Dorsal column disease (tabes dorsalis). (**D**) Amyotrophic lateral sclerosis. (**E**) Hemisection of the spinal cord (Brown-Séquard syndrome). (**F**) Complete ventral spinal artery occlusion of the spinal cord. (**G**) Subacute combined degeneration (vitamin B$_{12}$ neuropathy). (**H**) Syringomyelia.

- ○ Bilateral flaccid paralysis
- ○ Bilateral loss of pain and temperature sensation below the lesion
- ○ Bilateral Horner syndrome if the lesion is above T1
- • Vitamin B12 neuropathy or Friedreich's ataxia: Motor and sensory loss
  - ○ Bilateral spastic paresis with pyramidal signs below the lesion

- ○ Bilateral arm and leg dystaxia
- ○ Bilateral loss of tactile discrimination as well as position and vibration sense
- Syringomyelia: Combined motor and sensory loss
  - ○ Bilateral flaccid paralysis of the intrinsic hand muscles
  - ○ Bilateral loss of pain and temperature sense
- Multiple sclerosis: Combined motor and sensory loss; involves primarily white matter of the cervical cord; lesions are random and asymmetric

PERIPHERAL NERVE INJURY

Erb-Duchenne palsy	• Involves C5 and C6 ventral first-degree rami; caused by stretching between the head and shoulder (e.g., from falling on the shoulder or birth trauma) • Damages the musculocutaneous, suprascapular, axillary, and phrenic nerves • Signs and symptoms: Arm is pronated and medially rotated ("waiter's tip hand"), and ipsilateral paralysis of the diaphragm occurs
Klumpke's paralysis	• Involves C8 and T1 ventral first-degree rami; caused by a sudden upward pull of the arm (i.e., abduction injury) • Damages the median and ulnar nerves and the T1 spinal nerve sympathetics • Signs and symptoms: Loss of wrist and hand function; Horner's syndrome (miosis, ptosis, and hemianhydrosis)
Thoracic outlet syndrome	• May result from a cervical rib compressing the lower trunk of the brachial plexus or subclavian artery • Clinical findings include atrophy of thenar and hypothenar eminences, atrophy of the interosseous muscles, sensory deficits on the medial side of the forearm and hand, diminished radial artery pulse upon moving the head to the opposite side, and bruit over the subclavian artery
Anterior dislocation of the humerus	• Anterior direction is the most common. The humeral head lies anterior and inferior to the coracoid process of the scapula. This can damage the axillary nerve or artery. • Signs and symptoms: Loss of normal round contour of the shoulder; a depression under the acromion is palpable; the head of humerus is palpable in the axilla; cutaneous sensation over the deltoid muscle is impaired
Nursemaid's elbow	• Severe distal traction of the radius (e.g., a parent yanking the arm of a child) causing subluxation of the radial head from its encirclement by the annular ligament • Signs and symptoms: Child presents with flexed and pronated forearm held close to the body

Carpal tunnel syndrome	• Tendosynovitis caused by repetitive hand movements (e.g., data entry) that compresses the median nerve within the carpal tunnel
	• Signs and symptoms: Sensory loss on the palmar and dorsal aspects of the index, middle, and half of the ring fingers and palmar aspect of the thumb; flattening of thenar eminence ("ape hand")
	• Tinel test: Tapping of the palmaris longus tendon produces a tingling sensation
	• Phalen test: Forced flexion of the wrist reproduces symptoms; extension alleviates symptoms
Compartment syndrome	• Increased interstitial fluid pressure (> 30 mm of Hg) within an osseofascial compartment sufficient enough to compromise microcirculation, leading to muscle and nerve damage
	• Most frequent in the:
	◦ Anterior compartment of the thigh in crush injuries; involves the femoral artery and nerve
	◦ Anterior compartment of the leg caused by tibial fractures; involves the anterior tibial artery and deep peroneal nerve
	• Signs and symptoms: Swollen, tense compartment; pain upon stretching tendons within the compartment; pink color; warm; detectable pulse over the involved compartment

Topic **9**

Cytology

Must Knows

- Blood cells and their derivatives
- Cells' functioning in bone homeostasis
- Nervous system support cells
- Respiratory cells

BLOOD

Erythrocytes	• Possess no nuclei or mitochondria; perform glycolysis and hexose monophosphate (HMP) shunt for energy; biconcave shape maintained by spectrin; contain hemoglobin; lifespan is 100 to 120 days

- Erythropoietin (secreted by kidneys) regulates erythrocyte formation
- Membrane has band-3 protein for HCO_3/Cl cotransport

Neutrophils	• Most abundant peripheral leukocytes (50% to 70%); possess multilobed nucleus; contain first-degree azurophilic granules (i.e., lysosomes) that have acid hydrolases and myeloperoxidase
	• First to arrive at tissue damage; have a phagocytic role
	• Nuclei become hypersegmented in B12/folate deficiency
Eosinophils	• 0% to 4% of peripheral leukocytes; bilobed nucleus; eosinophilic granules; have role against parasitic infections
Basophils	• 0% to 2% of peripheral leukocytes; possess highly basophilic granules containing heparin, histamine, 5-hydroxytryptamine
	• Have a role in type 1 hypersensitivity reactions
Monocytes	• 2% to 9% of peripheral leukocytes
	• Members of monocyte–macrophage lineage: Kupffer cells, alveolar macrophages, histiocytes, microglia, Langerhans cells, osteoclasts
	• Called macrophages when they enter tissue
T lymphocytes	• Mediate cellular immunity
	• CD4+ helper T cells
	○ Differentiated in the thymus; possess CD4 and T-cell receptor
	○ Found in lymph node paracortex, periarterial lymphatic sheath of spleen, gut-associated lymphoid tissue (GALT)
	○ Functions: Antigen recognition in association with major histocompatibility complex (MHC) II; lymphokine release to stimulate B-cell and antibody production; stimulate T-cell proliferation
	• CD8+ cytotoxic T cell
	○ Differentiated in the thymus; possess CD8 and T-cell receptor
	○ Found in: Same as CD4+ helper T cells
	○ Functions: Antigen recognition in association with MHC I; kill allogeneic and virus-infected cells and fungi
B lymphocytes	• Mediate humoral immunity; undergo differentiation in bone marrow
	• Found in: Lymph node cortex, splenic lymphatic follicles, GALT
	• Functions: Antigen recognition, differentiation into plasma cells
Plasma cells	• Formed from B-cell differentiation; possess eccentric nucleus with clock-face chromatin, a perinuclear area containing Golgi

	bodies, and abundant rough endoplasmic reticulum (rER) for protein synthesis • Functions: Immunoglobulin synthesis and secretion
Mast cells	• Arise from bone marrow stem cells • Function in type I hypersensitivity reactions, inflammation, allergy • Possess IgE receptors, which bind antibody and stimulate release of heparin, histamine, leukotrienes, eosinophil chemotactic factor; similar to basophils
Macrophages	• Also known as histiocytes; reside in connective tissue; arise from circulating monocytes • Activated by lipopolysaccharide (LPS) and γ-interferon; secrete interleukin-1 (IL-1), IL-6, pyrogens, tumor necrosis factor-α (TNF-α), and granulocyte macrophage colony-stimulating factor (GM-CSF) • Phagocytic and antigen presenting; can form foreign body giant cells

BONE

Osteoblasts	• Derived from osteoprogenitor cells; secrete osteoid for osteogenesis, possess parathyroid hormone (PTH) and vitamin D receptors • Clinical markers of osteogenesis: Serum alkaline phosphatase and osteocalcin
Osteoclasts	• Derived from granulocyte and monocyte precursors; multinucleated cells that reside in Howship's lacunae; function in bone resorption; possess calcitonin receptors • Clinical markers of bone resorption: Urine hydroxyproline

NERVOUS SYSTEM

Oligodendrocytes	• Produce myelin sheaths in the central nervous system (CNS); one oligodendrocyte can myelinate several (up to 30) axons
Astrocytes	• Project foot processes that contribute to the blood–brain barrier • Have a role in the metabolism of neurotransmitters (e.g., glutamate, γ-aminobutyrate [GABA], serotonin) • Buffer the [K$^+$] of the CNS extracellular space • Form glial scars in a damaged area of the CNS (i.e., astrogliosis)
Schwann cells	• Derived from THE neural crest; produce myelin sheaths in the peripheral nervous system; one Schwann cell myelinates only one axon
Microglia	• Derived from monocytes; possess phagocytic function

LUNG	
Type I pneumocytes	• Make up the simple squamous epithelium that line THE alveoli • Involved in gas exchange; possess no mitotic capacity
Type II pneumocytes	• Secrete surfactant (dipalmitoylphosphatidylcholine) • Possess mitotic capacity; serve as stem cells to regenerate epithelium

Topic **10**

Microscopic Anatomy

Must **Knows**

● Functions of endoplasmic reticulum and Golgi apparatus

● Components of tissue architecture

● Renal filtration apparatus

● Histology of select organs

ENDOPLASMIC RETICULUM AND GOLGI APPARATUS

Rough endoplasmic reticulum (rER)	• A membranous organelle that contains ribosomes attached to its cytoplasmic surface
	• The function of the rER include:
	  ◦ Synthesis of secretory proteins (e.g., insulin), cell membrane proteins (e.g., hormone receptors), and lysosomal enzymes
	  ◦ Co-translational modification of proteins, including N-linked glycosylation (addition of sugars to asparagine begins in the rER and is completed in the Golgi complex); hydroxylation of proline and lysine during collagen synthesis; cleavage of the signal sequence; folding of the nascent protein into a three-dimensional configuration; and association of protein subunits into a multimeric complex

Golgi complex	• A stack of membranous cisternae that receives vesicles of newly synthesized proteins from the rER and that releases condensing vacuoles of posttranslationally modified proteins • The functions of the Golgi complex include: ◦ Posttranslational modification of proteins: Completion of N-linked glycosylation that began in the rER; O-linked

glycosylation (addition of sugars to serine by the enzyme glycosyltransferase); sulfation; and phosphorylation

○ Protein sorting and packaging: Secretory proteins (e.g., insulin) are packaged into clathrin-coated vesicles; cell membrane proteins (e.g., hormone receptors) are packaged into nonclathrin-coated vesicles; and lysosomal enzymes are packaged into clathrin-coated vesicles after phosphorylation of mannose to form mannose-6-phosphate

○ Membrane recycling

Smooth endoplasmic reticulum	• Membranous organelle with no ribosomes
	• The functions of the sER include:
	  ○ Synthesis of membrane phospholipids
	  ○ Synthesis of steroid hormones
	  ○ Drug detoxification using cytochrome P450 monooxygenase that catalyzes phase I reactions
	  ○ Drug detoxification using glucuronyl transferase that catalyzes phase II reactions
	  ○ Glycogen degradation; fatty acid elongation; lipolysis begins in the sER
	  ○ Lipoprotein assembly
	  ○ Ca^{2+} fluxes associated with muscle contraction

TISSUE FEATURES

Cilia	• Motile cell processes; contain a core of microtubules called the axoneme • The axoneme consists of nine doublet microtubules uniformly spaced around two central microtubules (9 + 2 arrangement). Nexin connects the nine doublet microtubules. • Each doublet has short arms that consist of dynein ATPase, which splits adenosine triphosphate (ATP) to provide energy for cilia movement
Zonula occludens	• Also known as tight junctions • Extends around the entire perimeter of cells; outer leaflets of the cell membrane of two adjoining cells fuse at various points • Prevents or retards the diffusion of material across an epithelium via the paracellular pathway (i.e., through the intercellular space)
Zonula adherens	• Also known as intermediate junctions • Completely encircles the cell; however, adjacent plasma membranes are separated by a gap of approximately 20 nm; provides rigidity and stability

Macula adherens	• Also known as desmosomes
	• Situated below zonula adherens; provides strong attachment between cells
	• Found in tissues subject to physical stress
	• Disc-shaped structure occurring in a row of discrete spots (similar to spot welds)
Hemidesmosomes	• Similar in morphology to halves of desmosomes
	• Anchoring junctions for attachment of a cell to underlying extracellular matrix
	• Defects in proteins integral to hemidesmosome function underlie skin-blistering pathology
Gap junction	• Occur at small discrete sites for metabolic and electrical coupling
	• Cell membranes of two adjoining cells are separated by an intercellular space bridged by connexons
	• Connexons contain central pores that allow passage of ions, cyclic adenosine monophosphate (cAMP), amino acids, steroids, and small molecules (< 1200 d) between cells
Collagen	• Contains hydroxyproline and hydroxylysine; synthesis by fibroblasts involves intracellular and extracellular events:
	○ Intracellular: Synthesis of preprocollagen within rER → hydroxylation of proline and lysine in rER (vitamin C is essential here) → glycosylation of hydroxylysine in rER → formation of triple helix procollagen in rER → addition of carbohydrates in Golgi → secretion of procollagen
	○ Extracellular: Cleavage of procollagen to form tropocollagen → self-assembly of tropocollagen into fibrils → cross-linking of adjacent tropocollagen molecules
	• Collagen types
	○ I (most abundant): Bone, tendon, skin, dentin, fascia, cornea
	○ II: Cartilage, vitreous body, nucleus pulposus
	○ III (reticulin): Skin, vessels, uterus, fetal and granulation tissue
	○ IV: Basement membrane
Skeletal muscle fiber types	• Type I fibers (red): Slow-twitch fibers; contain much myoglobin; comprise the antigravity muscles (i.e., muscles that can react more slowly and imprecisely but over long duration)
	• Type II fibers (white): Fast-twitch fibers; contain less myoglobin; comprise the extraocular muscles (i.e., muscles that act quickly and precisely and are easily fatigable)
Blood–air barrier	• The components of the blood–air barrier include surfactant, type I pneumocyte, basement membrane, and capillary endothelial cell
	• The rate of diffusion across is governed by the Fick law

RENAL HISTOLOGY

Renal glomerulus (Fig. II-22)	• A capillary network; receives blood from an afferent arteriole (site of blood flow autoregulation); drained by an efferent arteriole • Contains a mesangium (extracellular matrix) and mesangial cells, which have a phagocytic and contractile function. Mesangial cells have receptors for angiotensin II and atrial natriuretic peptide. • Contains juxtaglomerular (JG) cells, which are modified smooth muscle cells of the afferent arteriole
Juxtaglomerular apparatus	• Has a role in blood pressure regulation. JG cells secrete renin (a proteolytic enzyme): renin converts angiotensinogen (produced by the liver) to angiotensin I. • Extraglomerular mesangial cells (Lacis cells) between the afferent and efferent arterioles have receptors for angiotensin II and atrial natriuretic peptide • Macula densa (MD) cells are located in the wall of the distal straight tubule (DST); they monitor decreases in Na^+ in the DST fluid
Glomerular filtration barrier	• Glomerular capillary endothelium: A continuous, fenestrated endothelium • Basal lamina: Contains fibronectin, laminin, type IV collagen, and heparan sulfate (important in maintaining negative charge) • Podocytes filtration slits: Foot processes (or pedicles) contact the basal lamina surrounding the glomerular capillarie; gaps between pedicles are the slits

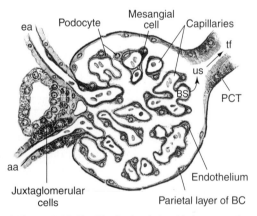

● **Figure II-22** The histologic relationship between the glomerulus and Bowman's capsule (BC), where filtration occurs through the glomerular filtration barrier from the blood space (BS) to the urinary space (US) to form tubular fluid (tf; see *arrow*). Note that the urinary space is continuous with the lumen of the proximal convoluted tubule (PCT). aa = afferent arteriole; ea = efferent arteriole.

SPECIAL TISSUES

Adrenal gland (Fig. II-23)

- Cortex
  - Angiotensin II, increased [K$^+$]: Zona glomerulosa: aldosterone
  - Adrenocorticotropic hormone (ACTH): Zona fasciculate: cortisol (negative feedback to pituitary and hypothalamus)
  - ACTH: Zona reticularis: androgens
- Medulla
  - Catecholamines (epinephrine, 80%; norepinephrine, 20%)

Spleen (Fig. II-24)

- White pulp: B lymphocytes surround a central artery; T lymphocytes are arranged into periarteriolar lymphatic sheaths (PALS)

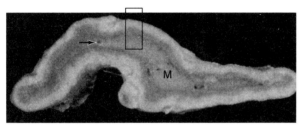

A.

● **Figure II-23** (**A**) Gross photograph of a sliced normal adrenal gland. The zona glomerulosa and zona fasciculata appear as a light area (yellow color in fresh gross specimens) because of the large amount of lipid of these cells. The zona reticularis appears as a dark area (dark brown color in fresh gross specimens) because of the eosinophilia and lipofuscin pigment of these cells. The medulla (M) appears as a gray area where dilated venules are observed (*arrows*). The boxed area is shown at higher magnification in B. (**B**) LM of a normal adrenal gland. A capsule is present on the exterior of the gland. The three zones of the adrenal cortex and the adrenal medulla are clearly apparent. (**C**) LM of the zona glomerulosa (ZG). The ZG is a narrow, inconstant band (15% of the cortical volume) of cortex situated immediately below the capsule (*cap*). The cells of the ZG have distinct cell membranes and are arranged in glomerular-like clusters surrounded by small amounts of connective tissue. The ZG cells have a round nucleus and a faintly eosinophilic, vacuolated cytoplasm. (**D**) LM of the zona fasciculate (ZF). The ZF is a broad band of cortex (78% of the cortical volume). The ZF lies between the ZG and the zona reticularis (ZR). The cells of the ZF have distinct cell membranes and are arranged as two-cell-wide vertical cords that run perpendicular to the capsule and are separated by parallel-running capillaries. The cells of the ZF have a round nucleus and a lipid-filled cytoplasm that give the ZF cells a vacuolated, clear appearance. The high lipid content of the ZF cells gives this zone a yellow color observed in fresh gross specimens. (**E**) LM of the ZR. The ZR is a band of cortex (7% of cortical volume). The ZR lies deep to the ZF and, in the head and body of the adrenal gland, abuts on the medulla. The cells of the ZR have a distinct cell membrane and are arranged as one-cell-wide anastomosing rows of cells separated by capillaries. The cells of the ZR have a round nucleus and a lipid-sparse, distinctly eosinophilic cytoplasm. The deepest-located cells next to the medulla usually contain a yellow-brown lipofuscin pigment. The eosinophilia and lipofuscin pigment of the ZR cells give this zone a dark brown color in fresh gross specimens. (**F** and **G**) LM of the medulla. The medulla is located deep to the ZR in the head and body of the adrenal gland. The medulla is usually absent in the tail of the adrenal. The boundary between the cortex and medulla is quite distinct. At low magnification (**F**), venules (*asterisk*) and nerve fibers (*arrows*) can be observed coursing through the medulla. At higher magnification (**G**), chromaffin cells have an indistinct cell membrane and are arranged in tight clusters. The chromaffin cells have variable-shaped nuclei and generally a finely granular basophilic cytoplasm, although some cells appear vacuolated, which gives the medulla a mottled appearance.

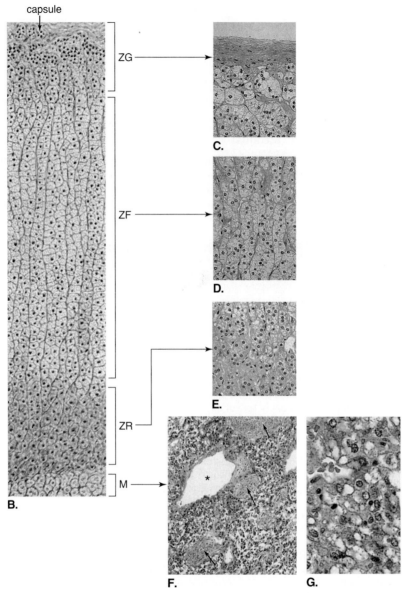

● **Figure II-23** (*Continued*)

- Marginal zone: Where blood meets the spleen parenchyma and antigen-presenting cells (APCs) and macrophages reside
- Red pulp: Contains Billroth cords separated by sinusoids with discontinuous basal laminae

Lymph node (Fig. II-25)

- Outer cortex: contains follicles composed of B lymphocytes
- Inner cortex (paracortex): Contains T lymphocytes
- Medulla: Contains B lymphocytes, plasma cells, macrophages

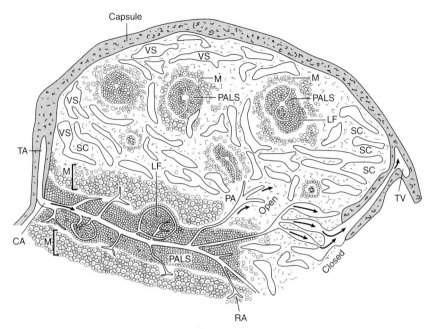

● **Figure II-24** Normal splenic architecture and vascular pattern. The trabecular artery (TA) branches into a central artery (CA), which becomes ensheathed by T cells forming the periarterial lymphatic sheath (PALS). Some branches of the CA, called radial arterioles (RA), terminate in the marginal zone (M), where the immune response in the spleen is initiated and where lymphocytes exit the bloodstream to repopulate the spleen. The CA branches into penicillar arterioles (PAs), which may open directly into the red pulp, forming an extensive extravascular compartment of blood (open circulation), or empty directly into splenic venous sinusoids (VS; closed circulation). Splenic venous sinusoids empty into trabecular veins (TVs). Along the central artery, lymphatic follicles (LFs) consisting of B cells are apparent. SC = splenic cord.

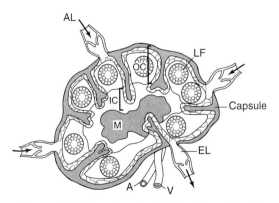

● **Figure II-25** A lymph node. Note the afferent lymphatic vessels (AL) along the convex surface; efferent lymphatic vessel (EL) at the hilus; outer cortex (OC) with lymphatic follicles (LF), many of which contain germinal centers; inner cortex (IC); and medulla (M).

Physiology

10 Top Tips

Physiology

Topic	Main Focus	USMLE Example
1 Cellular Physiology	Active transport, action potentials, and muscle contraction are the framework for higher level functions.	• A 32-year-old woman with myasthenia gravis is treated with an acetylcholinesterase inhibitor and has increased muscle strength. This improvement occurs because inhibition of acetylcholinesterase allows acetylcholine to persist in the synapse, triggering action potentials and increasing strength.
2 Neurophysiology	The autonomic nervous system (ANS) regulates smooth muscle, cardiac muscle, and glands to integrate involuntary functions.	• Prazosin is prescribed in an attempt to control a 58-year-old patient's hypertension. This agent acts to antagonize α_1 receptors on vascular smooth muscle, causing cutaneous and splanchnic vascular vasodilation, leading to decreased blood pressure.
3 Cardiac Physiology	Electrical properties of myocardium and autonomic control over variables such as cardiac output determine cardiac function.	• A 37- year old woman who reports episodes of lightheadedness and palpitations has a pulse of 190 bpm and a blood pressure of 72/42 mm Hg. In this patient, tachycardia has resulted in shortening of the duration of systole and even more shortening of the duration of diastole.
4 Circulatory Physiology	Both fast, neurally regulated, and slow, hormonally regulated, mechanisms are responsible for responding to changes in blood pressure.	• A 4-year-old boy who has been in a motor vehicle collision has a massive hemorrhage. Decreased blood volume and pressure trigger the baroreceptor reflex, increasing sympathetic outflow and reducing parasympathetic outflow, causing increased heart rate and peripheral vasoconstriction.

(Continued)

10 Top Tips

Physiology   *(Continued)*

Topic	Main Focus	USMLE Example
5 Respiratory Physiology	Balance between ventilation and perfusion allows for efficient gas exchange, hemoglobin saturation, and oxygenation of peripheral tissues.	• A 60-year-old man who has moved from Baltimore to Colorado develops an increased ventilation rate, higher hematocrit level secondary to erythropoietin production, increased 2,3-diphosphoglycerate (2,3-DPG), and relative pulmonary vasoconstriction. These changes have occurred in response to the lower O_2 partial pressures at the higher altitude characteristic of Colorado.
6 Renal Physiology	Renal function is defined by the necessity to maintain body water and electrolyte equilibria, excrete waste products, and preserve glucose and protein.	• As a 21-year-old man runs a marathon on a day with a temperature of 95°F. He drinks pure water to quench his thirst. By doing so, he has undergone a net loss in NaCl without a loss in water. As a result, his extracellular osmolarity decreases and water is shifted into the intracellular space. These changes cause increased hemoconcentration (Hct) because of a decrease in extracellular fluid and a shift of water into erythrocytes.
7 Acid–Base Physiology	Acid–base balance is maintained by buffers, ventilatory rate, and renal regulation of HCO_3^- and H^+ absorption and excretion.	• Blood gas studies are obtained from a 72-year-old patient. The results show a pH of 7.51, PCO_2 of 22 mm Hg, and HCO_3^- of 15 mEq/L. These values suggest that the patient has a respiratory alkalosis and that he was probably hyperventilating when the blood gas was drawn.
8 Gastrointestinal Physiology	The gastrointestinal tract is the portal for nutrient entry. Its primary function is to propel, digest, and absorb these substances to provide metabolic substrates.	• After gastrectomy, a 50-year-old man is told that he will need to take supplemental vitamin B_{12}. His physician explains that the parietal cells of the stomach responsible for making intrinsic factor and required for vitamin B_{12} absorption in the distal ileum are now largely gone as a result of the surgery.

(Continued)

10 Top Tips

Physiology   *(Continued)*

Topic	Main Focus	USMLE Example
9 Endocrine Physiology	The endocrine organs secrete hormones to maintain physiologic equilibrium. Negative feedback keeps endocrine systems in check.	• A 38-year-old man has noticed the development of coarse facial features, brow protrusion, and growth of his hands and feet over the course of his adult life. Tests identify a pituitary adenoma that is secreting growth hormone independently of its usual regulation by hypothalamic growth hormone releasing hormone.
10 Reproductive Physiology	Sex hormones govern the processes of male and female sexual maturation, gametogenesis, and the maintenance of pregnancy.	• A 49-year-old woman who stopped menstruating 3 months ago uses a home pregnancy test, which shows that she is not pregnant. Her physician finds that her luteinizing hormone and follicle-stimulating hormone levels are high as a result of inadequate estrogen secretion and negative feedback by her follicle-depleted ovaries. This finding confirms that she is in a menopausal state.

Topic **1**

Cellular Physiology

Must **Knows**

● Transport across cellular membranes

● Cellular potentials

● Synaptic neurotransmission

● Muscle contraction

TRANSPORT ACROSS CELLULAR MEMBRANES

Cell membranes	• Composed of a lipid bilayer with phospholipids (a glycerol backbone is the hydrophilic head, and two fatty acid chains are the hydrophobic tails)
	• Hydrophobic substances (O_2, CO_2, steroid hormones) cross easily
	• Hydrophilic substances (Na^+, glucose, H_2O) must pass through channels, pores, or via carrier proteins
	• Contain integral and peripheral proteins located on either side
Diffusion	• Simple: Not carrier mediated; down an electrochemical gradient; passive
	• Facilitated: Down the electrochemical gradient; passive; more rapid than simple diffusion; carrier mediated (e.g., glucose transport in muscle cells)
	• Flux equation
	○ $J = -PA(C_1 - C_2)$
	▪ J = flux (flow) (mmol/sec)
	▪ P = permeability
	▪ A = area (cm^2)
	▪ C_1 = concentration$_1$ (mmol/L)
	▪ C_2 = concentration$_2$ (mmol/L)
Active transport	• Primary: Against the electrochemical gradient; requires direct input of energy; active; carrier mediated (e.g., Na^+/K^+-ATPase)
	• Secondary: Coupled transport of two or more solutes: one goes uphill, the other downhill; energy is indirectly provided
	• Symport occurs when solutes move in the same direction; antiport is when solutes move in opposite directions

Osmosis	• Flow of H_2O across semipermeable membranes from high to low solute concentrations; solutions can be isotonic, hypotonic, or hypertonic
	• Oncotic pressure: Osmotic pressure created by proteins in solution
	• Osmolarity: Concentration of osmotically active particles in solution

CELLULAR POTENTIALS

Ion channels	• Integral membrane proteins; permit passage of selected ions; may be open or closed
	• Voltage gated: Opened or closed state determined by membrane potential
	• Ligand gated: Opened or closed state determined by ligand binding
Diffusion potential	• Potential difference created by ionic concentration differences across a membrane
Nernst equation	• $E = -2.3\ (RT/zF)\ \log_{10}\ [C_i]/[C_e]$
	○ E = equilibrium potential (mV)
	○ 2.3 RT/F = constants (60 mV at 37°C)
	○ z = charge on the ion
	○ C_i = intracellular concentration (mM)
	○ C_e = extracellular concentration (mM)
	• Calculates the equilibrium potential at a given concentration difference of a permeable ion across a cell membrane
Resting membrane potential	• Expressed by convention as the intracellular potential relative to the extracellular potential
	• Established by diffusion potentials that result from concentration differences in permeant ions
Basics of the action potential	• Depolarization makes the membrane potential less (−); the inside of the cell becomes less (−) because of the inward flow of positive charge (Na^+)
	• Hyperpolarization makes the membrane potential more (−), the inside of the cell becomes more (−) because of the flow of (+) charge outward
	• Threshold: Membrane potential at which the action potential is inevitable; the inward current must be sufficient to achieve the threshold potential
	• Propagation: Occurs via spread of local currents; velocity increases with increasing fiber size (decreased internal resistance); myelin acts as an insulator, and myelinated nerves demonstrate salutatory conduction

Ionic basis of the action potential

- Resting potential: Approximately −70 mV; results from high K^+ conductance (membrane is impermeable to Na^+ while K^+ leaks outward)

- Upstroke: Inward (+) current depolarizes to threshold; Na^+ channels open and Na^+ conductance increases; inside of the cell becomes more positive (tetrodotoxin [TTX] blocks these Na^+ channels)

- Repolarization: Depolarization closes the inactivation gates of Na^+ channels; Na^+ conductance stops; depolarization opens K^+ channels and increases K^+ conductance; outward K^+ current brings cells back to resting potentials

- Hyperpolarization: K^+ conductance remains higher than at rest for some time after Na^+ channels close

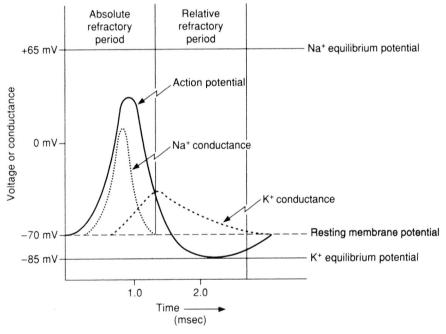

● **Figure III-1** Nerve action potential and associated changes in Na^+ and K^+ conductance.

Refractory periods

- Absolute: Another action potential cannot be triggered regardless of the stimulus strength (caused by closing of the Na^+-channel inactivation gates)

- Relative: An action potential can be elicited but requires a larger stimulus; inward high K^+ conductance keeps membrane potential farther away from threshold; begins after absolute refractory period

SYNAPTIC NEUROTRANSMISSION

Chemical synapses	• An action potential causes depolarization of the presynaptic terminal; Ca^{2+} enters the presynaptic terminal via voltage-gated Ca^{2+} channels, triggering release of neurotransmitter; neurotransmitter diffuses across the synapse and contacts receptors on postsynaptic membrane
	• Excitatory neurotransmitters: Depolarize postsynaptic cells (e.g., acetylcholine)
	• Inhibitory neurotransmitters: Hyperpolarize postsynaptic cells (e.g., γ-aminobutyric [GABA])
Neuromuscular junction	• Acetylcholine, synthesized from acetyl-CoA and choline by choline acetyltransferase, is the neuromuscular junction (NMJ) neurotransmitter
	• Postsynaptic membrane possesses nicotinic receptors (ligand gated); acetylcholine binds these receptors, causing them to open and allowing Na^+ and K^+ flow
Myasthenia gravis	• Caused by the presence of antibodies to the nicotinic acetylcholine receptor
	• Characterized by skeletal muscle weakness and fatigability attributable to decreased number of receptors
	• Treatment: Acetylcholinesterase inhibitors to prolong the time acetylcholine is in the synapse and exposed to receptors
Neurotransmitters	• Norepinephrine: Postganglionic sympathetic transmitter; binds α and β receptors on postsynaptic membranes; removed by reuptake and metabolism (monoamine oxidase [MAO] and catechol-O-methyltransferase [COMT])
	• Epinephrine: Secreted by the adrenal medulla
	• Dopamine: Prominent in midbrain neurons; inhibits prolactin secretion; Parkinson's disease involves degeneration of dopaminergic neurons, and schizophrenia involves increased levels of D_2 receptors
	• Serotonin: Present in high concentrations in the brain stem; synthesized from tryptophan; converted to melatonin in the pineal gland
	• Histamine: Synthesized from histidine; present in hypothalamic neurons (H_1 receptors are responsible for wakefulness; H_1 antagonists cause sedation)
	• Glutamate: Most prevalent excitatory neurotransmitter; kainate receptor for glutamate is a Na^+ and K^+ ion channel
	• GABA: Inhibitory neurotransmitter; $GABA_A$ receptor increases Cl^- conductance and is the site of action for benzodiazepines and barbiturates; $GABA_B$ increases K^+ conductance
	• Glycine: Inhibitory neurotransmitter; increases Cl^- conductance

MUSCLE CONTRACTION

Skeletal muscle

- Muscle fibers are multinucleated, containing bundles of myofibrils surrounded by sarcoplasmic reticulum and invaginated by transverse tubules; thick and thin filaments are arranged longitudinally in sarcomeres; sarcomeres run Z line to Z line

- Thick filaments: Present in the A band; contain myosin; the myosin head binds both actin and adenosine triphosphate (ATP) and is involved in cross-bridge formation

- Thin filaments: Anchored to Z line; present in I bands; contain actin, tropomyosin, and troponin; troponin binds Ca^{2+} and regulates cross-bridge formation

A

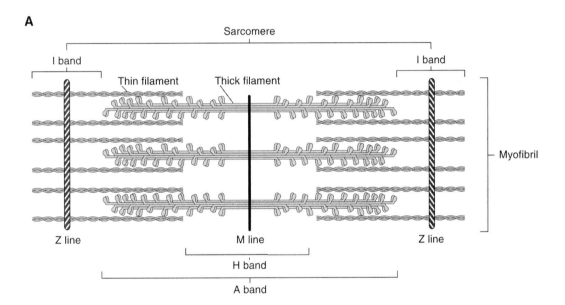

B

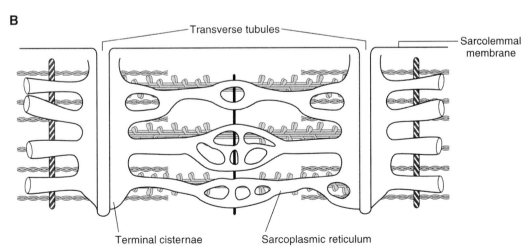

● **Figure III-2** Structure of the sarcomere in skeletal muscle. *(A)* Arrangement of thick and thin filaments. *(B)* Transverse tubules and sarcoplasmic reticulum (SR).

- T tubules: Carry depolarization from the sarcolemma membrane to the cell's interior; contain voltage-sensitive dihydropyridine receptors
- Sarcoplasmic reticulum: Site of Ca^{2+} storage; has terminal cisternae in intimate contact with T tubules; contains Ca^{2+} release channels called ryanodine receptors

---

Skeletal muscle contraction

- Action potentials initiate depolarization of T tubules
- Depolarization of the T tubules opens Ca^{2+} release channels in the nearby SR, causing Ca^{2+} release into the intracellular fluid
- Intracellular $[Ca^{2+}]$ increases
- Ca^{2+} binds troponin C on thin filaments, causing a conformational change in troponin that moves tropomyosin out of the way
- With no ATP bound to myosin, it is tightly bound to actin; during rapid contraction, this phase is brief; in the absence of ATP, this state is permanent (i.e., rigor mortis)
- ATP binds myosin, producing a conformational change that causes it to be released from actin
- Myosin is displaced toward the (+) end of actin; ATP is hydrolyzed to adenosine diphosphate (ADP), and P_i, ADP remains bound to myosin

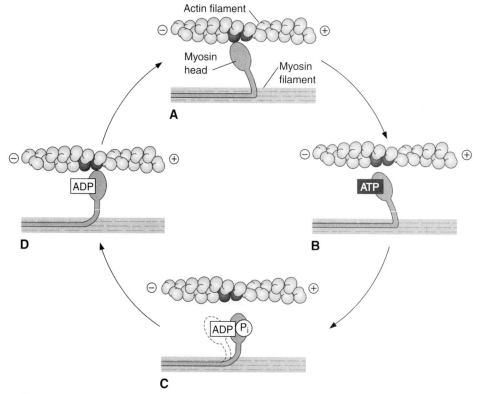

● **Figure III-3** Cross-bridge cycle. Myosin "walks" toward the plus end of actin to produce shortening and force-generation. *ATP* = adenosine triphosphate; *ADP* = adenosine diphosphate; P_i = inorganic phosphate.

- Myosin binds a new site on actin, which constitutes the power stroke; ADP is then released, returning myosin to the rigor state
- The cycle repeats as long as Ca^{2+} is bound to troponin C; each cross-bridge cycle "walks" myosin along the actin filament
- Relaxation: Occurs when $[Ca^{2+}]$ is reaccumulated by the SR and intracellular $[Ca^{2+}]$ decreases; $[Ca^{2+}]$ is released from troponin C, and tropomyosin again blocks the myosin binding site on actin

Smooth muscle	

- Excitation–contraction occurs via a distinct mechanism
- Depolarization of the cell membrane opens voltage-sensitive Ca^{2+}-channels and Ca^{2+} flows into the cell. Increased intracellular $[Ca^{2+}] \rightarrow Ca^{2+}$ binds calmodulin. This complex binds to and activates myosin light-chain kinase (MLCK), which phosphorylates myosin and allows it to bind actin, causing contraction

Topic **2**

Neurophysiology

Must **Knows**

- Autonomic nervous system
- Temperature regulation
- Nerve fiber types

AUTONOMIC NERVOUS SYSTEM

Receptor types	

- α_1: On vascular smooth muscle of skin and splanchnic regions, bowel and bladder sphincters, and radial eye muscles; produce excitation and act by forming inositol-1,4,5-trisphosphate (IP3) and increasing intracellular $[Ca^{2+}]$
- α_2: Located on presynaptic nerve terminals, platelets, fat cells, and walls of the gastrointestinal (GI) tract; produce inhibition, inhibit adenylate cyclase, and decrease cyclic adenosine monophosphate (cAMP)
- β_1: Located in the sinoatrial (SA) node, atrioventricular (AV) node, and ventricular muscle; produce excitation, activate adenylate cyclase, and increase cAMP
- β_2: Located on vascular smooth muscle of skeletal muscle beds, bronchial smooth muscle, and walls of the GI tract and bladder; produce relaxation and act via the same mechanism as β_1 receptors

- Nicotinic receptors: Located in autonomic ganglia, at the neuromuscular junction (NMJ), and in the adrenal medulla; activated by acetylcholine; produce excitation; acetylcholine binds α subunits of receptors (these are ion channels for Na^+ and K^+)

- Muscarinic receptors: Located in the heart, smooth muscle (except vascular smooth), and glands; activated by acetylcholine; are inhibitory in the heart and excitatory in smooth muscle and glands; mechanism (1) in SA node: inhibits adenylate cyclase, this opens a K^+ channel, slowing spontaneous depolarizations and decreasing heart rate; (2) in smooth muscle it triggers IP3 formation and increases intracellular Ca^{2+}

Effects of the autonomic nervous system (ANS) on organ systems	Refer to Table III-1

TEMPERATURE REGULATION

Heat-generating mechanisms	• Thyroid hormone: Increases metabolic rate and heat production by stimulation of the Na^+/K^+-ATPase • Cold temperatures: Activate the sympathetic nervous system; via β receptor activation in brown fat, metabolic rate and heat are increased

TABLE III-1	EFFECT OF THE AUTONOMIC NERVOUS SYSTEM ON ORGAN SYSTEMS

Organ	Sympathetic Action	Sympathetic Receptor	Parasympathetic Action (Receptors are Muscarinic)
Heart	Increases heart rate Increases contractility Increases AV node conduction	β_1 β_1 β_1	Decreases HR Decreases contractility (atria) Decreases AV node conduction
Vascular smooth muscle	Constricts blood vessels in skin; splanchnic	α_1	—
	Dilates blood vessels in skeletal muscle	β_2	—
GI tract	Decreases motility Constricts sphincters	α_2, β_2 α_1	Increases motility Relaxes sphincters
Bronchioles	Dilates bronchiolar smooth muscle	β_2	Constricts bronchiolar smooth muscle
Male sex organs	Ejaculation	α	Erection
Bladder	Relaxes bladder wall Constricts sphincter	β_2 α_1	Contracts bladder wall Relaxes sphincter
Sweat glands	Increases sweating	Muscarinic (sympathetic cholinergic)	—
Kidney	Increases renin secretion	β_1	—
Fat cells	Increases lipolysis	β_1	—

AV = atrioventricular; GI = gastrointestinal; HR = heart rate.

- Shivering: Most potent mechanism; cold temperatures activate shivering via the posterior hypothalamus; motor neurons are activated in response, and skeletal muscle contraction produces shivering

Heat loss mechanisms	• Orchestrated by the posterior hypothalamus; increased temperature causes decreased sympathetic tone to cutaneous blood vessels; increased blood flow through the arterioles causes arteriovenous shunting to the venous plexus near the skin surface • Evaporative heat loss occurs via sweat gland activity and H_2O evaporation under sympathetic muscarinic control
Body temperature set point	• Controlled by the anterior hypothalamus; when core temperature is below the set point, heat-generating mechanisms are triggered; when core temperature is above the set point, heat-losing mechanisms are triggered • Fever: Pyrogens increase IL-1 (interleukin-1) production, which acts on the anterior hypothalamus to increase production of prostaglandins; these increase the set point, triggering heat-generating mechanisms • Aspirin: Reduces fever by inhibiting cyclooxygenase and preventing prostaglandin synthesis, therefore reducing the set point • Steroids: Reduce fever by blocking the release of arachidonic acid, preventing prostaglandin synthesis

NERVE FIBER TYPES

Refer to Table III-2

TABLE III-2	CHARACTERISTICS OF NERVE FIBER TYPES		
General Fiber Type and Example	**Sensory Fiber Type and Example**	**Diameter**	**Conduction Velocity**
A-α Large α-motoneurons	**Ia** Muscle spindle afferents	Largest	Fastest
	Ib Golgi tendon organs	Largest	Fastest
A-β Touch, pressure	**II** Secondary afferents of muscle spindles; touch and pressure	Medium	Medium
A-γ γ-Motoneurons to muscle spindles (intrafusal fibers)	—	Medium	Medium
A-δ Touch, pressure, temperature, and pain	**III** Touch, pressure, fast pain, and temperature	Small	Medium
B Preganglionic autonomic fibers	—	Small	Medium
C Slow pain; postganglionic autonomic fibers	**IV** Pain and temperature (unmyelinated)	Smallest	Slowest

Topic **3**

Cardiac Physiology

Must
Knows

- Hemodynamics
- Cardiac electrophysiology
- Cardiac contractility

HEMODYNAMICS

Vessels	• Arterioles: Sites of highest resistance in the cardiovascular system; innervated by the autonomic nervous system; α_1 receptors are in skin and splanchnic regions; β_2 are on arterioles of skeletal muscle
	• Capillaries: Possess the largest cross-sectional and surface areas
	• Veins: Under low pressure, contain the highest proportion of the blood in the cardiovascular system
Pulse pressure	• Difference between systolic and diastolic pressures; most important determinant is stroke volume; decreased arterial capacitance (as occurs with aging) results in increased pulse pressure
Mean arterial pressure	• Is approximately diastolic pressure plus one third of the pulse pressure
Atrial pressure	• Lowest pressure in the system; left atrial pressure is estimated by the pulmonary capillary wedge pressure in which a catheter is inserted into the smallest branches of the pulmonary artery; the measured pressure is slightly higher than the left atrial pressure

CARDIAC ELECTROPHYSIOLOGY

Electrocardiography	• P wave: Atrial depolarization; atrial repolarization is buried in the QRS complex
	• PR interval: From the beginning of the P wave to the beginning of the Q wave; varies with conduction velocity through the atrioventricular (AV) node
	• QRS complex: Represents depolarization of the ventricles

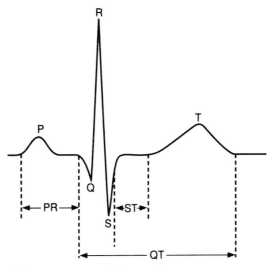

● **Figure III-4** Normal electrocardiogram measured from lead II.

- QT interval: From the beginning of the Q wave to the end of the T wave; represents the entire period of depolarization and repolarization of the ventricles

- ST segment: From the end of the S wave to the beginning of the T wave; this period is isoelectric, the period during which ventricles are depolarized

- T wave: Represents ventricular repolarization

Myocardial action potential
- Phase 0: The upstroke, caused by transient Na^+ conductance, this depolarizes the cell (makes inside more positive)

- Phase 1: Brief period of initial repolarization, caused by an outward current, partly attributable to K^+ conductance outward and decreased Na^+ conductance inward

- Phase 2: The plateau, caused by transient increase in Ca^{2+} conductance, movement of Ca^{2+} inward, and an increase in K^+ conductance; the inward and outward currents are approximately equal

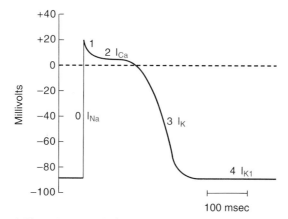

● **Figure III-5** Ventricular action potential.

- Phase 3: Repolarization; Ca^{2+} conductance decreases, K^+ increases and predominates, and high K^+ conductance produces large K^+ flow outward; this hyperpolarizes the cell
- Phase 4: Return to resting potential near the K^+ equilibrium potential

Pacemaker action potential	• Sinoatrial (SA) node: Normally the heart's pacemaker; no constant resting membrane potential; exhibits phase 4 depolarization (or automaticity); SA node has the fastest rate of phase 4 depolarization, so it overdrive suppresses lower potential pacemakers in atrial muscle, the AV node, the His-Purkinje system, and the ventricles

- ○ Phase 0: Upstroke; caused by Ca^{2+} conductance and inward current, making inside more positive; Na^+ drives phase 0 in the ventricles, atria, and Purkinje
- ○ Phase 3: Repolarization caused by K^+ conductance and outward K^+ current
- ○ Phase 4: Slow depolarization; accounts for pacemaker activity; caused by increased Na^+ conductance, resulting in inward Na^+ current called I_f
- ○ Phases 1 and 2 are not present

- • AV node: Upstroke is the result of inward Ca^{2+} current, just as in the SA node

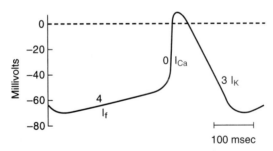

● **Figure III-6** Sinoatrial node action potential.

Autonomic effects on heart rate (HR) and conduction velocity	• Chronotropic effects: Negative = decreased HR; positive = increased heart rate

- • Dromotropic effects: Negative = decreased conduction velocity through the AV node; positive = increased conduction velocity
- • Sympathetic effects: Via β_1 receptors: (+) chronotropic effects; increases HR by increasing phase 4 depolarization; increases I_f; (+) dromotropic effects; increases conduction velocity via the AV node and decreases the PR interval; works via increased Ca^{2+} current inward
- • Parasympathetic effects: SA node, atria, and AV node, but not ventricles, have parasympathetic nervous system (PNS) vagal

innervation; acetylcholine acts on muscarinic receptors: (−) chronotropic effects by decreasing the rate of phase 4 depolarization; decreased I_f: (−) dromotropic effects at the AV node; increase the PR interval; occurs via decreased inward Ca^{2+} current and increased outward K^+ current

CARDIAC CONTRACTILITY

Contractility

- Intrinsic ability of muscle to develop force at a given length, called inotropism; estimated by ejection fraction (normally 50% to 55%)
- Positive inotropic factors:
  - Increased HR: More Ca^{2+} enters the cell, causing more to be released from intracellular stores, providing greater tension
  - Sympathetic stimulation: Catecholamines via β_1 receptors: increase inward Ca^{2+} during the plateau phase; increases activity of the Ca^{2+} pump at the SR, so more Ca^{2+} accumulates and more is available for contraction
  - Cardiac glycosides: Increase contraction force by inhibition of the Na^+/K^+-ATPase; intracellular Na^+ increases, and the force driving the Na^+/Ca^{2+}-exchange (Ca^{2+} outward) is diminished, causing increased Ca^{2+} available for contraction
- Negative inotropic factors:
  - Parasympathetic stimulation: Via acetylcholine and muscarinic receptors; decrease atrial contraction force by decreasing Ca^{2+} entry during the plateau phase of the action potential

Ventricular length–tension relationship

- Preload: = End-diastolic volume (EDV); related to right atrial pressure; increased venous return increases EDV, which lengthens ventricular fibers

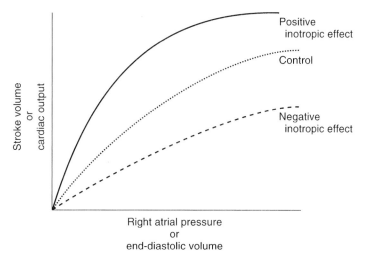

● **Figure III-7** Frank-Starling relationship and the effect of positive and negative inotropic agents.

- Afterload: For the left ventricle (LV), this = aortic pressure; for the right ventricle (RV), this = pulmonary artery pressure; therefore, increased arterial pressure increases afterload

- Sarcomere length: Determines the maximum number of cross-bridges that can form and determines the maximum tension

- Frank-Starling relationship: Describes increases in cardiac output (or systolic volume [SV]) that occur in response to an increase in venous return or EDV: increases in EDV increase ventricular fiber length and increase developed tension; increased contractility shifts the curve upward; decreased contractility shifts the curve downward

Ventricular pressure–volume loops

- Steps 1 to 2: Isovolumetric contraction; diastole ends at point 1; LV is filled with blood (approximately 140 cc); on excitation, LV contracts, increasing pressure; all valves are closed; no blood is ejected

- Steps 2 to 3: Ventricular ejection; aortic valve opens at point 2 when LV pressure is greater than aortic pressure; blood is ejected, and volume decreases; volume ejected is the stroke volume (measured by width of pressure volume loop); the remaining volume is the end-systolic volume (ESV)

- Steps 3 to 4: Isovolumetric relaxation, LV < aortic pressure so the aortic valve closes, all valves are closed so volume does not change

- Steps 4 to 1: Ventricular filling; LV pressure is less than left atrial pressure; the mitral valve opens, and filling begins

- Effects of increased preload: Refers to increased EDV from venous return; causes increased stroke volume, reflected in the width of the loop

- Effects of increased afterload: Refers to increased aortic pressure; LV ejects blood against higher pressure; results in decreased stroke volume, reflected in the decreased width of the loop; causes an increase in ESV

- Effects of increased contractility: The LV develops greater tension than usual during systole; causes increased stroke volume; this causes a decrease in ESV

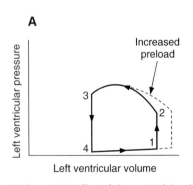 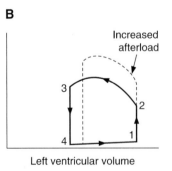 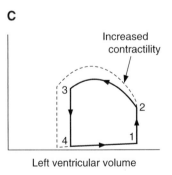

● **Figure III-8** Effect of changes in (*A*) preload, (*B*) afterload, and (*C*) contractility on the ventricular pressure-volume loop.

CARDIAC CYCLE

Stages of the cardiac cycle
• (A) Atrial systole: Preceded by a P wave; contributes to but not essential for ventricular filling; the *a* wave on the venous pulse curve is caused by increased atrial pressure with atrial systole;

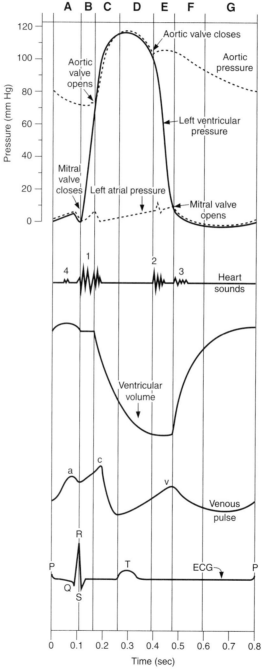

● **Figure III-9** The cardiac cycle. *ECG* = electrocardiogram; *A* = atrial systole; *B* = isovolumetric ventricular contraction; *C* = rapid ventricular ejection; *D* = reduced ventricular ejection; *E* = isovolumetric ventricular relaxation; *F* = rapid ventricular filling; *G* = reduced ventricular filling.

filling of the ventricle by atrial systole causes the fourth heart sound, which is not normally audible, but heard with decreased LV compliance

- (B) Isovolumetric ventricular contraction: Begins after onset of the QRS, when ventricular pressure is greater than atrial pressure; the AV valves close; this corresponds to the first heart sound (S1), the mitral valve (MV) closes before the tricuspid valve (TV); the S1 may be split; no blood leaves the ventricles as the aortic valve is closed

- (C) Rapid ventricular ejection: Ventricular pressure reaches its maximum; LV is greater than aortic pressure; the aortic valve opens; rapid ejection of blood into the aorta because of the pressure gradient between the ventricle and the aorta; volume decreases dramatically as most of the stroke volume is ejected during this phase; atrial filling begins; onset of T wave (ventricular depolarization) marks the end of this phase

- (D) Reduced ventricular ejection: Ejection is slower; ventricular pressure decreases; aortic pressure decreases as blood runs off into smaller arteries; atrial filling continues

- (E) Isovolumetric ventricular relaxation: Repolarization of ventricles completed; aortic valve closes; pulmonic closes next, which corresponds to the second heart sound (S2); inspiration causes splitting of S2; ventricular pressure decreases further; volume is constant as all valves are closed; the blip on aortic pressure curve is the dicrotic notch, which occurs after closure of aortic valve; when ventricular pressure becomes less than atrial, the mitral valve opens

- (F) Rapid ventricular filling: The MV is open, and filling begins; aortic pressure decreases further; rapid flow of blood from atria into ventricles causes third heart sound (S3)

- (G) Reduced ventricular filling: The longest phase of the cardiac cycle; filling is slower; the time required for this phase and filling depends on HR; increased HR decreases time for filling

Topic **4**

Circulatory Physiology

Must **Knows**

- Blood pressure regulation
- Fluid exchange across capillary walls

BLOOD PRESSURE REGULATION

Baroreceptor reflex

- Fast neural mechanism; controls arterial blood pressure (BP) on a minute-to-minute scale; produces vasoconstrictor activity tonically, which accounts for vasomotor tone
- Baroreceptors are stretch receptors in the walls of the carotid sinus near the bifurcation of carotids; others are located at the aortic arch but only respond to increases in pressure
- Steps in baroreceptor reflex:
  - Decreased arterial pressure decreases the stretch of the walls; the receptors are most sensitive to changes in arterial pressure; decreasing pressure produces more response than constant low pressure
  - Decreased stretch decreases firing rate of carotid sinus nerve (CN IX), which carries signals to vasomotor area in the brainstem
  - Setpoint for mean arterial pressure (MAP) is about 100 mm Hg; thus, MAP less than that triggers series of autonomic responses by the vasomotor center to increase BP
  - Responses are decreased parasympathetic (vagal) outflow to the heart and increased sympathetic outflow to the heart and vessels
- The baroreceptor mechanism is a negative feedback system; increased stretch on the carotid sinus equals decreased signal to the vasomotor center

Chemoreceptors

- Cerebral ischemia: When the brain is ischemic, CO_2 and H^+ increase in brain tissue; chemoreceptors in the vasomotor center respond by increasing both sympathetic and parasympathetic outflow
- Ventricular contractility and total peripheral resistance (TPR) are increased; heart rate (HR) is decreased (because of overriding parasympathetic outflow); with increased TPR and peripheral vasoconstriction, blood flow to other organs is decreased to preserve flow to the brain
- Cushing reaction: Occurs as described above because of increased intracranial pressure causing compression of cerebral blood vessels; MAP is elevated (increased contractility and TPR) with decreased HR (parasympathetic)
- Chemoreceptors in carotid and aortic bodies have high rates of O_2 consumption; they are very sensitive to hypoxia; a decrease in arterial BP decreases O_2 delivery, and signals are sent to the vasomotor center that activates mechanisms to increase BP

Response to hemorrhage

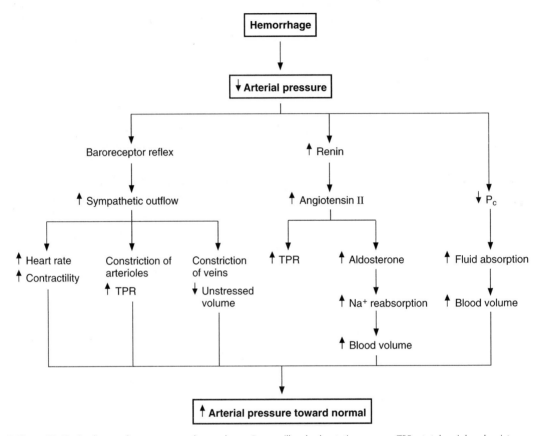

● **Figure III-10** Cardiovascular responses to hemorrhage. P_c = capillary hydrostatic pressure; *TPR* = total peripheral resistance.

FLUID EXCHANGE ACROSS CAPILLARY WALLS

The Starling equation

- $J_v = K_f [(P_c - P_i) - (\pi_c - \pi_i)]$
  - J = fluid movement (cc/min); K_f = hydraulic conductance (cc/min × mm Hg); P_c = capillary hydrostatic pressure; P_i = interstitial hydrostatic pressure; π_c = capillary oncotic pressure; π_i = interstitial oncotic pressure
- J_v = net fluid movement out of the capillary, (+) with filtration, (−) with absorption
- K_f = filtration coefficient, the water permeability of the capillary wall
- P_c = an increase favors filtration out; is determined by arterial/venous pressures and resistances; venous pressure increases have a great effect
- P_i = an increase opposes filtration, normally 0 mm Hg or negative

- π_c = an increase opposes filtration out; is increased by increases in blood protein concentration (e.g., dehydration) and decreased by decreases in blood protein concentration (e.g., nephrotic syndrome, protein malnutrition)
- π_i = an increase favors filtration out; depends on the protein concentration in the interstitial fluid; normally low as little protein is filtered
- Increased P_c, decreased P_i, decreased π_c, and increased π_i all increase filtration

Topic **5**

Respiratory Physiology

Must Knows

- Lung volumes and capacities
- Gas exchange
- Ventilation/perfusion
- Control of breathing

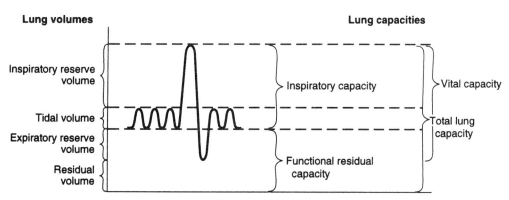

● **Figure III-11** Lung volumes and capacities.

LUNG VOLUMES AND CAPACITIES

Volumes	• Tidal volume (TV): Inspired and expired with each normal breath
	• Inspiratory reserve volume (IRV): Volume that can be inspired above the TV
	• Expiratory reserve volume (ERV): Volume that can be expired after the expiration of TV
	• Residual volume (RV) remains in lungs after maximum expiration (cannot be measured)
Capacities	• Inspiratory capacity = TV + IRV
	• Function residual capacity = ERV + RV, includes RV, so it cannot be measured with spirometry
	• Vital capacity = TV + IRV + ERV, amount expired after maximal inspiration
	• Forced vital capacity = amount forcibly expired after maximal inspiration
	• TLC = sum of all four lung volumes; volume after maximal inspiration
FEV$_1$	• Volume that can be expired in 1 second after max inspiration, normally 80% of the forced vital capacity (FEV$_1$/FVC) = 0.8
	• Restrictive disease (e.g., fibrosis): FEV$_1$ and FVC are reduced; ratio stays the same or increases
	• Obstructive disease (e.g., asthma, COPD), FEV$_1$ decreases more than FVC, so ratio decreases
Dead space	• Anatomic dead space: Volume of conducting airways, approximately 150 cc
	• Physiologic dead space: Volume that does not participate in gas exchange; approximately equal to the anatomic dead space, may be greater than anatomic in lung disease with V/Q mismatches
	• Calculated by the following equation:
	○ $V_D = V_T \times (Pa_{CO2} - PE_{CO2})/Pa_{CO2}$
	○ $Pa_{CO2} = P_{CO2}$ of arterial blood; $PE_{CO2} = P_{CO2}$ of expired air; V_D = physiologic dead space; V_T = tidal volume
Alveolar ventilation	• Alveolar ventilation equals (TV − Dead space) × Breaths/min

GAS EXCHANGE

Surfactant	• Surface tension results from attractive forces between molecules of liquid lining the alveoli; creates a collapsing pressure proportional to surface tension and inversely proportional to alveolar radius

- Surfactant: Synthesized by type II alveolar cells; consists primarily of the phospholipid dipalmitoyl phosphatidylcholine. In the fetus, it may be present as early as 24 weeks, but it is always present by 35 weeks; a lecithin:sphingomyelin ratio greater than 2:1 in amniotic fluid reflects mature levels of surfactant
- Neonatal respiratory distress syndrome: Occurs in premature infants who lack surfactant. The infant exhibits atelectasis during expiration and has difficulty reinflating the lungs. Hypoxemia results because of a V/Q mismatch

Oxygen transport

- O_2 is carried in two forms, dissolved and hemoglobin (Hgb) bound
- Hgb: Composed of 2 α and 2 β subunits; each has an iron-containing heme moiety; ferrous iron binds O_2; ferric (methemoglobin) cannot
- HgbF (fetal): β Chains are replaced by γ; O_2 affinity of fetal Hgb is greater than adult Hgb because 2,3- diphosphoglycerate (2,3-DPG) is bound less avidly; this facilitates movement of O_2 from the mother to the fetus

Hgb-O_2 dissociation curve

- Sigmoid shape reflects positive cooperativity of O_2 binding
- Arterial blood: P_{O_2} of 100 mm Hg; Hgb is almost 100% saturated

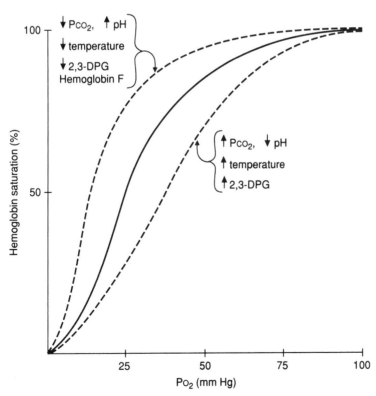

● **Figure III-12** Changes in the hemoglobin-O_2 dissociation curve. Effects of P_{CO_2}, pH, temperature, 2,3-diphosphoglycerate (DPG), and fetal hemoglobin (hemoglobin F) on the hemoglobin-O_2 dissociation curve.

- Mixed venous: P_{O_2} of 40 mm Hg; Hgb is 75% saturated
- P_{O_2} of 25 mm Hg; Hgb is 50% saturated
- Shifts to the right occur when Hgb affinity for O_2 is decreased, P_{50} is increased, and O_2 unloading to tissues is enhanced
  - Increases in P_{CO_2}; decreases in pH (Bohr effect)
  - Increases in temperature
  - Increases in 2,3-DPG: Binds β chains of deoxy-Hgb and decreases O_2 affinity (high-altitude adaptation increases 2,3-DPG synthesis)
- Shifts to the left occur when Hgb affinity increases; P_{50} is decreased
  - Decreased P_{CO_2}, increased pH, decreased temperature, decreased 2,3-DPG
  - HgbF: 2,3-DPG binds this Hgb less avidly, increasing its O_2 affinity
  - Carbon monoxide (CO) poisoning: Hgb affinity for CO is 200× that for O_2; this decreases O_2 binding capacity and give remaining binding sites with higher affinity for O_2, causing left shift

CO$_2$ transport	<ul><li>Forms of CO_2: Dissolved, carbaminohemoglobin, HCO_3^- (makes up 90%)</li><li>Transport of CO_2 as HCO_3^-<ul><li>In erythrocytes, CO_2 combines with H_2O for form H_2CO_3 (catalyzed by carbonic anhydrase); this dissociates into H^+ and HCO_3^-; HCO_3^- leaves erythrocyte in exchange for Cl^- and goes to the lungs in plasma</li></ul></li></ul>

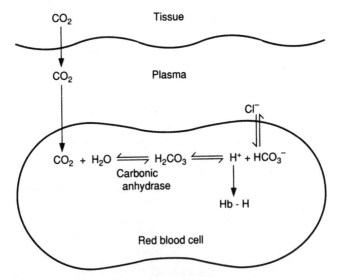

● **Figure III-13** Transport of CO_2 from the tissues to the lungs in venous blood. H^+ buffered by hemoglobin (Hb-H).

- ○ H^+ in erythrocytes is buffered by deoxyhemoglobin
- ○ In the lungs, all these processes reverse, and CO_2 is generated to be expired after diffusion into the lung

VENTILATION/PERFUSION

Pulmonary circulation

- Zone 1: Blood flow is the lowest; alveolar pressure > arterial > venous; alveolar pressure can compress capillaries with decreased arterial pressure (hemorrhage) or increased alveolar pressure (positive pressure ventilation)
- Zone 2: Arterial pressure > alveolar > venous; arterial pressure increases because of a gravitational increase in hydrostatic pressure
- Zone 3: Arterial pressure > venous > alveolar

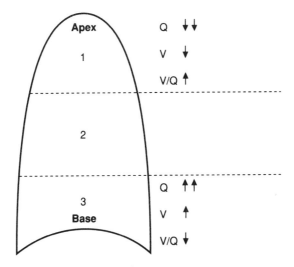

● **Figure III-14** Variation of ventilation (V) and blood flow [perfusion (Q)] in different regions of the lung.

Regulation of pulmonary blood flow

- Hypoxia causes vasoconstriction, the opposite of other organs; this diverts blood away from poorly ventilated hypoxic regions to other well-ventilated regions; this also explains the high fetal pulmonary vascular resistance: with the first breath of a neonate, oxygenation increases, so pulmonary vascular resistance decreases

Shunts

- Right to left: A very small normal right-to-left shunt occurs as approximately 2% of cardiac output bypasses the lungs; large shunts occur with congenital abnormalities (i.e., tetralogy of Fallot); these always produce a decrease in arterial P_{O_2} because of mixture between arterial and venous blood; shunt magnitude can be estimated by having the patient breathe 100% O_2 and measuring the degree of dilution

- Left to right: More common than right to left because of higher left-sided cardiac pressures, usually caused by congenital defects (e.g., ventricular septal defect) or injury; do not decrease arterial P_{O_2}; instead, P_{O_2} is higher on the right side of the heart because of mixture of left- and right-sided blood

V/Q defects	<ul><li>V/Q ratio: Ratio of alveolar ventilation (V) to pulmonary blood flow (Q); matching of V and Q is important for ideal gas exchange; if frequency, TV, and cardiac output are normal, V/Q is approximately 0.8; this produces arterial P_{O_2} of approximately 100 mm Hg and P_{CO_2} of approximately 40 mm Hg</li><li>Changes in V/Q:<ul><li>Airway obstruction: Ventilation decreases; can go to 0 with complete obstruction. When blood flow is normal, V/Q goes to 0 and there is no gas exchange; arterial P_{O_2} and P_{CO_2} will approach levels in venous blood</li><li>Blood flow obstruction: When blood flow is blocked (i.e., with a pulmonary embolism), then blood flow goes to 0 with normal ventilation, V/Q becomes infinite, and then P_{O_2} and P_{CO_2} of alveolar gas approach levels of inspired air</li></ul></li><li>V/Q ratios at different areas of the lungs:<ul><li>Blood flow is lowest at the apex and highest at the base</li><li>Ventilation is lowest at the apex and highest at the base, but differences in ventilation are not as great as for perfusion</li><li>V/Q at the apex is > 1.0; at the base < 0.8</li></ul></li></ul>
Causes of hypoxia	Refer to Table III-3

CONTROL OF BREATHING

Central control	<ul><li>Medullary respiratory center:<ul><li>Dorsal respiratory group: Primarily responsible for inspiration; generates basic rhythm of breathing; input via cranial nerve (CN) X (peripheral chemoreceptors and mechano-</li></ul></li></ul>

TABLE III-3	CAUSES OF HYPOXIA
Cause	**Mechanisms**
Decreased cardiac output	Decreased blood flow
Hypoxemia	Decreased Pa_{O_2} causes decreased % saturation of hemoglobin
Anemia	Decreased hemoglobin concentration causes decreased O_2-carrying capacity of blood
Carbon monoxide poisoning	Decreased O_2-binding capacity of hemoglobin
Cyanide poisoning	Decreased O_2 utilization by tissues

Pa_{O_2} = arterial P_{O_2}.

receptors in the lung) and CN IX (peripheral chemo-receptors); output via the phrenic nerve

   ○ Ventral group: Primarily responsible for expiration; not active during normal breathing when expiration is passive

- Apneustic center: In the lower pons, stimulates inspiration, producing deep and prolonged inspiratory gasp

- Pneumotaxic center: In the upper pons, inhibits inspiration; therefore, regulates inspiratory volume and respiratory rate

- Cerebral cortex: Controls the voluntary component of breathing (i.e., a person can voluntarily hold breath or hyperventilate)

Chemoreceptors for CO_2, H^+, and O_2	• Central chemoreceptors in the medulla:
	
	   ○ Sensitive to cerebrospinal fluid (CSF) pH: Decreased CSF pH causes hyperventilation; H^+ does not cross the blood–brain barrier (BBB) as well as CO_2; CO_2 (lipid soluble) crosses the BBB and combines with H_2O to yield H^+ and HCO_3^-; H^+ acts directly on chemoreceptors; increased H^+ stimulates breathing, and decreased H^+ inhibits breathing
	
	• Peripheral chemoreceptors: Carotid and aortic bodies
	
	   ○ Decreased arterial P_{O_2} stimulates peripheral chemoreceptors and increases breathing rate; P_{O_2} must be < 60 mm Hg; when below this pressure, rate is extremely sensitive to P_{O_2}
	
	   ○ Increased arterial P_{CO_2} stimulates peripheral chemoreceptors and increases breathing rate; less important than the response of the central chemoreceptors to H^+
	
	   ○ Increased arterial H^+ directly stimulates carotid bodies, independent of CO_2 change; with metabolic acidosis, breathing rate increases because arterial H^+ increases and pH decreases

Adaptation to high altitude	• Alveolar P_{O_2} is decreased at high altitudes; arterial P_{O_2} is decreased (hypoxemia) • This stimulates peripheral chemoreceptors and triggers hyperventilation, which produces respiratory alkalosis (this can be treated by an acetazolamide-carbonic anhydrase inhibitor) • Hypoxemia also triggers renal production of erythropoietin to increase erythrocyte production and increase Hgb concentration, which increases O_2-carrying capacity • 2,3-DPG concentration increases: Shifts Hgb-O_2 dissociation curve to the right, causing decreased O_2 affinity of Hgb, and facilitates O_2 unloading to tissues • Pulmonary vasoconstriction occurs, causing increased pulmonary arterial pressure, increased work of the right ventricle (RV), and RV hypertrophy

Topic **6**

Renal Physiology

Must Knows

- Body fluids
- Clearance, blood flow, glomerular filtration rate
- Regulation of ion homeostasis
- Hormones that act on the kidney

BODY FLUIDS

Total body water	• Total body water is approximately 60% of total body weight (TBW); higher for newborns and males; lowest in women and elderly individuals as adipose collects
	• Intracellular fluid (ICF) is two thirds of TBW; major cations are K^+ and Mg^{2+}; anions are protein and organic phosphates (i.e., adenosine triphosphate [ATP])
	• Extracellular fluid (ECF) is one third of TBW; major cation is Na^+; major anions are Cl^- and HCO_3^-
	○ Plasma is one fourth of the ECF; major plasma proteins are albumin and globulins
	○ Interstitial fluids are three fourths of the ECF; composition is similar to plasma except it has little protein; thus, the interstitial fluid is the ultra filtrate of the plasma
	• 60-40-20 rule: TBW = 60% of body weight; ICF = 40%; ECF = 20%
Shifting body water	• At steady state, ECF and ICF osmolarity are approximately equal; this is achieved via shifting of water between the two
	• Infusion of isotonic sodium chloride (NaCl; addition of isotonic fluid)
	○ ECF volume increases, but no change in osmolarity occurs between ECF and ICF; therefore, no water is shifted
	○ Plasma protein concentration and hematocrit decrease
	○ Arterial blood pressure (BP) increases
	• Diarrhea: Loss of isotonic fluid
	○ ECF volume decreases, but no change in osmolarity occurs and water does not shift

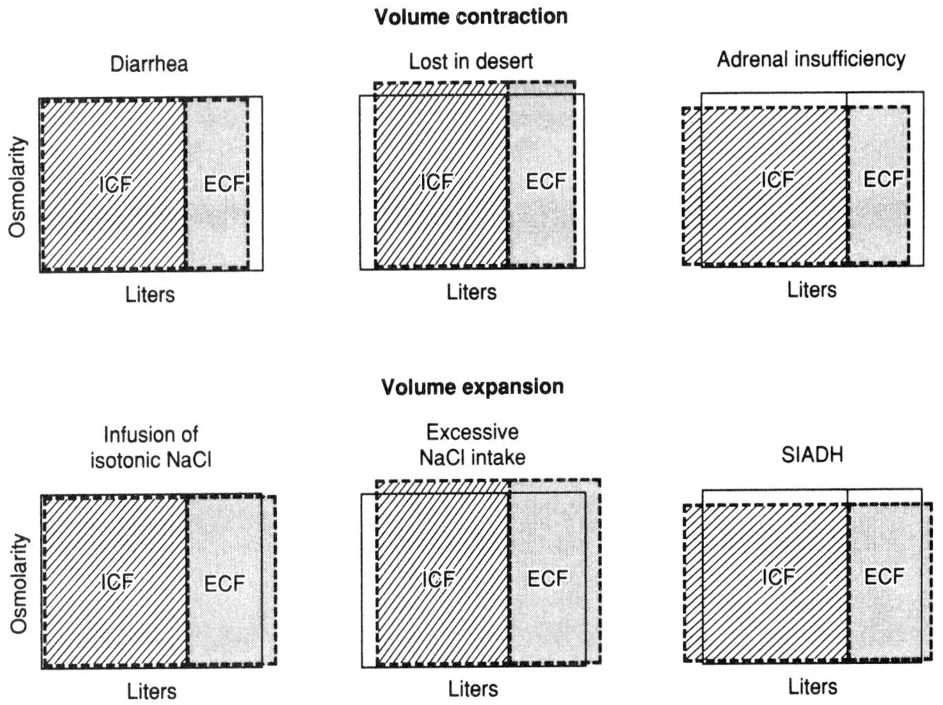

Volume contraction

Volume expansion

● **Figure III-15** Shifts of water between body fluid compartments. Volume and osmolarity of normal extracellular fluid (ECF) and intracellular fluid (ICF) are indicated by the *solid lines*. Changes in volume and osmolarity in response to various situations are indicated by the *dashed lines*. SIADH = syndrome of inappropriate antidiuretic hormone.

- ○ Plasma protein concentration and hematocrit increase
- ○ Arterial BP decreases
- Excessive NaCl intake: Hyperosmotic volume expansion
  - ○ Osmolarity of ECF increases, water shifts from ICF to ECF, and ICF osmolarity increases until it is equal to ECF
  - ○ ECF volume increases and ICF volume decreases
  - ○ Plasma protein concentration and hematocrit decrease
- Sweating in the desert: Hyperosmotic volume contraction
  - ○ Osmolarity of ECF increases because sweat is hyposmotic, ECF volume decreases, water shifts out of the ICF, ICF osmolarity increases to equal ECF, and ICF volume decreases
  - ○ Plasma protein concentration increases, hematocrit remains largely unchanged as water shifts out of the erythrocytes, and their volume is decreased as well
- Syndrome of inappropriate antidiuretic hormone (SIADH): Hyposmotic volume expansion
  - ○ Osmolarity of ECF decreases, ECF volume increases, water shifts into cells, ICF osmolarity decreases to equal ECF, and ICF volume increases
  - ○ Plasma protein concentration decreases and hematocrit remains unchanged as water shifts into the erythrocytes, increasing their volume

- Adrenocortical insufficiency (aldosterone deficiency): Hyposmotic volume contraction
  - Osmolarity of ECF decreases with NaCl excretion > H_2O excretion, ECF volume decreases, water shifts into cells, ICF osmolarity decreases until equal to ECF, and ICF volume increases
  - Plasma protein concentration increases and hematocrit increases with ECF volume loss as erythrocytes take up water
  - Arterial BP decreases with a decrease in ECF

CLEARANCE, BLOOD FLOW, AND GLOMERULAR FILTRATION RATE

Clearance Equation	• $C = UV/P$ • C = clearance (mL/min or mL/24 hr); P = plasma concentration (mg/mL); U = urine concentration (mg/mL); V = urine volume/time (mL/min)
Renal blood flow	• 25% of cardiac output; directly proportional to the pressure difference between renal artery and vein; inversely proportional to resistance of renal vasculature • Autoregulation: Via changing renal vascular resistance, renal blood flow remains constant of arterial pressures from 80 to 200 mm Hg • Myogenic: Renal arterioles contract in response to stretch • Tubuloglomerular feedback: Increased renal arterial pressure leads to increased delivery of fluid to the macula densa. It senses increased load and triggers constriction of the efferent arteriole to maintain constant flow.
Renal plasma flow (RPF)	• RPF is based on the clearance of para-aminohippuric acid (PAH) • PAH: Filtered and secreted, measures effective RPF; underestimates by approximately 10% ◦ $RPF = C_{PAH} = [U]_{PAH} V/[P]_{PAH}$ • Measure of renal blood flow: $RBF = RPF/1 - Hct$ (hematocrit)
Glomerular filtration rate (GFR)	• Measurement of GFR is based on the clearance of inulin (filtered, not secreted or reabsorbed) • $GFR = [U]_{inulin} V/[P]_{inulin}$

Determining GFR via Starling forces	• Filtration is always favored because net ultrafiltration pressure always favors movement of fluid out of the capillary
	• $GFR = K_f [(P_{GC} - P_{BS}) - (\pi_{GC} - \pi_{BS})]$
	   ◦ K_f = filtration coefficient; the filtration barrier consists of capillary endothelium, basement membrane, and podocyte filtration slits; anionic glycoproteins line the filtration barrier, which restricts filtration of plasma protein
	   ◦ P_{GC} = glomerular capillary hydrostatic pressure; increased by dilation of the afferent arteriole or constriction of the efferent arteriole

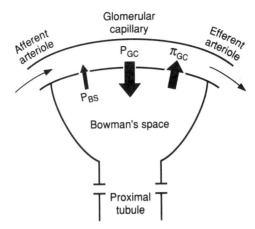

● **Figure III-16** Starling forces across the glomerular capillaries. *Heavy arrows* indicate the driving forces across the glomerular capillary wall. P_{BS} = hydrostatic pressure in Bowman's space; P_{GC} = hydrostatic pressure in the glomerular capillary; π_{GC} = colloidosmotic pressure in the glomerular capillary.

- ○ P_{BS} = Bowman's space hydrostatic pressure; increased by constriction of the ureters
- ○ π_{GC} = glomerular capillary oncotic pressure; increases along the length of the glomerular capillary; increased by protein concentration
- ○ π_{BS} = Bowman's space oncotic pressure; usually 0 because very little protein is filtered

Filtration fraction	• The fraction of RPF filtered across the glomerular capillaries • FF = GFR/RPF; normally about 0.20 • Increases in filtration fraction produce increases in the protein concentration of the peritubular capillary blood
TF/P$_X$ ratio	• Compares the concentration of a substance in tubular fluid at any point along the nephron with the concentration in plasma • TF/P < 1.0: Reabsorption of a substance has been greater than that of H_2O • TF/P > 1.0: reabsorption of a substance has been less than than that of H_2O, or it has been secreted • TF/P = 1.0: reabsorption of a substance is equal to that of H_2O

Free water clearance (C$_{H2O}$)	• Free water clearance (C_{H_2O}) is used to estimate the ability to concentrate or dilute urine; free water is produced by the diluting segments; in the absence of antidiuretic hormone (ADH), this solute free water is secreted and C is positive; in the presence of ADH this solute-free water is not excreted but is absorbed in the distal tubule and collecting duct, and C is negative; the calculation is:
	  ○ $C_{H_2O} = V - C_{osm}$
	  ○ C_{osm} = osmolar clearance ($U_{osm}V/P_{osm}$); V = urine flow rate

- ○ Isosmotic urine = C_{H_2O} of 0; produced by treatment with loop diuretic, which inhibits NaCl reabsorption in the thick ascending limb, inhibiting the diluting segment and the corticopapillary osmotic gradient; therefore, urine cannot be diluted or concentrated
- ○ Hyposmotic urine (low ADH) = produced with high H_2O intake, diabetes insipidus; C_{H_2O} is positive
- ○ Hyperosmotic urine (high ADH) = H_2O deprivation or SIADH

REGULATION OF IONIC HOMEOSTASIS

NaCl regulation

- • Proximal tubule reabsorbs 67% of filtered Na^+ and H_2O; is the site of glomerulotubular balance; process is isosmotic with the TF/P = 1.0
  - ○ Early proximal tubule reabsorbs Na^+ and H_2O via co-transport with HCO_3^-, glucose, amino acids, lactate, phosphate; this accounts for reabsorption of all filtered glucose and amino acids; Na^+ is also reabsorbed through countertransport via the Na^+- H^+-exchange, which is linked directly to the reabsorption of filtered HCO_3^-
  - ○ Middle and late proximal: Na^+ is reabsorbed with Cl^-

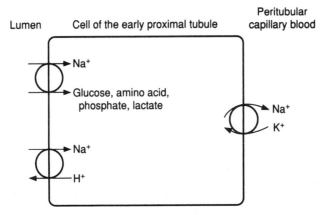

● **Figure III-17** Mechanism of Na^+ reabsorption in the cells of the early proximal tubule.

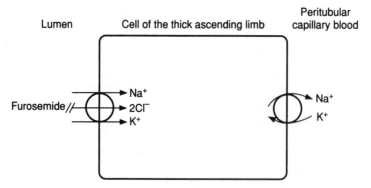

● **Figure III-18** Mechanism of ion transport in the thick ascending limb of the loop of Henle.

- Thick ascending limb of the loop of Henle reabsorbs 25% of filtered Na^+; contains Na^+-K^+-$2Cl^-$ co-transporter; site of action of loop diuretics; impermeable to water (TF/P for Na^+ becomes < 1.0); is the diluting segment
- Distal tubule and collecting duct reabsorbs 8% of filtered Na^+
  - Early distal tubule reabsorbs NaCl via Na^+-Cl^- co-transporter; the site of action of thiazide diuretics; is impermeable to H_2O, as is the thick ascending limb; NaCl absorption occurs without H_2O, further diluting portion, called the cortical diluting segment
  - Late distal tubule and collecting duct have two cell types (1) principal cells, which reabsorb Na^+ and H_2O and secrete K^+; aldosterone increases Na^+ reabsorption and K^+ secretion; ADH increases H_2O permeability by triggering insertion of H_2O channels in the luminal membrane; K^+-sparing diuretics act here; (2) α-intercalated cells, which secrete H^+ by an H^+-ATPase that is stimulated by aldosterone; reabsorb K^+ by a H^+/K^+-ATPase

K^+ regulation

- Shifts of K^+ between ICF and ECF (e.g., insulin, acidosis, cell lysis); shift out causes hyperkalemia, and shift in causes hypokalemia
- K^+ is filtered, reabsorbed, and secreted; balance is achieved with urinary excretion equaling dietary intake; excretion can vary from 1% to 110% of filtered load depending on intake, aldosterone levels, and acid–base status
- Proximal tubule reabsorbs 67% of filtered K^+ with Na^+ and H_2O
- Thick ascending limb of loop of Henle reabsorbs 20% of K^+ via Na^+-K^+-$2Cl^-$ co-transporter
- Distal tubule and collecting duct reabsorb or secrete K^+, depending on intake
  - Reabsorption involves H^+, K^+-ATPase of intercalated cells; occurs only with low K^+ diet; K^+ secretion can be as low as 1% of filtered load

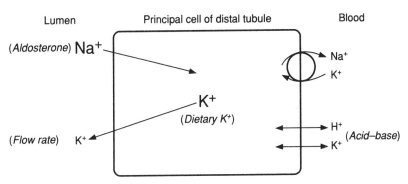

● **Figure III-19** Mechanism of K^+ secretion in the principal cell of the distal tubule.

- Secretion via principal cells; depends on diet, aldosterone, acid–base status, urine flow rate
  - Basolateral Na^+- K^+-ATPase increases intracellular K^+; at luminal membrane, K^+ is passively secreted based on electrochemical driving force (i.e., increased outward movement with increased intracellular K^+ or decreased tubular K^+)

Urea, phosphate, Ca^{2+}, and Mg^{2+}	• Urea: 50% of filtered is reabsorbed in proximal tubule passively; the distal tubule, cortical, and outer medullary collecting duct are impermeable

- Urea: 50% of filtered is reabsorbed in proximal tubule passively; the distal tubule, cortical, and outer medullary collecting duct are impermeable
  - ADH increases urea permeability of inner medullary collecting duct; urea absorption here causes urea recycling in the inner medulla to develop the corticopapillary osmotic gradient
- Phosphate: 85% of filtered is reabsorbed in the proximal tubule by Na^+-phosphate co-transport; the remaining nephron is impermeable
  - PTH inhibits phosphate reabsorption in the proximal tubule by activating adenylate cyclase, increasing cyclic adenosine monophosphate (cAMP), and inhibiting the Na^+-phosphate co-transporter; parathyroid hormone (PTH) causes phosphaturia and increased urine cAMP; phosphate is a urinary H^+ buffer
- Ca^{2+}: 60% of plasma Ca^{2+} is filtered; the proximal tubule and thick ascending limb reabsorb more than 90% of filtered Ca^{2+} via a passive process coupled to Na^+ reabsorption
  - Loop diuretics increase urinary Ca^{2+} excretion because Ca^{2+} reabsorption is linked to Na^+ reabsorption in the loop of Henle; with volume replacement, loop diuretics can be used to treat hypercalcemia
  - Distal tubule and collecting duct reabsorb 8% of filtered Ca^{2+} via active processes; PTH increases Ca^{2+} reabsorption via adenylate cyclase activation
  - Thiazide diuretics increase Ca^{2+} reabsorption in the distal tubule and decrease its excretion; they can be used to treat idiopathic hypercalciuria
- Mg^{2+} is reabsorbed in the proximal tubule, thick ascending limb, and distal tubule; in the thick ascending limb, Mg^{2+} and Ca^{2+} compete for reabsorption; thus, hypercalcemia increases Mg^{2+} secretion and hypermagnesemia increases Ca^{2+} excretion

HORMONES THAT ACT ON THE KIDNEYS

Regulatory hormones	Refer to Table III-4

TABLE III-4			**SUMMARY OF HORMONES THAT ACT ON THE KIDNEYS**	
Hormone	Stimulus for Secretion	Time Course	Mechanism of Action	Actions on Kidneys
PTH	Decreased plasma [Ca^{2+}]	Fast	Basolateral receptor Adenylate cyclase cAMP → urine	Decreases phosphate reabsorption (proximal tubule) Increases Ca^{2+} reabsorption (distal tubule) Stimulates 1α- hydroxylase (proximal tubule)
ADH	Increased plasma osmolarity Decreased blood volume	Fast	Basolateral V$_2$ receptor Adenylate cyclase cAMP (Note: V$_1$ receptors are on blood vessels; mechanism is Ca^{2+}–IP$_3$)	Increase H$_2$O permeability (late distal tubule and collecting duct principal cells)
Aldosterone	Decreased blood volume (via renin–angiotensin II) Increased plasma [K$^+$]	Slow	New protein synthesis	Increases Na$^+$ reabsorption (distal tubule principal cells) Increases K$^+$ secretion (distal tubule principal cells) Increases H$^+$ secretion (distal tubule α-intercalated cells)
ANF	Increased atrial pressure	Fast	Guanylate cyclase cGMP	Increases GFR Decreases Na$^+$ reabsorption
Angiotensin II	Decreased blood volume (via renin)			Increases Na$^+$–H$^+$ exchange and HCO$_3^-$ reabsorption (proximal tubule)

ADH = antidiuretic hormone; ANF = atrial natriuretic factor; cAMP = cyclic adenosine monophosphate; cGMP = cyclic guanosine monophosphate; GFR = glomerular filtration rate; PTH = parathyroid hormone.

Topic **7**

Acid–Base Physiology

Must **Knows**

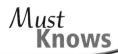

● Renal regulation of acid–base balance
● Acid–base disorders

RENAL ACID–BASE BALANCE

Reabsorption of HCO$_3^-$

- In the proximal tubule cells, CO_2 and H_2O form carbonic acid (via carbonic anhydrase), which dissociates to HCO_3^- and H^+; H^+ is secreted into the lumen via Na^+- H^+ exchange, HCO_3^- is reabsorbed; in the lumen, H^+ combines with HCO_3^-, which dissociates to CO_2 and H_2O; these enter cells, and the cycle repeats; this process produces net reabsorption of HCO_3^- but not net secretion of H^+

- Regulated by changes in filtered load, P_{CO_2}, extracellular fluid (ECF) volume, and angiotensin II

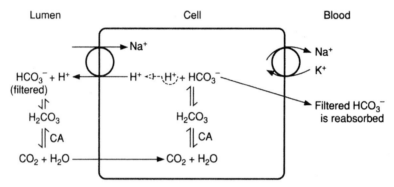

● **Figure III-20** Mechanism of reabsorption of filtered HCO_3^- in the proximal tubule. *CA* = carbonic anhydrase.

Excretion of fixed H$^+$

- Via titratable acid and NH_4
- Luminal H^+ combines with H_2PO_4 and is excreted as a titratable acid, causing net H^+ secretion and HCO_3^- reabsorption; urine pH becomes lower (minimum = 4.4)
- NH_3 is produced by luminal cells and diffuses into the lumen down its gradient; H^+ combines with NH_3 to trap it in the lumen; the lower the urinary pH, the more NH_3 moves into the lumen to increase H^+ excretion
- Hyperkalemia inhibits NH_3 synthesis and causes a decrease in H^+ excretion; hypokalemia does the opposite

Henderson-Hasselbalch equation

- $pH = pK + \log([A^-]/[HA])$
  - $pH = -\log_{10}[H^+]$
  - $pK = -\log_{10}$ equilibrium constant
  - $[A^-]$ = base form of buffer (mM)
  - $[HA]$ = acid form of buffer (mM)

ACID–BASE DISORDERS

Serum anion gap	• Anion gap = $[Na^+] - ([Cl^-] + [HCO_3^-])$ ○ Represents unmeasured anions in serum; these include phosphate, citrate, sulfate, and protein; normally approximately 12 mEq/L

Metabolic acidosis	• Overproduction or ingestion of fixed acid or loss of base; this increases arterial H^+, HCO_3^- and buffers extra acid, decreasing arterial HCO_3^-
	
	   ○ Respiratory compensation = Hyperventilation
	
	   ○ Renal correction consists of increased excretion of excess fixed H^+ as a titratable acid and NH_4^+ and increased new reabsorption of HCO_3^-

Metabolic alkalosis	• Loss of fixed H^+ or gain of base produces decreased arterial H^+; arterial HCO_3^- increases (i.e., vomiting causes loss of H^+ from the stomach; HCO_3^- remains)
	
	   ○ Respiratory compensation = Hypoventilation
	
	   ○ Renal correction consists of increased excretion of HCO_3^- as filtered load exceed ability of the tubule to reabsorb it
	
	   ○ If metabolic alkalosis is accompanied by ECF volume contraction, the reabsorption of HCO_3^- increases (secondary to contraction), worsening the alkalosis

Respiratory acidosis	• The primary disturbance is decreased respiratory rate and retention of CO_2, which causes increased arterial P_{CO_2} and increased H^+ and HCO_3^- by mass action ○ Renal compensation consists of increased excretion as a titratable acid and NH_4^+ and increased absorption of new HCO_3^-; the increased P_{CO_2} aids this by providing more H^+ to renal cells, resulting in an increase in serum HCO_3^- • Acute respiratory acidosis: Renal compensation has not occurred yet • Chronic respiratory acidosis: Renal compensation (increased HCO_3^-) has occurred; arterial pH has increased toward normal
Respiratory alkalosis	• Caused by increased respiratory rate and decreased CO_2; decreased arterial P_{CO_2} causes decreased H^+ and HCO_3^- ○ Renal compensation: Decreased excretion of H^+ as a titratable acid and NH_4+, and decreased reabsorption of HCO_3^-; this is aided by the decreased P_{CO_2}, which provides less H^+ to tubular cells for secretion, the decreased HCO_3^- helps normalize pH • Acute respiratory alkalosis: No renal compensation yet • Chronic respiratory alkalosis: Renal compensation with decreased HCO_3^-; absorption has occurred; arterial pH is decreased toward normal • Hypocalcemia: H^+ and Ca^{2+} compete for binding of plasma proteins; with decreased H^+, more Ca^{2+} can bind, causing decreased free ionized Ca^{2+} • Refer to Figure III-1

Acid–base map

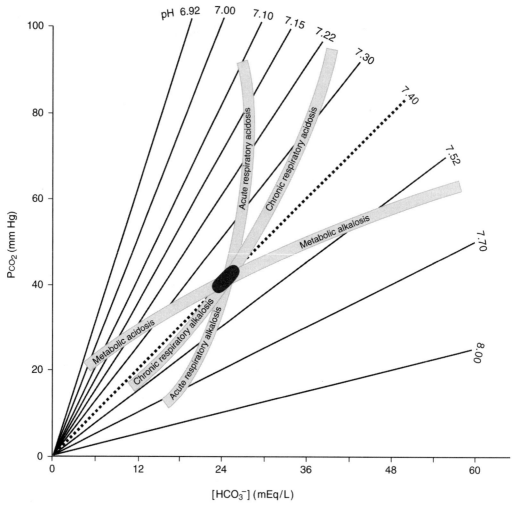

● **Figure III-21** Acid-base map with values for the simple acid-base disorders superimposed. The relationships are shown between arterial P_{CO2}, $[HCO_3^-]$, and pH. The *ellipse* in the center shows the normal range of values. *Shaded areas* show the range of values associated with simple acid-base disorders. Two shaded areas are shown for each respiratory disorder: one for the acute phase and one for the chronic phase.

Topic **8**

Gastrointestinal Physiology

Must Knows

- Regulatory substances
- Gastrointestinal secretion
- Digestion and absorption

REGULATORY SUBSTANCES

Gastrin	• Increases H^+ secretion by gastric parietal cells; stimulates growth of gastric mucosa
	
	• Stimuli for gastrin release: Secreted from G cells of the gastric antrum in response to:
	  ○ Small peptides and amino acids (most potently by tryptophan and phenylalanine)
	  ○ Stomach distention
	  ○ Vagal stimulation, which is mediated by release of gastrin-releasing peptide
	
	• Inhibition of gastrin secretion:
	  ○ H^+ in the lumen of the stomach; negative feedback
	
	• Zollinger-Ellison syndrome (gastrinoma): Occurs when gastrin is secreted by non–β-cell tumors of the pancreas

Cholecystokinin (CCK)	• Stimulates gallbladder contraction and relaxation of the sphincter of Oddi for bile secretion; stimulates pancreatic enzyme secretion; potentiates secretin-induced stimulation of pancreatic HCO_3^-; stimulates growth of the exocrine pancreas; inhibits gastric emptying • Stimuli for release: Released from I cells of the duodenal and jejunal mucosa ○ Small peptides and amino acids; fatty acids and monoglycerides
Secretin	• Actions are coordinated to reduce the amount of H^+ in the lumen of the small intestine; stimulates pancreatic HCO_3^- secretion and increases growth of the exocrine pancreas; stimulates HCO_3^- and H_2O secretion by the liver and increases bile secretion; inhibits H^+ secretion by gastric parietal cells

- Stimuli for release: Released from S cells of the duodenum in response to:
  - H^+ and fatty acids in the lumen of the duodenum

Gastric inhibitory peptide (GIP)	• Stimulates insulin release (e.g., oral glucose is better at triggering insulin release than intravenous); inhibits H^+ secretion by gastric parietal cells • Stimuli for release: Secreted by the duodenum and jejunum ◦ GIP is the only hormone released in response to fat, protein, and carbohydrate; its release is stimulated by fatty acids, amino acids, and orally administered glucose
Paracrine hormones	• Somatostatin: Secreted by cells throughout the gastrointestinal (GI) tract in response to H^+ in the lumen; its secretion is inhibited by vagal stimulation; it inhibits the release of all GI hormones and inhibits gastric H^+ secretion • Histamine: Secreted by mast cells of the gastric mucosa; increases gastric H^+ secretion directly by potentiating the effects of gastrin and vagal stimulation
Neurocrine hormones	• Vasoactive intestinal peptide (VIP): Produces relaxation of GI smooth muscle, including lower esophageal sphincter ◦ Stimulates release of HCO_3^- from the pancreas; inhibits gastric H^+ release • Gastrin-related peptide (GRP, or bombesin): Released from vagus nerves that innervate G cells; stimulates gastrin release from G cells • Enkephalins: Stimulates contraction of GI smooth muscle (lower esophageal, pyloric, ileocecal sphincters); inhibits intestinal secretion of fluid and electrolytes,, which forms the basis for the usefulness of opiates in the treatment of diarrhea

GASTROINTESTINAL SECRETION

Salivary secretion	• Functions of saliva: Initial starch digestion by ptyalin; triglyceride digestion by lingual lipase; lubrication by mucus; protection by dilution and buffering
	
	• Composition: High K^+ and HCO_3^-, low Na^+ and Cl^-, hypotonic, ptyalin, lingual lipase, kallikrein
	  ◦ Varies with flow rate: Low flow = low osmolarity with low Na^+, Cl^- and HCO_3^-, high K^+; high flow = composition is closest to plasma
	
	• Formed in parotid, submaxillary, sublingual glands
	  ◦ Saliva is produced in the acinus with composition similar to plasma, it is isotonic; ducts modify saliva via Na^+ and Cl^- reabsorption, secretion of K^+ and HCO_3^-
	  ◦ Aldosterone: Acts on ductal cells to increase Na^+ reabsorption and K^+ secretion

- Regulation of saliva production
  - Increased by autonomic nervous system (ANS) activity; parasympathetics are more important
  - Parasympathetic (cranial nerves (CNs) VII and IX) stimulation increases saliva production; cholinergic receptors are muscarinic; anticholinergic drugs cause dry mouth
  - Sympathetic stimulation: Receptors on acinar cells are β-adrenergic
  - Production is increased by food in the mouth, smells, conditioned reflexes, and nausea; it is decreased by sleep, dehydration, fear, and anticholinergic drugs

Gastric secretion

- Parietal cells: Located in the gastric body; secrete HCl and intrinsic factor
- Chief cells: Located in the gastric body; secrete pepsinogen
- G cells: Located in the gastric antrum; secrete gastrin
- Mechanisms of gastric H^+ secretion:
  - Parietal cells secrete HCl into the lumen and absorb HCO_3^- into the bloodstream; in the parietal cells, CO_2 and H_2O are converted to H^+ and HCO_3^- by carbonic anhydrase; H^+ is secreted into the lumen by the H^+, K^+-ATPase; Cl^- is secreted along with H^+; omeprazole inhibits the H^+, K^+-ATPase and thus blocks H^+ secretion
  - HCO_3^- produced is absorbed into the bloodstream in exchange for Cl^- (Cl^--HCO_3^- exchange); as HCO_3^- is added to venous blood, the pH increases ("alkaline tide"); if vomiting occurs, gastric H^+ never arrives to the small intestine and thus there is no stimulus for HCO_3^- secretion, and blood pH becomes alkaline
- Stimulation:
  - Vagus nerve: Increases H^+ secretion directly and indirectly; direct = vagus innervates parietal cells and directly stimulates H^+ secretion; the neurotransmitter is acetylcholine and the receptor is muscarinic; indirect = vagus innervates G cells and stimulates gastrin release; the neurotransmitter is GRP

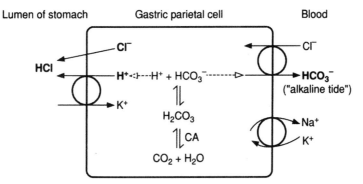

● **Figure III-22** Simplified mechanism of H^+ secretion by gastric parietal cells.

- ○ Histamine: Released from mast cells; diffuses to parietal cells; stimulates H^+ secretion by activating H_2 receptors (target for drugs such as cimetidine)
- ○ Gastrin: Released in response to eating a meal; stimulates H^+ release via interaction with an unknown receptor
- Inhibition: Via negative feedback
  - ○ Low pH (< 3.0); chyme in the duodenum (via GIP and secretin)

Pancreatic secretion

- Composition: Similar $[Na^+]$ and $[K^+]$ as plasma; higher $[HCO_3^-]$ than plasma; lower $[Cl^-]$ than plasma, isotonic, lipase, amylase, and proteases
  - ○ Low flow: Secretion is isotonic, composed mostly of Na^+ and Cl^-
  - ○ High flow: Secretion is isotonic, composed mostly of Na^+ and HCO_3^-
  - ○ Regardless of flow rate, fluid is always isotonic
- Formation
  - ○ Acinar cells produce a small volume of fluid with mostly Na^+ and Cl^-
  - ○ Ductal cells modify fluid by secreting HCO_3^-, absorbing Cl^- via Cl^- and HCO_3^- exchange; water then moves into the lumen to make secretion isosmotic
- Stimulation:
  - ○ Secretin is secreted by S cells of the duodenum in response to H^+ in the lumen; acts on ductal cells to increase HCO_3^- secretion
  - ○ Cholecystokinin (CCK) is secreted by I cells in response to small peptides, amino acids, and fatty acids in the lumen; acts on acinar cells to increase enzyme secretion
  - ○ Acetylcholine: Via vasovagal reflexes; released in response to H^+, small peptides, amino acids, and fatty acids; stimulates enzyme secretion by acinar cells and potentiates the effects of secretin on HCO_3^- secretion

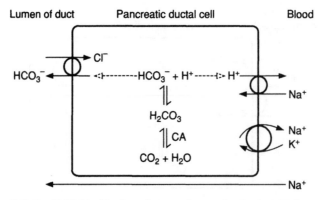

● **Figure III-23** Modification of pancreatic secretion by ductal cells.

- Cystic fibrosis: Results from a defect in Cl^- channels caused by a mutation in the cystic fibrosis transmembrane conductance regulator (CFTR) gene; associated with a deficiency of pancreatic enzymes resulting in malabsorption and steatorrhea

Bile secretion	- Composition: Contains bile salts, phospholipids, cholesterol, bile pigments
	
	- Bile salts: Amphipathic with hydrophobic and hydrophilic portions; orient themselves around lipid droplets for emulsification; solubilize lipids in micelles
	
	- During interdigestive periods: Gallbladder is relaxed and sphincter of Oddi is closed, so bile fills the gallbladder; bile is concentrated via isosmotic absorption of solutes and H_2O
	
	- Gallbladder contraction
	   ○ CCK causes contraction of gallbladder and relaxation of the sphincter of Oddi
	   ○ Acetylcholine also causes gallbladder contraction
	
	- Recirculation of bile acids: Terminal ileum contains Na^+-bile acid co-transporter

Secretion of electrolytes and H_2O	- H_2O and electrolytes are secreted from the blood to lumen; secretory mechanisms are in the crypts; absorptive mechanisms are in the villi - Cl^- is the primary ion secreted via Cl^- channels regulated by cyclic adenosine monophosphate (cAMP) - Na^+ is secreted passively following Cl^-; H_2O follows to maintain isosmotic conditions - *Vibrio cholera* toxin causes diarrhea by stimulating Cl^- secretion, binding to luminal membrane receptors and activating adenylate cyclase on basolateral membrane; intracellular cAMP increases, resulting in luminal membrane Cl^- channels opening; Na^+ and H_2O follow Cl^- into lumen

DIGESTION AND ABSORPTION

Carbohydrates	- Digestion: Only monosaccharides are absorbed; polysaccharides are broken down by a number of enzymes (e.g., amylase, sucrase, lactase)
	
	- Absorption
	   ○ Glucose and galactose are transported into cells via Na^+-dependent co-transport (SGLT 1) in the luminal membrane; sugar is transported uphill, and Na^+ is transported downhill; Na^+- K^+-ATPase keeps the intracellular Na^+ concentration low
	   ○ Fructose is transported exclusively by facilitated diffusion
	
	- Lactose intolerance results from absence of brush border lactase, an inability to hydrolyze lactose; non-absorbed lactose causes osmotic diarrhea

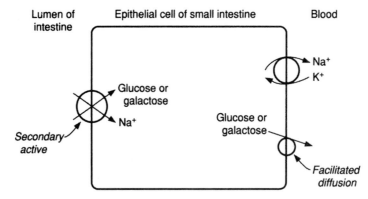

Lumen of intestine   Epithelial cell of small intestine   Blood

● **Figure III-24** Mechanism of absorption of monosaccharides by intestinal epithelial cells. Glucose and galactose are absorbed by Na⁺-dependent cotransport (secondary active), and fructose (not shown) is absorbed by facilitated diffusion.

Proteins

- Digestion: Endopeptidases degrade proteins by hydrolyzing interior peptide bonds; exopeptidases hydrolyze one amino acid at a time from the C terminus; pepsin is not essential for protein digestion; it is secreted as a zymogen by chief cells, activated at low pH, and denatured above pH of 5
  - Pancreatic proteases: Trypsin(ogen) enterokinase; converts chymotrypsinogen, proelastase, and procarboxypeptidase A and B to active forms; after their work is done they digest each other
- Absorption can be absorbed as amino acids, di- and tripeptides
  - Free amino acids: Na⁺-dependent amino acid co-transport occurs at the luminal membrane; amino acids are then transported by facilitated diffusion into the blood; there are four separate carriers (neutral, acidic, basic, imino)
  - Di- and tripeptides; Absorbed faster than amino acids; H⁺-dependent co-transport of di- and tripeptides occurs on luminal membrane; after transported into cells, they are hydrolyzed by intracellular peptidases and then transported into the blood by facilitated diffusion

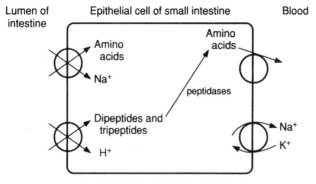

Lumen of intestine   Epithelial cell of small intestine   Blood

● **Figure III-25** Mechanism of absorption of amino acids, dipeptides, and tripeptides by intestinal epithelial cells.

Lipids	• Digestion
	  ○ Stomach: Mixing breaks lipids into droplets to increase surface area; lingual lipases digest triglycerides to monoglycerides and fatty acids; most are digested by pancreatic lipase; CCK slows gastric emptying to allow for adequate digestion and absorption in the intestine
	  ○ Small intestine: Bile acids emulsify lipids, increasing surface area for absorption; pancreatic lipase hydrolyzes lipids; hydrophobic products are solubilized in micelles by bile acids
	• Absorption of lipids
	  ○ Micelles bring digestive products into contact with absorptive surfaces; digestive products diffuse across luminal surface
	  ○ In intestinal cells, digestive products are re-esterified to triglycerides, cholesterol ester, phospholipids (with apolipoproteins, these form chylomicrons); lack of apoprotein B results in the inability to transport chylomicrons out of intestinal cells (abetalipoproteinemia)
	  ○ Chylomicrons are transported out of intestinal cells by exocytosis into lymphatics and are added to the blood via the thoracic duct
	• Causes of malabsorption include: pancreatic disease, gastrin hypersecretion, ileal resection, bacterial overgrowth, decreased number of intestinal cells, failure to synthesize apolipoprotein-B

NaCl	• Na^+ moves into luminal membrane down its gradient via:
	  ○ Passive diffusion (Na^+ channels); Na^+-glucose or Na^+-amino acid co-transport; Na^+-Cl^- co-transport; Na^+-H^+ exchange (co-transport is most important in small intestine; passive diffusion via Na^+ channels is most important in colon and is stimulated by aldosterone)
	  ○ Na^+ is pumped out of basolateral surface via Na^+-K^+-ATPase against its gradient
	  ○ Cl^- absorption accompanies Na^+ absorption via passive diffusion via paracellular route, Na^+-Cl^- co-transport, and Cl^--HCO_3^- exchange

K⁺	• Absorbed in the small intestine by passive diffusion via a paracellular route • K^+ is actively secreted in the colon by a mechanism similar to that in the renal tubule: secretion is stimulated by aldosterone; in diarrhea, K^+ secretion is increased via a flow rate–dependent mechanism similar to the renal tubule
H₂O	• Absorption is secondary to solute absorption; isosmotic absorption in the small intestine and gallbladder; in the colon, H_2O permeability is much lower
Absorption of other substances	• Fat-soluble vitamins (A, E, D, K) are absorbed along with lipids in micelles

- Water-soluble vitamins are absorbed via Na^+-dependent co-transport
- Vitamin B_{12} is absorbed in the ileum; requires intrinsic factor
- Ca^{2+} absorption in the small intestine depends on adequate amounts of active vitamin D produced by the kidney
- Iron is absorbed as heme or free-iron Fe^{2+}; free Fe^{2+} is bound in blood to transferrin, which transports it from the small bowel to storage sites (e.g., liver)

Topic **9**

Endocrine Physiology

Must Knows

- Pituitary gland
- Thyroid gland
- Adrenal gland
- Endocrine pancreas
- Calcium metabolism

PITUITARY GLAND

Anterior pituitary	• Linked to hypothalamus via the hypothalamic–hypophysial portal system
	• Thyroid-stimulating hormone (TSH), luteinizing hormone (LH), and follicle-stimulating hormone (FSH): Members of the same protein family; contain α and β subunits; α subunits are identical
	• Adrenocorticotropic hormone (ACTH), melanocyte-stimulating hormone, β-lipotropin, and β-endorphin: All derived from precursor proopiomelanocortin
	• Prolactin and growth hormone
Growth hormone (somatotropin)	• Release is pulsatile; secretion is increased by sleep, stress, puberty hormones, starvation, exercise, and hypoglycemia; secretion is decreased by somatostatin, somatomedins, obesity, hyperglycemia, and pregnancy

- Hypothalamic control: Growth hormone–releasing hormone (GHRH) stimulates synthesis and secretion; somatostatin inhibits secretion by blocking GHRH response of anterior pituitary
- Somatomedins (negative feedback): Produced by target tissues; inhibit growth hormone (GH) secretion by acting on the anterior pituitary and stimulating somatostatin secretion
- GHRH inhibits its own secretion, and GH inhibits its own secretion by stimulating somatostatin secretion
- Actions of GH: Decreases glucose uptake into cells, increases lipolysis, increases protein synthesis in muscle and lean body mass, and increases insulin-like growth factor (IGF) production
- Actions via IGF: In the liver, GH generates production of somatomedins (IGFs); increases protein synthesis by chondrocytes and linear growth; increases protein synthesis in muscle and lean body mass; increases protein synthesis in most organs and increases organ size
- Pathophysiology:
  - Deficiency: Caused by lack of GH, hypothalamic dysfunction (decreased GHRH), failure of liver to generate IGF, and receptor deficiency; causes short stature, obesity, and delayed puberty
  - Excess: Can be treated with somatostatin analogs (octreotide); hypersecretion causes acromegaly and before puberty can cause gigantism; after puberty, can cause increased bone growth, increased organ size, and glucose intolerance

Prolactin	- Responsible for lactogenesis; participates in breast development
	- Regulation: Tonically inhibited by dopamine secreted by the hypothalamus; thyrotropin-releasing hormone increases prolactin secretion; prolactin feeds back negatively by stimulating hypothalamic dopamine release
	- Actions: Milk production and breast development; inhibits ovulation (by decreased gonadotropin-releasing hormone [GnRH]); inhibits spermatogenesis
	- Pathophysiology
	○ Deficiency: Destruction of anterior pituitary; failure to lactate
	○ Excess: From hypothalamic destruction or from prolactinoma, causes galactorrhea and decreased libido, failure to ovulate, and amenorrhea by inhibiting GnRH; can be treated with bromocriptine via actions as a dopamine agonist
Posterior pituitary	- Derived from neural tissue, nerve cell bodies located in hypothalamic nuclei; hormones are synthesized in cell bodies and travel down axons for release
	- Antidiuretic hormone (ADH): Originates primarily from the supraoptic nuclei; regulates serum osmolarity by increased H_2O permeability of late distal tubules and collecting ducts (factors

increasing secretion: increased serum osmolarity, volume contraction, pain, nausea, hypoglycemia, nicotine, opiates, antineoplastic drugs; decreasing factors: decreased serum osmolarity, ethanol, α-agonists, atrial natriuretic peptide)

- Oxytocin: Originates primarily in paraventricular nuclei; causes ejection of milk from the breast when stimulated by suckling
  - Regulation: Major stimulus is suckling; afferent fibers carry impulses from the nipple to the spinal cord; relays in the hypothalamus trigger the release; dilation of the cervix and orgasm also stimulate release
  - Actions: Contraction of myoepithelial cells in the breast; contraction of the uterus; can be used exogenously to induce labor and reduce postpartum bleeding

THYROID GLAND

Thyroid hormone synthesis
- Stimulated by TSH
- Iodide pump: Present on follicular cells; pumps I^- into cells; inhibited by thiocyanate or perchlorate; Wolff-Chaikoff effect = high I^- inhibits pump
- Oxidation of I^- to I_2: Catalyzed by peroxidase enzyme; I_2 can be organified; peroxidase is inhibited by propylthiouracil (PTU)

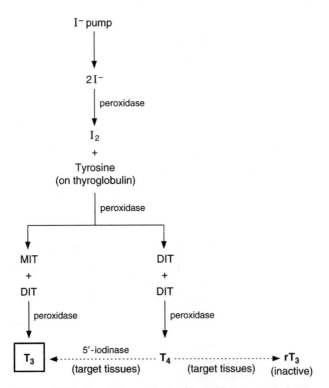

● **Figure III-26** Steps in the synthesis of thyroid hormones. Each step is stimulated by thyroid-stimulating hormone (TSH). *DIT* = diiodotyrosine; *I⁻* = iodide; *MIT* = monoiodotyrosine; *rT₃* = reverse T₃; *T₃* = triiodothyronine; *T₄* = thyroxine.

- Organification: Tyrosine is incorporated into thyroglobulin; thyroglobulin is extruded into follicular lumen; at the luminal border, tyrosine residues react with I_2 to form monoiodotyrosine (MIT) and diiodotyrosine (DIT)
- Coupling: 2 DITs make thyroxine (T_4); one DIT and one MIT make triiodothyronine (T_3)
- Iodinated thyroglobulin: Stored in follicular lumen until secretion is stimulated
- Stimulation of thyroid cells by TSH: Iodinated thyroglobulin is taken up by follicular cells; lysosomal enzymes digest thyroglobulin releasing T_3 and T_4 into circulation; remaining MIT and DIT are deiodinated so I_2 can be reutilized
- Binding of T_3 and T_4: Most is bound to thyroxine-binding globulin (TBG)
  - TBG levels decrease in liver failure, leading to decreased bound levels but normal free; therefore, decreased total; pregnancy causes increased TBG levels, leading to increased total thyroid hormone but normal free
- Conversion of T_4 to T_3 and rT_3: Occurs in peripheral tissues, T_3 activity $>T_4$; rT_3 is inactive

Regulation of hormone secretion	<ul><li>TRH: Secreted by hypothalamus; stimulates TSH secretion by pituitary</li><li>TSH: Increases synthesis and secretion of thyroid hormones via cyclic adenosine monophosphate (cAMP) mechanism; chronic elevated TSH causes hypertrophy of gland</li><li>T_3: Downregulates TRH receptors in anterior pituitary</li><li>Thyroid-stimulating immunoglobulin (Igs): Igs that are antibodies to TSH receptors on gland stimulate the thyroid gland–like TSH; present in high concentrations in patients with Grave's disease (high thyroid hormones but low TSH)</li></ul>
Thyroid hormone actions	<ul><li>Growth: Attainment of adult stature; acts synergistically with GH to promote bone growth; stimulates bone maturation</li><li>Central nervous system: Maturation in the perinatal period is dependent on thyroid hormones<ul><li>Hyperthyroidism in adulthood causes hyperexcitability and irritability</li><li>Hypothyroidism causes listlessness, slowed speech, somnolence, impaired memory, and decreased mental capacity</li></ul></li><li>Autonomic nervous system (ANS) has many of the same actions as the sympathetic nervous system; upregulates β1-adrenergic receptors in the heart; therefore, β-blockers are useful in hyperthyroidism</li><li>Basal metabolic rate: O_2 consumption and basal metabolic rate (BMR) are increased; increased the synthesis of Na^+-K^+-ATPase and therefore O_2 consumption</li></ul>

TABLE III-5	PATHOPHYSIOLOGY OF THE THYROID GLAND	
	Hyperthyroidism	**Hypothyroidism**
Symptoms	Increased metabolic rate Weight loss Negative nitrogen balance Increased heat production (sweating) Increased cardiac output Dyspnea Tremor and weakness Exophthalmos Goiter	Decreased metabolic rate Weight gain Positive nitrogen balance Decreased heat production (cold sensitivity) Decreased cardiac output Hypoventilation Lethargy and mental slowness Drooping eyelids Myxedema Growth and mental retardation (perinatal) Goiter
Causes	Graves' disease (antibodies to TSH receptor) Thyroid neoplasm	Thyroiditis (autoimmune thyroiditis; Hashimoto's thyroiditis) Surgical removal of thyroid I^-deficiency Cretinism (congenital) Decreased TRH or TSH
TSH levels	Decreased (because of feedback inhibition on anterior pituitary by high thyroid hormone levels)	Increase (because of decreased feedback inhibition on anterior pituitary by low thyroid hormone levels) Decreased (if primary defect is in hypothalamus or anterior pituitary)
Treatment	Propylthiouracil (inhibits thyroid hormone synthesis by blocking peroxidase) Thyroidectomy ^{131}I (destroys thyroid) β-blockers (adjunct therapy)	Thyroid hormone replacement

TRH = thyrotropin-releasing hormone; TSH = thyroid-stimulating hormone.

- Cardiovascular and respiratory systems: Increase cardiac output and ventilation rate to ensure that more O_2 are delivered to tissues; heart rate and systolic volume are increased
- Metabolic effects: Metabolism is increased to meet demand; glucose absorption in the gastrointestinal tract is increased; glycogenolysis, gluconeogenesis, and glucose oxidation are increased; lipolysis and protein metabolism are increased

Pathophysiology   See Table III-5

ADRENAL GLAND

Cortex

- Zona glomerulosa = aldosterone; zona fasciculate = mostly glucocorticoids (cortisol); zona reticularis = mostly androgens

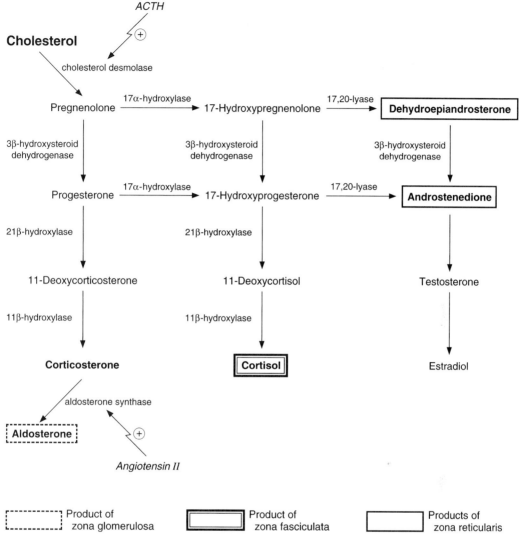

● **Figure III-27** Synthetic pathways for glucocorticoids, androgens, and mineralocorticoids in the adrenal cortex. *ACTH* = adrenocorticotropic hormone.

Regulation	• Glucocorticoids: Secretion oscillates with circadian rhythm; cortisol levels are highest in the a.m. and lowest in the p.m., for those who sleep at night

- Glucocorticoids: Secretion oscillates with circadian rhythm; cortisol levels are highest in the a.m. and lowest in the p.m., for those who sleep at night

- Hypothalamic control (corticotrophin-releasing hormone [CRH]): Neurons in paraventricular nuclei, when stimulated, release CRH to the anterior pituitary; stimulates synthesis of proopiomelanocortin (POMC) and secretion of ACTH

- ACTH increases steroid hormone synthesis in the adrenal cortex by stimulating cholesterol desmolase; also upregulates its own receptor; chronically increased levels cause gland hypertrophy

  ○ Negative feedback via cortisol: Cortisol inhibits CRH secretion and ACTH secretion; dexamethasone suppression test is based on its ability to inhibit ACTH secretion

- Aldosterone: Under tonic control of ACTH, also regulated by the renin–angiotensin system and K^+ levels
  - Renin–angiotensin: Decreased blood volume causes decreased renal perfusion, which increases renin secretion; renin catalyzes conversion of angiotensinogen to angiotensin I (ATI); ATI is converted to angiotensin II (ATII) by angiotensin-converting enzyme (ACE); ATII acts on the zona glomerulosa to increase aldosterone synthesis; aldosterone increases renal Na^+ absorption to restore extracellular fluid (ECF) volume
  - Hyperkalemia increases aldosterone secretion, which increases renal K^+ secretion

Actions of glucocorticoids	<ul><li>Essential for the stress responses</li><li>Stimulation of gluconeogenesis: Increase protein catabolism in muscle, providing more amino acids to liver for gluconeogenesis; decrease glucose utilization and insulin sensitivity of adipose; increase lipolysis</li><li>Anti-inflammatory effects: Induce synthesis of lipocortin, an inhibitor of phospholipase A2, thus inhibiting formation of arachidonic acid; inhibit production of interleukin-2 (IL-2) and thus inhibit proliferation of T lymphocytes; inhibit release of histamine and serotonin from mast cells and platelets</li><li>Suppression of the immune response: Via the above mechanism involving IL-2; at pharmacologic doses, glucocorticoids are used to prevent rejection of transplanted organs</li><li>Maintenance of vascular responsiveness to catecholamines: Cortisol upregulates α_1 receptors on arterioles; with cortisol excess, arterial pressure increases; with deficiency, it decreases</li></ul>
Actions of mineralocorticoids	<ul><li>Increase renal Na^+ reabsorption and K^+ secretion</li><li>Increase renal H^+ secretion via action on α-intercalated cells</li></ul>
Pathophysiology	<ul><li>Adrenocortical insufficiency<ul><li>Primary: Addison's disease, which is most commonly caused by immune-mediated destruction of the cortex</li><li>Result is decreased glucocorticoids, androgens, mineralocorticoids; increased ACTH; hypoglycemia; weight loss, weakness; nausea and vomiting; hyperpigmentation; decreased pubic and axillary hair in women; ECF volume contraction; hypotension; hyperkalemia; and metabolic acidosis</li><li>Secondary: Caused by deficiency of ACTH; no hyperpigmentation; no volume contraction, hyperkalemia or metabolic acidosis because aldosterone levels are normal</li></ul></li><li>Adrenocortical excess: Cushing's syndrome<ul><li>Most commonly iatrogenic; less commonly via adrenal hyperplasia (Cushing's disease is caused by overproduction of ACTH)</li><li>Characterized by increased cortisol and androgens; increased ACTH or decreased ACTH (if caused by adrenal or iatro-</li></ul></li></ul>

genic); hyperglycemia; increased protein catabolism and muscle wasting; central obesity; poor wound healing; virilization in women; hypertension; osteoporosis; striae (ketoconazole inhibits steroid hormone synthesis and can be used to treat Cushing's syndrome)

- Hyperaldosteronism: Conn's syndrome; caused by hypersecreting tumor
  - Characterized by hypertension, hypokalemia, metabolic alkalosis, and decreased renin
- 21-β-hydroxylase deficiency: Most common biochemical abnormality of steroidogenic pathway
  - Characterized by decreased cortisol and aldosterone levels; increased 17-hydroxyprogesterone and progesterone levels; increased ACTH; hyperplasia of zona fasciculate and reticularis caused by high ACTH levels; increased adrenal androgens; virilization in women; suppression of gonadal function

ENDOCRINE PANCREAS

Glucagon

- Secreted by α cells at outer rim of islets
- Regulation: Decreased blood glucose stimulates secretion
- Actions: Acts on liver and adipose tissue
  - Increases blood glucose: Increases glycogenolysis and prevents recycling of glucose to glycogen; increases gluconeogenesis; decreases production of fructose 2,6-bisphosphate, decreasing phosphofructokinase
  - Increases blood fatty acid and ketoacid concentration: Increases lipolysis; ketoacids are produced from acetyl coenzyme A (CoA) via fatty acid degradation
  - Increases urea production: Amino groups from amino acids used for gluconeogenesis

Insulin

- Contains α and β chains joined by two disulfide bridges; proinsulin synthesized as a single peptide chain; the connecting C peptide is removed and secreted along with insulin; its level can be used to monitor β cell function
- Regulation: The major regulating factor is increased blood glucose
- Secretion: Glucose binds Glut2 receptor; glucose is oxidized inside β cells to adenosine triphosphate (ATP), which closes K^+ channels, causing depolarization (sulfonylurea drugs close these channels), thus opening Ca^{2+} channels, increasing intracellular Ca^{2+}, and promoting secretion of insulin
- Insulin receptor: A tetramer of 2 α and 2 β subunits; the β subunits have tyrosine kinase activity; insulin downregulates its own receptors on target tissue; therefore, the insulin receptor number goes up in starvation and down in obesity
- Actions: Acts on liver, adipose, and muscle
  - Decreases blood glucose: Increases uptake of glucose by directing insertion of glucose transporters into membrane;

promotes glycogenesis; inhibits glycogenolysis; decreases gluconeogenesis (via increased fructose 2,6-bisphosphate)

- ○ Decreases blood fatty acid and ketoacid concentration: Stimulates fat deposition and inhibits lipolysis; inhibits ketoacid formation because of decreased fatty acid degradation

- ○ Decreases blood amino acid concentration: Stimulates amino acid uptake, increases protein synthesis, and inhibits protein degradation (anabolic)

- ○ Decreases blood K^+: Increases K^+ uptake into cells

Diabetes mellitus	• Hyperglycemia : Caused by insulin deficiency; glucose uptake and glycogen synthesis are decreased
	• Hypotension: Caused by ECF volume contraction; high level of glucose overwhelms kidneys ability to reabsorb it; it acts as an osmotic diuretic
	• Metabolic acidosis: Caused by overproduction of ketoacids (β-hydroxybutyrate and acetoacetate); this increases the ventilation rate as a respiratory compensation
	• Hyperkalemia: Insulin normally promotes K^+ uptake into cells

CALCIUM METABOLISM

Ca^{2+} homeostasis	• 40% of total Ca^{2+} is bound to plasma proteins; 60% is unbound and is ultrafilterable; free, ionized Ca^{2+} is biologically active; serum Ca^{2+} is determined by balance of absorption, excretion, and bone remodeling

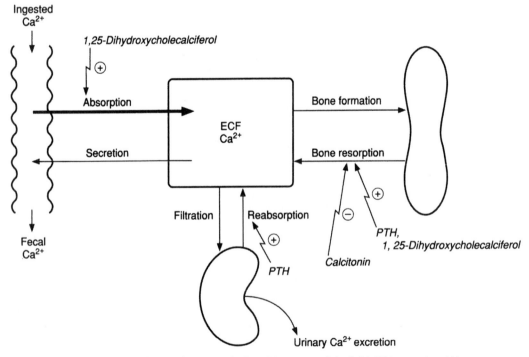

● **Figure III-28** Hormonal regulation of Ca^{2+} metabolism. *ECF* = extracellular fluid; *PTH* = parathyroid hormone.

- Positive balance: Seen in growing children; intestinal absorption exceeds urinary excretion; excess is deposited in bones
- Negative balance: Seen during pregnancy and lactation; absorption is less than excretion; deficit comes from maternal bones

Parathyroid hormone	- Major hormone that regulates serum Ca^{2+}; synthesized by chief cells of parathyroid glands
	
	- Secretion: Controlled by serum Ca^{2+} through negative feedback; decreased serum Ca^{2+} increases PTH secretion; mild decreases in Mg^{2+} also increase parathyroid hormone (PTH) secretion; severe decreases in Mg^{2+} inhibit PTH secretion and produce symptoms of hypoparathyroidism
	
	- Actions: Produce increases in serum Ca^{2+} and decreases in serum phosphate
	   ○ Increases bone resorption; Brings both Ca^{2+} and phosphate from bone into ECF; these complex together; thus, no immediate increase in ionized free Ca^{2+} results
	   ○ Inhibits renal phosphate reabsorption in the proximal tubule, thus increasing excretion; phosphate resorbed from bone is excreted while serum Ca^{2+} increases
	   ○ Increases renal reabsorption of Ca^{2+} in the distal tubule
	   ○ Increases intestinal Ca^{2+} absorption by stimulating production of 1,25-dihydroxycholecalciferol in the kidney

PTH pathophysiology	- Primary hyperparathyroidism: Commonly caused by a parathyroid adenoma
	   ○ Characterized by hypercalcemia, hypophosphatemia, increased urinary phosphate, increased urinary Ca^{2+}, increased urinary cAMP, and increased bone resorption
	
	- Hypercalcemia of malignancy: Caused by a PTH-related peptide secreted by some tumors; has all of the physiological actions of PTH
	   ○ Characterized by all the same as primary PTH, but with decreased PTH levels
	
	- Hypoparathyroidism: Most commonly secondary to thyroid surgery or congenital (DiGeorge's)
	   ○ Characterized by hypocalcemia and tetany, hyperphosphatemia, and decreased urinary phosphate excretion
	
	- Pseudohypoparathyroidism type Ia: Albright's hereditary osteodystrophy
	   ○ Results from a defective G protein in PTH signaling; causes end-organ resistance
	   ○ Hypocalcemia and hyperphosphatemia occur that do not respond to PTH administration; circulating PTH levels are high
	
	- Chronic renal failure: Decreased GFR leads to decreased phosphate filtration, phosphate retention, and increased serum phosphate levels; phosphate and Ca^{2+} complex to decrease

ionized Ca^{2+}; decreased renal 1,25-vitamin D caused by dis-
eased renal tissue; decreased Ca^{2+} causes hyperparathyroidism;
the increased PTH and decreased vitamin D produce renal
osteodystrophy with bone resorption and osteomalacia

Vitamin D

- Provides Ca^{2+} and phosphate to ECF for bone mineralization;
  deficiency in children causes rickets; in adults, deficiency
  causes osteomalacia

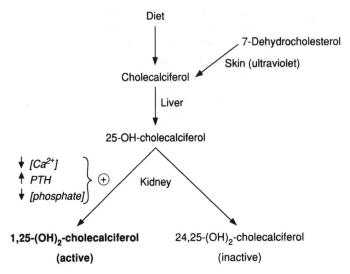

● **Figure III-29** Steps and regulation in the synthesis of 1,25-dihydroxychole-
calciferol. *PTH* = parathyroid hormone.

- Metabolism: Active form is 1,25-(OH)2D3 form; production of
  this occurs in kidney by 1α-hydroxylase (the activity of which
  increases with decreased serum Ca^{2+}, increased PTH, and
  decreased serum phosphate)
- Actions of 1,25-vitamin D
  ○ Increase intestinal absorption of Ca^{2+}, calbindin D produc-
    tion is induced; PTH increases intestinal Ca^{2+} absorption
    indirectly by stimulating 1α-hydroxylase
  ○ Increases intestinal phosphate absorption
  ○ Increases renal reabsorption of Ca^{2+} and phosphate
  ○ Increases bone resorption and provides Ca^{2+} and phosphate
    from old bone

Calcitonin

- Synthesized by parafollicular cells of thyroid; secretion stimulated by increase in serum Ca^{2+}; acts primarily to inhibit bone
  resorption; can be used to treat hypercalcemia

Topic **10**

Reproductive Physiology

Must Knows

- Male reproduction
- Female reproduction
- Menstrual cycle
- Pregnancy

MALE REPRODUCTION

Testosterone	• Major androgen synthesized and secreted by Leydig cells; these cells cannot secrete glucocorticoids or mineralocorticoids
	• Luteinizing hormone (LH) increases testosterone synthesis by stimulating cholesterol desmolase; accessory sex organs contain 5α-reductase to convert testosterone to DHT (dihydro-testosterone), the active form; 5α-reductase inhibitors (finasteride) may be used to treat benign prostatic hypertrophy via blocking activation of testosterone
Regulation of testes	• Hypothalamic control via gonadotropin-releasing hormone (GnRH); arcuate nuclei of hypothalamus secrete GnRH to the portal system; this stimulates anterior pituitary follicle-stimulating hormone (FSH) and LH secretion
	• FSH: Acts on Sertoli cells to maintain spermatogenesis; Sertoli cells secrete inhibin, which feeds back negatively to inhibit FSH secretion
	• LH: Acts on Leydig cells to promote testosterone synthesis; testosterone also acts in the testes on Sertoli cells to reinforce FSH effects
	• Negative feedback: Testosterone and inhibin; testosterone feeds back to inhibit GnRH release at the hypothalamus and LH at the anterior pituitary; inhibin inhibits FSH secretion from the anterior pituitary
Actions of androgens	• Cause prenatal differentiation of Wolffian ducts and external genitalia, development of secondary sexual characteristics at puberty, and pubertal growth spurt; maintain spermatogenesis in the Sertoli cells; increase size and secretory activity of the epididymis, vas, prostate, and seminal vesicles; increase libido

FEMALE REPRODUCTION

Estrogen and progesterone synthesis	• Theca cells produce testosterone in response to LH; testosterone diffuses to nearby granulosa cells that contain aromatase and convert it to 17β-estradiol (stimulated by FSH) • Progesterone is synthesized by theca cells from cholesterol via pregnenolone; this is in response to LH

Regulation of the ovaries	• Hypothalamic GnRH: Pulsatile GnRH stimulates FSH and LH
	
	• Anterior pituitary: FSH and LH stimulate steroidogenesis in ovarian follicles and corpus luteum, follicular development past the antral stage, ovulation, and luteinization
	
	• Negative and positive feedback of estrogen and progesterone
	   ◦ Follicular phase: Estrogen feeds back negatively on the anterior pituitary
	   ◦ Mid-cycle: Estrogen feeds back positively to the anterior pituitary
	   ◦ Luteal phase: Estrogen and progesterone feed back negatively on the anterior pituitary and hypothalamus, respectively

Actions of estrogen	• Has both negative and positive feedback on FSH and LH release • Causes maturation and maintenance of the fallopian tubes, uterus, cervix, and vagina; development of female secondary sex characteristics; development of breasts; upregulates estrogen, LH, and progesterone receptors; proliferation and development of ovarian granulose cells; maintains pregnancy; lowers the uterine threshold to contractile stimuli during pregnancy; stimulates prolactin secretion (but then blocks its action on the breasts)
Actions of progesterone	• Has negative feedback effects on FSH and LH release during the luteal phase • Maintains secretory activity of the uterus during the luteal phase; maintains pregnancy; raises the uterine threshold to contractile stimuli during pregnancy; participates in the development of breasts

MENSTRUAL CYCLE

Follicular phase (days 1 to 14)	• A primordial follicle develops to the graafian stage with atresia of other follicles • LH and FSH receptors are upregulated in theca and granulosa cells • Estradiol levels increase and cause proliferation of the uterus • FSH and LH levels are suppressed by the negative feedback effect of estradiol on the anterior pituitary • Progesterone levels are low

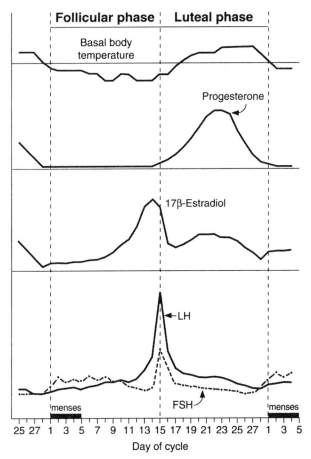

● **Figure III-30** The menstrual cycle. *FSH* = follicle-stimulating hormone; *LH* = luteinizing hormone.

Ovulation (day 15)	• Occurs 14 days before menses, regardless of cycle length • Burst of estradiol synthesis at end of follicular phase has a positive feedback effect on secretion of FSH and LH, with an LH surge • Ovulation occurs as a result of the estrogen-stimulated LH surge • Estrogen levels decrease just after ovulation but increase again during the luteal phase • Cervical mucus increases in quantity and becomes less viscous and more penetrable by sperm
Luteal phase (days 15 to 28)	• The corpus luteum begins to develop and synthesizes estrogen and progesterone • The vascularity and secretory activity of endometrium increase in preparation for receipt of a fertilized egg • Basal body temperature increases because of the effect of progesterone on the hypothalamic thermoregulatory center • In the absence of fertilization, the corpus luteum regresses at the end of the luteal phase; thus, estradiol and progesterone levels decrease

Menses (days 1 to 4)	• The endometrium is sloughed off because of the abrupt withdrawal of estradiol and progesterone

PREGNANCY

Hormonal regulation	• Pregnancy is characterized by increasing levels of estrogen and progesterone to maintain the endometrium for the fetus, suppress ovarian follicular function (via FSH and LH inhibition), and stimulate development of the breasts
Human chorionic gonadotropin (HCG)	• Upon fertilization, the corpus luteum is preserved by HCG, which is produced by the placenta
First trimester	• The corpus luteum produces estradiol and progesterone via HCG stimulation; peak HCG levels occur at gestational week 9 and then decline
Second and third trimesters	• Progesterone is produced by the placenta • Estrogens are produced by the interplay of the fetal adrenal gland and the placenta. The fetal adrenal synthesizes dehydroepiandrosterone-sulfate (DHEA-S), which is hydroxylated in the fetal liver, these intermediates are transferred to the placenta, where sulfate is removed, and they are aromatized to estrogens • The major placental estrogen is estriol • Human placental lactogen is produced throughout pregnancy, with actions similar to GH and prolactin
Parturition	• During pregnancy, progesterone increases the threshold for uterine contraction • Near term, the estrogen/progesterone ratio increases, making the uterus more sensitive to contractile stimuli

Lactation	• Estrogens and progesterone stimulate growth and development of the breasts; prolactin levels increase steadily throughout pregnancy as estrogen stimulates prolactin secretion from the anterior pituitary; lactation does not occur during pregnancy because estrogen and progesterone block prolactin's effects
	
	• With parturition, estrogen/progesterone levels decrease and lactation occurs; it is maintained by suckling, which stimulates oxytocin and prolactin secretion
	
	• Ovulation is suppressed as long as lactation continues as prolactin:
	  ○ Inhibits hypothalamic GnRH secretion
	  ○ Inhibits action of GnRH on the anterior pituitary and thus FSH and LH secretion
	  ○ Antagonizes the actions of LH and FSH on the ovaries

Pathology

10 *Top Tips*
Pathology

Topic	Main Focus	USMLE Example
1 Inflammation	Inflammation	• The legs of a 75-year-old man with diabetes show the cardinal signs of inflammation: calor, dolor, rubor, and tumor. These signs indicate that the patient has cellulitis.
2 Neoplasia	Markers of neoplasia	• The pap smear of a 34-year-old noncompliant woman with a history of multiple sexual partners and complaints of sporadic vaginal bleeding demonstrates pleomorphism and hyperchromatic and large nuclei with prominent mitotic figures throughout the squamous cervical epithelium. The patient is diagnosed with carcinoma in situ.
3 Cardiovascular System and Hematology	Complications of myocardial infarction (MI)	• After a 54-year-old man with hypercholesterolemia has had an acute MI, he undergoes emergent angioplasty. The patient is doing well for 3 days and then develops sudden shortness of breath and an apical holosystolic murmur. An echocardiogram demonstrates papillary muscle rupture and consequent mitral insufficiency.
4 Respiratory System	Chronic obstructive pulmonary disease	• 65-year-old woman with a 50-pack-year history of smoking complains of shortness of breath. When laboratory studies reveal a decreased forced expiratory volume in 1 second ($FEV_{1.0}$): forced vital capacity (FVC), increased total lung capacity (TLC), and respiratory acidosis; she is diagnosed with emphysema.

(Continued)

10 Top Tips

Pathology   (Continued)

Topic	Main Focus	USMLE Example
5 Gastrointestinal System	Colon cancer	• A 60-year-old man complains to his doctor of increasingly narrowed stools, episodes of constipation, and severe fatigue and is found to be anemic. A colonoscopy demonstrates cancer of the descending colon.
6 Genitourinary System and Diseases of the Breast	Breast tumors	• A 28-year-old woman complains to her doctor about a mass in her left breast that is tender yet round and movable. She is afraid it is cancer, but a biopsy proves it is a fibroadenoma, a benign tumor common in women younger than age 30 years.
7 Rheumatology and the Musculoskeletal System	Rheumatoid arthritis	• A 45-year-old woman complains of painful swollen joints in her wrists and fingers that are worse in the morning. Her doctor begins treatment for rheumatoid arthritis.
8 Dermatology	Bullous diseases	• A 22-year-old woman is started on sulfamethoxasole-trimethoprim for a urinary tract infection. After 2 days of therapy, she develops a fever and diffuse, round, erythematous skin lesions. Her doctor suspects Stevens-Johnson syndrome and immediately stops treatment.
9 Endocrine System	Hyperthyroidism	• A 45-year-old woman develops irritability, heat intolerance, tremors, diarrhea, and protruding eyes. Her thyroid-stimulating hormone level is low, and her T_4 is high. She is diagnosed with Graves' disease.
10 Nervous System	Guillain-Barré syndrome	• A 34-year-old man recovering from a mild respiratory tract infection develops sudden weakness and paresthesias that began in his legs and are spreading upward. A lumbar puncture shows albumino-cytologic dissociation, and he is diagnosed with Guillain-Barré syndrome.

Topic **1**

Inflammation

Must Knows

- Cellular changes associated with hypoxia, cell death, and apoptosis
- Necrosis
- Fundamentals of inflammation
- Key inflammatory mediators

HYPOXIC CELL INJURY AND DEATH

Early cellular changes	• Hypoxia leads to a failure of aerobic metabolism, which leads to anaerobic metabolism, decreased adenosine triphosphate (ATP) production, and increased lactate; this leads to failure of Na^+K^+-ATPase and decreased intracellular pH
	• Cytoplasmic swelling (hydropic change of endoplasmic reticulum, vacuoles, and mitochondria)
	• Dissociation of ribosomes
Late cellular changes	• Accumulation of reactive oxygen species, membrane and organelle damage, and cell membrane blebbing
Irreversible damage	• Further membrane damage: Calcium influx, activation of hydrolytic enzymes, and cell death

NECROSIS (FIG. IV-1)

Coagulative necrosis	• Caused by ischemia
	• Cell appears opaque and acidophilic
Liquefactive necrosis	• Occurs in brain tissue as result of powerful hydrolytic enzymes
Fat necrosis	• Caused by release of lipases from dead cells, which act on triglycerides and react with Ca^{2+}; leads to the formation of calcium soaps (Ca^{2+} + free fatty acids)
	• Occurs with acute pancreatitis and breast trauma

Coagulative necrosis

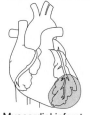

Myocardial infarct

Liquefactive necrosis

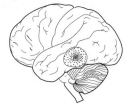

Brain infarct

Caseous necrosis

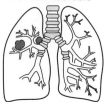

Pulmonary granulomas
(e.g., tuberculosis,
fungal infections)

Fat necrosis

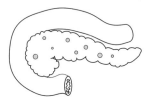

Pancreatitis

Fibrinoid necrosis

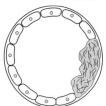

Arteries, arterioles, glomerular capillaries
(autoimmune disease)

● **Figure IV-1** Forms of necrosis.

Caseous necrosis	• Induced by cell-mediated immunity (T lymphocytes, macrophages, inflammatory cytokines) to infections with *Mycobacterium tuberculosis* or fungi such as *Histoplasma capsulatum* • Combination of coagulation and liquefactive necrosis • The necrotic area appears cheesy or milky
Gangrenous necrosis	• Occurs with ischemic coagulative necrosis and infection

Apoptosis	• Controlled cell death without inflammation
	  ◦ Cell shrinkage
	  ◦ Nuclear chromatin condensation
	• Fragmentation of nucleus
	• Fragmentation of cell into apoptotic bodies
	• Controlled by TP53, which regulates the balance between apoptosis related genes *bcl-2* (inhibits) and *bax* (stimulates)

FUNDAMENTALS OF INFLAMMATION

Clinical manifestations	• Calor (heat), dolor (pain), rubor (redness), tumor (swelling), functio laesa (loss of function)

Cellular events leading to accumulation of leukocytes	• Margination (leukocytes approach capillary walls)
	• Rolling (leukocytes receptors start contacting receptors on endothelial cells)
	• Adhesion
	• Transmigration (diapedesis)
	• Chemotaxis (stimuli include bacterial products, C5a, leukotriene B_4 [LTB_4], chemokines)
	• Phagocytosis
	   ◦ Recognition (opsonins IgG and C3b)
	   ◦ Engulfment into the phagolysosome
	   ◦ Killing by lysosomal enzymes (lactoferrin, lysozyme, defensins, myeloperoxidase)
	   ◦ Respiratory burst

Components of the respiratory burst	• Nicotinamide adenosine dinucleotide phosphate (NADPH) oxidase creates reactive oxide intermediates (free radicals) • Nitric oxide synthase (NOS) creates nitrogen oxide intermediates • These free radical species are destructive and are very effective at killing microorganisms. When out of control, they also damage healthy tissue
Chronic granulomatous disease	• Deficient NADPH oxidase results in an inability to kill microorganisms; clinical findings include repeated pyogenic infections

INFLAMMATORY MEDIATORS

Neurogenic vasoconstriction	• Vasoconstriction followed by vasodilation (initiates margination process and primary hemostasis)
Arachidonic acid metabolites	• Prostaglandins: Vasodilation and increased capillary permeability • Leukotrienes: Chemotaxis and increased capillary permeability
Platelet-activating factor (PAF)	• Vasodilation • Increases capillary permeability • Stimulates platelets and leukocytes • Stimulates platelet aggregation
Histamine	• Released by mast cells after stimulated by physical, immunologic, complement C3a and C5a, causing vasodilation and increased capillary permeability

Serotonin (5-HT)	• Large role in pain sensation
The kinin system	• Kininogen: Bradykinin and kininogen • Functions of bradykinin: Vasodilation, increased capillary permeability, smooth muscle contraction, pain
Complement system	• Increased capillary permeability (causes edema) • Neutrophil chemotaxis (mediates inflammation) • Opsonization (facilitates phagocytosis) • Cell lysis (mediates hemolysis or killing of tumor cells)

Topic **2**

Neoplasia

Must **Knows**

● Difference between dysplasia and neoplasia

● Difference between benign and malignant tumors

● Clinical manifestation of malignancy

● Environmental and viral causes of malignancy

● Role of protooncogenes and tumor suppressor genes

Dysplasia	• Disorderly cell proliferation that is reversible if the cause is removed (e.g., if one stops smoking). In some cases, it may progress to carcinoma in situ and invasive neoplasia. • Irregular maturation of the epithelium (e.g., cervix, bronchus) • Nuclear pleomorphism, irregularities, hyperchromasia • Mitotic figures found in upper layers of the epithelium
Neoplasia	• Disorderly uncontrollable cell proliferation; related to irreversible genetic changes typically found in malignant tumors • Disorderly layering of cells and loss of cellular polarity and orientation • Nuclear pleomorphism, hyperchromasia, prominent nucleoli • Increased nuclear:cytoplasm ratio • Numerous and atypical mitoses, distributed at random

Carcinoma in situ	• When dysplasia involves the entire thickness of epithelium

Benign vs. malignant	**Benign**	**Malignant**
	• Well differentiated	• Poorly differentiated
	• Circumscribed	• Locally invasive (Note that the word *cancer* is derived from the Latin word for *crab*; it claws onto surrounding tissue and will not let go)
	• Slow rate of growth	• Slow to rapid rate of growth
	• No metastasis	• Distant metastasis

Tumor kinetics	• Tumor cells do not grow faster than normal cells (normal doubling time) • Growth fraction: Percentage of cells in the proliferation pool (high)
Epidemiology of cancer	• Frequency increases with age • Most mortality is between ages 55 to 75 years; when the individual is older than age 75 years, the risk returns to the population base
Cancers common in patients younger than age 15 years	• Acute lymphoblastic leukemia • Lymphoma • Central nervous system (CNS) tumors • Soft tissue sarcomas • Bone sarcomas
Metastasis	• Carcinomas metastasize via lymphatics • Sarcomas metastasize via blood • Common targets for metastasis: Liver, lungs, brain, bone

Clinical manifestations of malignancy	• Cachexia
	• Mass effects: CNS (seizures, mental status changes), lung (pneumonia, Horner syndrome from Pancoast tumor)
	• Paraneoplastic syndromes
	   ○ Endocrine (Cushing, syndrome of inappropriate antidiuretic hormone secretion [SIADH]): Small cell lung carcinoma
	   ○ Hypercalcemia: Squamous cell carcinoma, multiple myeloma
	   ○ Polycythemia: Renal cell carcinoma
	   ○ Skin (acanthosis nigricans): Visceral malignancies
	   ○ Hypercoagulable state (Trousseau syndrome): Disseminated cancer, pancreatic adenocarcinoma

Environmental causes of malignancy	• Smoking: Lung, oropharyngeal, laryngeal, bladder, pancreatic • Asbestos: Mesothelioma • Radon: Lung

- Nitrosamine: Stomach
- Aflatoxin: Hepatocellular carcinoma
- Polyvinyl chloride: Hepatic angiosarcoma
- Aniline dyes: Transitional cell carcinoma of bladder
- Arsenic: Squamous cell carcinoma, basal cell carcinoma of skin
- Benzene: Leukemia

Viral causes of malignancy	<ul><li>Hepatitis B virus (HBV), hepatitis C virus (HCV): Hepatocellular carcinoma</li><li>Human papillomavirus (HPV): Cervical carcinoma (HPV 16 and 18)</li><li>Epstein-Barr virus (EBV): Burkitt lymphoma, nasopharyngeal carcinoma</li><li>Human T-lymphotropic virus (HTLV): Adult T-cell leukemia</li></ul>
The three molecular mechanisms to tumor genesis	<ul><li>Activation of protooncogenes</li><li>Inactivation of tumor suppressor genes</li><li>Mutations of genes that regulate apoptosis</li></ul>
Protooncogenes	<ul><li>Genes present in the normal human genome that have a role in normal cell physiology. They encode for proteins that promote growth. A somatic mutation of these genes may result in uncontrolled proliferation secondary to excessive amount of the gene's products.</li><li>*RAS:* Colon cancer, chronic lymphocytic leukemia</li><li>Cyclin-D: Breast cancer</li><li>*MYCN:* Neuroblastoma</li><li>*MYC:* Burkitt's lymphoma</li><li>*ABL:* Chronic myelogenous leukemia</li></ul>
Tumor suppressor genes	<ul><li>The products of these genes apply brakes to cellular proliferation:</li><li>*DCC:* Deleted on colon cancer</li><li>*APC:* Adenomatosis polyposis coli</li><li>*WT1, WT2:* Wilm's tumor</li><li>*NF1:* Neurofibromatosis I</li><li>*RB1:* Retinoblastoma, osteosarcoma</li><li>*TP53:* Li Fraumeni syndrome</li><li>*BRCA1:* Breast cancer, ovarian cancer</li></ul>
Knudson two-hit hypothesis	<ul><li>Two mutations ("hits") on the *RB1* gene (13q14) are required to produce retinoblastoma. Therefore, if a child receives one defective *RB1*, the child is more likely to develop retinoblastoma as a result of damage to the remaining *RB1* gene.</li><li>Sporadic cases may also occur to a person conceived with two normal copies if both copies are damaged</li></ul>

- Similarly, this hypothesis may also be applied to any of the tumor suppressor genes. Therefore, it is possible to screen patients for cancer susceptibility in cases with family history by looking for faulty tumor suppressor genes.

Detection	• Prostate specific antigen (PSA) • Carcinoembryonic antigen (CEA): Colon cancer • Alpha fetoprotein (AFP): Liver cancer, seminoma
Staging	• TNM (tumor, node, metastasis) system: Tumor size (1–4), nodal metastasis (0–3), distant metastasis (0 or 1)
Basic treatment concepts	• Surgery (best for local well demarcated Ca) • Radiation • Hormone therapy (breast cancer, prostate cancer) • Chemotherapy (can be single agent or combination)

Topic **3**

Cardiovascular System and Hematology

Must Knows

- Vascular pathology
- Cardiac pathology
- Causes of anemia
- Disorders of coagulation
- Myeloproliferative diseases, leukemias, and lymphomas

VASCULAR PATHOLOGY

Hypertension (HTN)	• 90% to 95% idiopathic (essential HTN) • 5% to 10% secondary to renal disease, primary aldosteronism, Cushing's disease, pheochromocytoma
Atherosclerosis	• Pathology: Endothelial injury → migration of circulating monocytes and other inflammatory cells, which engulf lipo-proteins and oxidized LDL → production of inflammatory mediators → continued inflammation and buildup of cholesterol → formation of plaques

	• Risk factors: HTN, diabetes mellitus, hypercholesterolemia, smoking, older age, male gender
	• Treatment: Blood pressure control, diabetic control, statins, *quit smoking!*
Hyperplastic arteriolosclerosis	• Pathology: Associated with malignant HTN
	• Causes concentric laminated thickening of arteriole walls with luminal narrowing from hypertrophy and hyperplasia of smooth muscle
Aneurysms	• Atherosclerotic aneurysms
	• Pathology: Atherosclerosis : Destruction of underlying tunica media leading to weakening of the aortic wall
	• Clinical features: Usually form in abdominal aorta below renal arteries; pulsating mass that may cause abdominal and back pain
	• Syphilitic aortitis
	• Pathology: 3° syphilis results in endarteritis obliterans → damages vasa vasorum → thoracic aortitis → aneurysmal dilation
	• Clinical features: Affects the ascending aorta and may result in dilation of aortic valve ring leading to aortic valve insufficiency
Aortic dissection	• Pathology: Intimal tears that originate 10 cm from the aortic valve (90%) or descending aorta just distal from subclavian artery; blood penetrates media and accumulates between the outer and middle third of media
	• Epidemiology: 40 to 60 years old with HTN; connective tissue disease (Marfan syndrome)
	• Marfan syndrome results in cystic medial necrosis leading to loss of elastica and smooth muscle without inflammation
	• Clinical features: Sudden onset of excruciating pain that propagates from the anterior chest or back and down the abdomen
Raynaud disease	• Recurrent vasospasm of arterioles usually in the hands or feet resulting in pallor or cyanosis and cold sensation
	• Seen in young women
Vasculitides	• May be local or systemic
	• Causes include immune complexes and antineutrophil cytoplasmic antibodies; these are also diagnostically useful
Polyarteritis nodosa	• Pathology: Transmural inflammation of small or medium arterioles
	○ Heart: Coronary artery disease leading to ischemia
	○ Kidneys: Hypertension, glomerulonephritis, hematuria

- Gastrointestinal (GI) system: Abdominal pain, diarrhea, melena
- Musculoskeletal: Myalgia or arthralgia, weakness
- Diagnosis: Perinuclear antineutrophil cytoplasmic autoantibodies (p-ANCA); may also be associated with hepatitis B surface antigen (HbsAg) (30%)

Wegener granulomatosis	• Pathology: Necrotizing granulomas of upper or lower respiratory tract and glomerulonephritis • Clinical features: Recurrent inflammatory sinusitis; ulcers of nose, palate, and larynx • Diagnosis: Cytoplasmic antineutrophil cytoplasmic autoantibodies (c-ANCA)
Temporal arteritis	• Epidemiology: Elderly persons, 50% have polymyalgia rheumatica • Pathology: Segmental granulomatous inflammation along the temporal artery • Clinical features: Headache, jaw claudication, amaurosis fugax • Diagnosis: Temporal artery biopsy, severely elevated erythrocyte sedimentation rate (ESR)
Hypersensitivity vasculitis	• Clinical features: Constitutional, palpable purpura, hemoptysis, GI pain, hematuria • Pathology: Acute inflammation of small vessels usually caused by an offending antigen such as medications, microorganisms, or heterologous proteins • Treatment: Removal of offending agent
Takayasu arteritis (pulseless disease)	• Pathology: Chronic vasculitis affecting aorta and its branches. May result in aortic root dilation → aortic valve insufficiency • Clinical features: Vascular insufficiency of upper extremities with cold/numb fingers
Kawasaki disease (mucocutaneous lymph node syndrome)	• Epidemiology: Children • Pathology: 2 phases: Acute: Vasculitis of arterioles, venules, and capillaries; chronic: Involves larger arteries including coronaries → CAD and coronary aneurysms • Clinical features: Fever, conjunctivitis, mucous membrane ulcers, lymphadenopathy • Treatment: Large doses of aspirin
Buerger disease (thromboangiitis obliterans)	• Epidemiology: Male smokers in Israel, Japan, India • Pathology: Segmental vasculitis of small to medium arteries • Clinical features: Painful ischemia usually in extremities resulting in chronic ulcers on toes, feet, and fingers • Treatment: Abstinence from smoking

Thrombophlebitis	• Associated with Virchow triad:
	• Endothelial injury (trauma)
	• Stasis (cardiac failure, prolonged immobilization)
	• Hypercoagulable state (neoplasm, pregnancy)
	• Clinical features: Pain over site (usually lower extremities), pulmonary emboli (chest pain, shortness of breath, tachycardia)

CARDIAC PATHOLOGY

Coronary artery disease	• Pathology: Atherosclerosis → development of cholesterol plaques → stenosis of the coronary vessels → ischemia (>75% luminal stenosis is critical)
	• Clinical features: Angina, MI, congestive heart failure (CHF)
	• Treatment: Reduction of risk factors (hypercholesterolemia, smoking, HTN, diabetes mellitus), nitrates for angina, angioplasty, coronary artery bypass graft (CABG)
Prinzmetal angina	• Epidemiology: Young women, associated with Raynaud disease
	• Pathology: Coronary artery vasospasm
	• Treatment: calcium channel blockers
Myocardial infarction (MI)	• Pathology: Thrombosis of coronary arteries leading to ischemia and necrosis of myocardial tissue. Necrosis begins in the first 20 to 30 minutes of thrombosis and is reversible during this time. After 1 hour, the damage becomes irreversible.
	○ Left anterior descending artery infarct: Damage to anterior and apical areas of the left ventricle and interventricular septum
	○ Right coronary artery: Sinoatrial (SA) node, atrioventricular (AV) node, posterior and basal portion of the left ventricle

Diagnostic enzymes for MI	Enzyme	Time positive	Time negative
	Troponin-I or troponin-T	4 to 6 hours	7 to 10 days
	Creatine kinase (CK-MB)	6 to 8 hours	3 days

Complications of MI	• Arrhythmias: Irregular rhythm, tachycardia, fibrillation, flutter, cardiac conduction blocks, and so on; the most common early complication but may occur later as well; the most common cause of death
	• Papillary muscle dysfunction: Results in severe mitral regurgitation; occurs approximately 3 days after MI
	• Ventricular rupture: Results in cardiac tamponade (hematopericardium with compression of the ventricles and atria); occurs during first week, 4 to 7 days after MI
	• Mural thrombus: Thrombus forms on the damaged endocardium; may result in emboli
	• Dressler syndrome: Autoimmune pericarditis that occurs in response to MI

- Congestive heart failure (CHF): Occurs when heart tissue is severely damaged and can no longer adequately meet systemic needs

---

Cardiomyopathy (Fig. IV-2)
- Dilated: Caused by ischemia, alcohol, HIV, coxsackie virus, trypanosomiasis, doxorubicin, beriberi
- Restrictive: Caused by amyloidosis, hemochromatosis, sarcoidosis
- Hypertrophic: Autosomal dominant; attributable to a gene mutation (e.g., myoglobin gene)

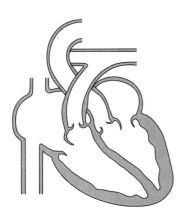

A. Normal

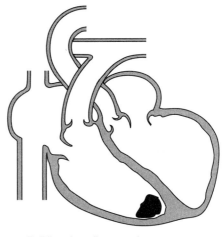

B. Dilated cardiomyopathy
- Mural thrombus
- Dilated ventricles

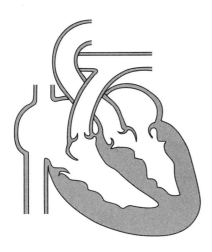

C. Hypertrophic cardiomyopathy
- Asymmetrically thickened septum
- Hypertrophy of the ventricular myocardium

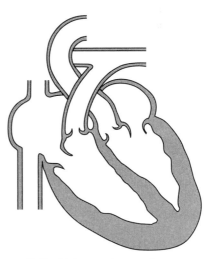

D. Restrictive cardiomyopathy
- Thickened myocardium
- Interstitial deposits (fibrosis, amyloid)

● **Figure IV-2** The three major clinicopathological forms of cardiomyopathy. (**A**) Normal heart. (**B**) Dilated cardiomyopathy. (**C**) Hypertrophic cardiomyopathy. (**D**) Restrictive cardiomyopathy. (Modified with permission from Damjanov I: *Histopathology A Color Atlas and Textbook*. Baltimore, Williams & Wilkins, 1996, p. 108.)

CHF	• *CHF is the manifestation of many heart diseases!!*
	• CHF always occurs secondary to underlying cardiac pathology: CAD, MI, cardiomyopathy, valvular heart disease, myocarditis
	• Morphologic changes: Heart failure cells, "nutmeg liver"
	• Clinical features according to system:
	◦ General: Fatigue
	◦ Neck: Jugular venous distention (JVD)
	◦ Cardiovascular system: Tachycardia
	◦ Respiratory: Dyspnea, PND, orthopnea, cough, pulmonary edema
	◦ GI: Hepatomegaly
	◦ Extremities: Pitting edema, cyanosis
Cor pulmonale	• Right heart disease secondary to pulmonary HTN secondary to disease of pulmonary parenchyma or vasculature
	• Etiology
	◦ Parenchymal lung disease: chronic obstructive pulmonary disease, interstitial fibrosis
	◦ Diseases of vasculature: pulmonary emboli or vasculitis
	◦ Causes of hypoxia: Sleep apnea, altitude sickness, Pickwickian syndrome, neuromuscular disease
	• Clinical features: Dyspnea, right chest heave, JVD, hepato-megaly, "nutmeg liver", lower extremity pitting edema
Valvular heart disease	• Calcific aortic stenosis
	◦ Epidemiology: Common in elderly
	◦ Pathology: Degenerative calcification of aortic valve
	◦ Clinical features: Usually asymptomatic; may cause angina, syncope, CHF
	◦ Treatment: Surgical valve replacement
	• Mitral valve prolapse
	◦ Pathology: Valve cusps are soft; chordae tendinea are loose and allow the valves to become floppy and incompetent during systole
	◦ Clinical features: Midsystolic click followed by late systolic murmur; symptoms usually asymptomatic but may result in palpitations, fatigue, chest pain, and increased risk of infective endocarditis
Rheumatic fever	• Pathology: Complication of *Streptococcus pyogenes* pharyngitis
	• Clinical features: Chorea, subcutaneous nodules, erythema marginatum, migrating polyarthritis, pancarditis (endocarditis, myocarditis with Aschoff nodules, pericarditis), mitral valve stenosis ("fishmouth deformity") or insufficiency
	• Treatment: Penicillin

Infective endocarditis	<ul><li>Acute: *Staphylococcus aureus*</li><li>Chronic: *Streptococcus viridans*, HACEK group (*Haemophilus parainfluenzae, Actinobacillus, Cardiobacter, Eikenella, Kingella*)</li><li>Clinical features: Fever, Roth spots, conjunctival petechiae, Osler nodes, Janeway lesions, splinter hemorrhages, splenomegaly, embolic disease</li></ul>
Myocarditis	<ul><li>Etiology (ETI): Coxsackie virus, trypanosomiasis</li><li>Clinical features: Fever, cardiac failure</li></ul>
Pericarditis	<ul><li>ETI: Viral infection, rheumatic fever, systemic lupus erythematosus (SLE), rheumatoid arthritis, uremia, nephrotic syndrome, Dressler syndrome</li><li>Clinical features: Fever, chest pain</li></ul>
Congenital heart disease	<ul><li>Ventricular septal defects (VSDs): Initially the shunt is left-to-right. As the pulmonary pressure increases, the shunt reverses and becomes right to left.</li><li>Atrial septal defects: Usually caused by defective septum formation; left-to-right shunt</li><li>Tetralogy of Fallot: Pulmonary stenosis, overriding of aorta, VSD, right ventricular hypertrophy; right-to-left shunt</li><li>Patent ductus arteriosus (PDA): Failure of closure after birth; left-to-right shunt; treat with indomethacin (inhibits synthesis of prostaglandins; maintains duct patency)</li><li>Coarctation of the aorta: Two forms, infantile and adult<ul><li>Infantile type involves the arch of the aorta, usually causing death in infancy</li><li>Adult type involves aorta distal to left subclavian artery → upper extremity HTN. Associated with development of collateral circulation through intercostals–may appear as rib notching on chest radiograph</li></ul></li><li>Transposition of the great vessels: The aorta comes off the right ventricle, and the pulmonary artery comes off the left ventricle with separate circulation; not compatible with life without surgery, which is curative in 90% cases</li></ul>

ANEMIA

Categorizing anemia	<ul><li>Hypochromic microcytic (mean corpuscular volume [MCV] < 82)<ul><li>Inadequate delivery of iron (iron deficiency anemia, anemia of chronic disease)</li><li>Inadequate hemoglobin synthesis (sideroblastic anemia, thalassemia)</li></ul></li><li>Macrocytic anemia (MCV > 100)<ul><li>Defective DNA synthesis (megaloblastic anemias)</li><li>Accelerated erythropoiesis</li></ul></li></ul>

- ○ Increased erythrocytes membrane area (liver disease, postsplenectomy)
- ○ Nonhematologic (alcohol abuse)
- Hemoglobinopathies (thalassemias, sickle cell anemia)
- Hemolytic anemia
  - ○ Inherited (abnormal hemoglobin, membrane abnormalities, erythrocytes enzyme defects, immune mediated)
  - ○ Acquired (mechanical hemolysis, hemolytic-uremic syndrome, thrombotic thrombocytopenic purpura)

Iron deficiency anemia	• ETI: Dietary deficiency, blood loss, increased requirement (pregnancy) • Clinical features: Fatigue, pallor, dyspnea, chest pain, glossitis, koilonychia • Diagnosis: Decreased hemoglobin/hematocrit (Hb/HCT) levels, hypochromic microcytic erythrocytes on smear, increased total iron-binding capacity (TIBC), decreased ferritin
Anemia of chronic disease	• ETI: Usually underlying chronic inflammation, infection, malignancy • Pathology: Thought to be secondary to inability to utilize circulating iron • Diagnosis: Mild decreased Hb/HCT, increased ferritin, decreased TIBC
Sideroblastic anemia	• ETI: X-linked recessive mitochondrial defect, drugs, heavy metals (lead) • Pathology: Decreased activity of *ALA synthase* or *ferrochelatase;* iron accumulates in ring-forming "ringed sideroblast" seen on blood smear
Sickle cell anemia	• ETI: Substitution of valine for glutamate in β chain; homozygotes have sickle cell disease (HbS), and heterozygotes are carriers • Pathology: Abnormal protein folding leads to polymerization of HbS on deoxygenation, which leads to sickling of erythrocytes, microvascular obstruction, and ischemic damage • Clinical features: Vasoocclusive painful crisis (abdomen, chest, joints), stroke, aplastic crisis triggered by parvovirus B19, autosplenectomy, *Salmonella sp.* osteomyelitis • Diagnosis: Electrophoresis

The thalassemias	1. α-Thalassemia
	  ○ ETI: Deletion of one or more genes for α chain synthesis
	  ○ Pathology and clinical features: According to how many genes are deleted:
	    1. --/--: Hydrops fetalis
	    2. --/-α: Hb H = β tetramers
	    3. -α/-α,--/αα: α thal minor = microcytic anemia
	    4. -α/αα: Asymptomatic carrier

1. β-Thalassemia

   a. ETI: Mutations of β genes

   b. Pathology: Mutation causes absence or deficiency of β chains

      1. Decreased HbA: Hypochromic anemia

      2. Precipitation of α-chains: Formation of inclusion bodies leading to cellular damage and hemolysis

      3. Ineffective erythropoiesis: Increased Fe absorption leading to Fe overload and hemochromatosis

         ○ Clinical features: Microcytic, hypochromic erythrocytes; target cells; poikilocytosis, anisocytosis, and reticulocytosis; hepatosplenomegaly secondary to extramedullary erythropoiesis; hemosiderosis; cardiac failure

Megaloblastic anemias	Pernicious anemia
	
	  a. Epidemiology: Most common cause of megaloblastic anemia
	
	  b. Pathology: An autoimmune disease; antibodies against intrinsic factor or parietal cell components lead to parietal cell death and chronic atrophic gastritis
	
	  c. Clinical features: Hypersegmented neutrophils, macrocytes, dorsal column degeneration of the spinal cord leading to peripheral neuropathy
	
	  d. Diagnosis: Schilling test
	
	Folate deficiency
	
	  a. ETI: Alcoholism, pregnancy, malabsorption syndromes
	
	  b. Clinical features: Macrocytes; not associated with neuropathy

Hereditary spherocytosis	• ETI: Defect in erythrocyte membrane. autosomal dominant • Pathology: Mutation in ankyrin gene → deficiency of spectrin → decreased membrane stability → takes on spherocyte shape → decreased plasticity → splenic sequestration and destruction • Clinical features: Anemia, spherocytes on blood smear, splenomegaly, cholelithiasis, jaundice • Diagnosis: Osmotic fragility test • Treatment: Splenectomy
Glucose-6-phosphate dehydrogenase deficiency	• ETI: X-linked recessive • Epidemiology: Most common erythrocyte enzyme deficiency causing anemia, most prevalent in African Americans and persons of Mediterranean origin (Italians, Greeks or Arabs) • Pathology: Decreased flux through oxidative portion of pentose phosphate pathway leads to decreased nicotinamide adenosine dinucleotide phosphate (NADPH), reduced glutathione, increased vulnerability of erythrocyte to oxidative stress, accumulation of ROS (reactive oxygen species), denaturation of Hb, hemolysis or precipitation of Hb (formation of Heinz bodies), splenic phagocytosis of Heinz bodies → "bite cells"

- Clinical features: Symptoms occur when erythrocytes are exposed to stresses:
  - Drugs: Antimalarials, sulfonamides, aspirin
  - Infections

Pyruvate kinase deficiency	- ETI: autosomal recessive (AR) - Epidemiology: Second most common erythrocyte enzyme deficiency causing anemia - Pathology: Failure of glycolytic pathway leads to decreased adenosine triphosphate (ATP), failure of ATPase, loss of osmotic/volume balance, and hemolysis
Immunologic hemolytic anemias	- Warm autoimmune hemolytic anemia (WAIHA) - ETI: Idiopathic or secondary to lymphoma, CLL, SLE, drugs - Pathology: IgG autoantibodies bind to erythrocyte at 37°C, opsonization by splenic macrophages, extravascular hemolysis - Clinical features: Fever, tachycardia, malaise, mild jaundice - Cold agglutinin disease - ETI: Idiopathic; secondary to mononucleosis, *Mycoplasma pneumonia* infection - Pathology: Anti-RBC (red blood cell) IgM antibodies bind < 30°C (in extremities), which leads to fixation of complement, increased temperature as erythrocytes move back toward core; IgM releases, C_{3b} remains (opsonin), and phagocytosis occurs - Clinical features: Mottling and numbness in the extremities; hemoglobinuria after exposure to cold
The Coombs test	- Indirect Coombs: Detects antibodies in the patient's serum - Direct Coombs: Detects presence of antibodies or complement on the patient's erythrocyte
Causes of hemolytic anemia and thrombocytopenia (TCP)	Thrombotic thrombocytopenic purpura (TTP) - Pathology: Formation of microvascular thrombi, TCP, micro-angiopathic hemolytic anemia leading to helmet cells and schistocytes - Clinical features: Pentad = fever, neurologic deficits, hemolytic anemia, renal failure, TCP, increased bleeding time Idiopathic thrombocytopenic purpura (ITP) - Epidemiology: Children; associated with upper respiratory infections (URIs, especially mycoplasma) - Pathology: Antiplatelet antibodies leading to opsonization of platelets - Clinical features: TCP, increased bleeding time Hemolytic uremic syndrome (HUS) - Epidemiology: Children; post-infection by *E. coli* O157:H7 - Clinical features: Bloody diarrhea, abdominal pain, acute renal failure, seizures, TCP, hemolytic anemia, increased bleeding time

DISORDERS OF COAGULATION

Disseminated intravascular coagulopathy (DIC)	• ETI: Sepsis, marked hemorrhage, amniotic fluid emboli, disseminated cancer • Pathology: Diffuse thrombogenesis leading to consumption of platelets and factors and diffuse thrombolysis; cycle continues • Clinical features: Uncontrolled profuse bleeding, especially from intravenous and central lines • Diagnosis: Increased fibrin split products, prolonged prothrombin time (PT), partial thromboplastin time (PTT), and bleeding time
Von Willebrand disease	• ETI: Deficiency of von Willebrand factor (vWF) • Pathology: Two pathways: 　○ Decreased vWF → decreased platelet adhesion → decreased primary hemostasis →increased bleeding time 　○ factor VIII → decreased secondary hemostasis → increased PTT • Diagnosis:increased bleeding time, increased PTT
Hemophilia	• Hemophilia A 　○ ETI: X-linked recessive; factor VIII deficiency 　○ Clinical features: Hemarthrosis, hematomas, ecchymoses 　○ Diagnosis: Increased PTT, normal PT, normal bleeding time • Hemophilia B 　○ ETI: Factor IX deficiency 　○ Clinical features: Same as hemophilia A

MYELOPROLIFERATIVE DISEASES, LEUKEMIAS, AND LYMPHOMAS

Polycythemia vera	• ETI: Primary polycythemia that must be differentiated from secondary polycythemia from chronic hypoxia (altitude sickness, chronic obstructive pulmonary disease), or increased erythropoietin from renal cell carcinoma • Pathology: Increased erythrocytosis leads to increased Hb/HCT and thrombotic phenomenon • Clinical features: Headache, diplopia, stroke, splenomegaly, decreased erythropoietin, may progress to leukemia or myelofibrosis (burn out)
Idiopathic myelofibrosis	• Pathology: Replacement of marrow with fibrotic tissue • Clinical features: Anemia, teardrop erythrocytes, splenomegaly (extramedullary erythropoiesis)

Acute lymphoblastic leukemia (ALL)	• Epidemiology: Children
	• Pathology: Lymphoblasts
	• Clinical features: Anemia, fever, fatigue. Good prognosis in children
Acute myelogenous leukemia (AML)	• Epidemiology: Adults
	• Pathology: Subdivided according to the French-American-British (FAB) classification into several variants (M0–M7); myeloblasts that may have Auer rods (M3 variant)
	• Clinical features: Anemia, fever, fatigue; M3 variant responds well to all-trans-retinoic acid
Chronic lymphocytic leukemia (CLL)	• Epidemiology: Elderly individuals
	• Pathology: Usually B-cell leukemia with increased mature lymphocytes that may express B-cell markers (CD19, CD20)
	• Clinical features: Indolent course with leukocytes from 50,000 to 200,000; splenomegaly; lymphadenopathy; warm autoimmune hemolytic anemia
Hairy cell leukemia	• Epidemiology: Men
	• Pathology: B-cell chronic leukemia with marked splenomegaly
	• Clinical features: Hairlike projections on the surface of tumor cells; cells also contain tartrate resistant acid phosphatase (TRAP)
Chronic myelogenous leukemia (CML)	• Epidemiology: Elderly individuals
	• Pathology: 9:22 translocation (Philadelphia chromosome); increased expression of myeloid stem cells
	• Clinical features: Increased leukocytosis with 50,000 to 200,000 leukocytes; may accelerate to AML blast crisis, severe splenomegaly, decreased leukocyte alkaline phosphatase
Non-Hodgkin's lymphoma (NHL)	• Follicular lymphoma
	◦ B-cell lymphoma with t(14:18) positive for CD19, CD20, but no CD5
	◦ Indolent course, survival without treatment is 7 to 9 years
	• Small lymphocytic lymphoma
	◦ B-cell lymphoma positive for CD19, CD10, CD5
	◦ Indolent course
	◦ Diffuse lymph node involvement with effacement of nodal architecture
	• Mantle cell lymphoma
	◦ Similar to small lymphocytic lymphoma with t(11:14)
	◦ Aggressive and rapidly disseminates
	• Diffuse large B-cell lymphoma
	◦ Large nuclei and prominent nucleoli
	◦ Aggressive and rapidly disseminates

- T-cell lymphoma
  - Children or adults
  - Nuclei appear convoluted
  - Clinically low grade or aggressive
- Burkitt lymphoma
  - B-cell lymphoma with t(8:14)
  - Endemic form (in Africa) affects lymph nodes and mandible/maxilla and is linked to EBV
  - Sporadic form (United States and other Western countries) involves intra-abdominal organs and lymph nodes
  - Histologically, starry sky appearance of affected lymph nodes
  - Responds well to chemotherapy

Hodgkin lymphoma (HL)	• Epidemiology: Bimodal age distribution: young men and elderly people
	• Pathology: Reed-Sternberg (RS) cells; binucleated giant cells with "owl eye" appearance
	• Clinical features: B symptoms are night sweats, fevers and chills, weight loss, pruritus
	• Lymphocyte predominant
	  ○ Minimal RS cells
	  ○ Good prognosis
	• Mixed cellularity
	  ○ Most frequent in older men
	• Lymphocyte depletion
	  ○ Least common
	  ○ Extensive fibrosis
	  ○ Poorest prognosis
	• Nodular sclerosis
	• Most frequent in women
	• Presence of fibrous bands and lacunar cells
	• Good prognosis

Multiple myeloma (Fig. IV-3)	• Pathology: Malignant monoclonal plasma cell tumor produces monoclonal antibodies (M protein) that are most often IgG • Clinical features: Lytic "punched-out" bone lesions, bone pain, hypercalcemia, renal failure, increased infections, anemia, amyloidosis • Diagnosis: Monoclonal immunoglobulin spike with electro-phoresis, Bence Jones proteins in urine, rouleaux formation on blood smear (stacked erythrocytes)
Waldenström macroglobulinemia	• Pathology: Lymphoplasmacytic lymphoma that produces monoclonal IgM • Clinical features: Hyperviscosity syndrome causing thrombosis and stroke, increased bleeding time

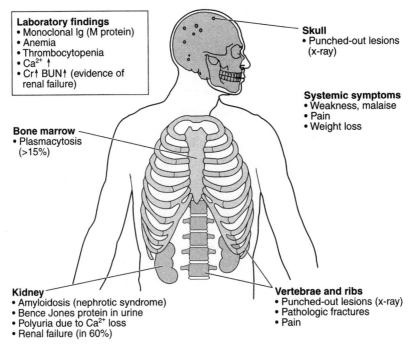

Laboratory findings
• Monoclonal Ig (M protein)
• Anemia
• Thrombocytopenia
• Ca^{2+} ↑
• Cr↑ BUN↑ (evidence of renal failure)

Skull
• Punched-out lesions (x-ray)

Systemic symptoms
• Weakness, malaise
• Pain
• Weight loss

Bone marrow
• Plasmacytosis (>15%)

Kidney
• Amyloidosis (nephrotic syndrome)
• Bence Jones protein in urine
• Polyuria due to Ca^{2+} loss
• Renal failure (in 60%)

Vertebrae and ribs
• Punched-out lesions (x-ray)
• Pathologic fractures
• Pain

● **Figure IV-3** Pathologic findings, and clinical signs and symptoms of multiple myeloma. BUN = blood urea nitrogen; Cr = creatinine.

Topic **4**

Respiratory System

Must
Knows

● Cystic fibrosis

● Obstructive lung diseases

● Restrictive lung diseases

● Pulmonary vascular disease

● Pneumonia and tuberculosis

● Lung cancer

Cystic fibrosis	• Epidemiology: 1:2500 whites; less common in other races
	• ETI: Defective cystic fibrosis transmembrane conductance regulator (CFTR) on chromosome 7, AR
	• Pathology: Defective CFTR protein found in the respiratory system, pancreas, gastrointestinal system, reproductive tract, sweat glands; inability to release Cl^-; Cl^- stays sequestered in cell; Na^+ and H_2O also stay in cell to maintain osmotic balance; this process leads to viscous secretions
	• Clinical features: Recurrent pneumonia (especially *Pseudomonas aeruginosa* infection), recurrent sinusitis, meconium ileus (pathognomonic), fat malabsorption (pancreatic insufficiency), salty skin

OBSTRUCTIVE LUNG DISEASE

Asthma	• ETI: Two types:
	○ Extrinsic: Mediated by type I hypersensitivity reaction
	○ Intrinsic: Trigger is nonimmune and may include aspirin, cold, exercise, psychogenic, or infection
	• Pathology: Bronchial wall edema and development of inflammatory infiltrate with increased number of eosinophils, thickening of basement membrane, bronchial smooth muscle hypertrophy and hyperplasia, and hypertrophy of submucosal mucous glands
	• Microscopic features include mucous plugs, Curschmann's spirals, and Charcot-Leyden crystals
	• Clinical features: Episodic dyspnea and wheezing
Emphysema (pink puffer)	• ETI: Smoking, hereditary α_1-antitrypsin deficiency
	• Pathology: Excess activity of protease and elastase resulting in permanent enlargement of distal airspaces with destruction of alveolar walls
	• Three patterns of emphysema:
	○ Centriacinar (centrilobar): Dilation of respiratory bronchials, common in apical segments
	○ Panacinar (panlobar): Acini are uniformly enlarged (associated with α_1-antitrypsin deficiency)
	○ Distal acinar (paraseptal): Common adjacent to pleura, resulting in bullae and blebs which may result in spontaneous pneumothorax
	• Clinical features: Dyspnea, decreased forced expiratory volume in 1 second ($FEV_{1.0}$), decreased forced vital capacity (FVC), increased total lung capacity, barrel chest, hypoxia, respiratory acidosis, pulmonary hypertension, cor pulmonale
Chronic bronchitis (blue bloater)	• ETI: Smoking
	• Pathology: Hypertrophy of submucosal mucous glands

- Clinical features: Productive cough for more than 3 consecutive months in 2 years, wheezing, cyanosis, rales, cor pulmonale

Bronchiectasis	• ETI: Chronic bronchial infection; associated with Kartagener syndrome (ciliary dysfunction), cystic fibrosis • Pathology: Chronic infection, inflammation, necrosis of bronchial wall, and bronchial dilation • Clinical features: Copious purulent sputum, hemoptysis

RESTRICTIVE LUNG DISEASE

Adult respiratory distress syndrome (ARDS)	• ETI: Diffuse alveolar damage (DAD) from shock, sepsis, inhalation injury, pancreatitis, oxygen toxicity • Pathology: Increased alveolar capillary permeability; accumulation of proteinaceous fluid; impaired gas exchange; hypoxia • Clinical features: Dyspnea, hypoxia resistant to supplemental O_2, diffuse infiltrates on chest radiograph
Neonatal respiratory distress syndrome (hyaline membrane disease)	• ETI: Deficiency of surfactant secondary to prematurity • Pathology: Decreased lung compliance leading to atelectasis, leakage of fluid into alveoli, formation of hyaline membrane, and impaired gas exchange • Clinical features: Dyspnea, cyanosis, tachypnea; consequences include bronchopulmonary dysplasia, necrotizing enterocolitis, intraventricular hemorrhage
Pneumoconioses	• Anthracosis: Caused by inhalation of carbon dust and has no clinical consequences • Coal workers: Inhalation of coal dust, which may result in progressive diffuse fibrosis, bronchiectasis, pulmonary hypertension, and cor pulmonale • Asbestosis: Fibers are engulfed by macrophages, leading to fibrosis; occurs in lower lobes; strong association with bronchogenic carcinoma and mesothelioma
Hypersensitivity pneumonitis	• ETI: Inhaled antigens (actinomycetes, bird dander) • Pathology: Acute: activation of complement and formation of immune complexes; chronic: delayed hypersensitivity • Clinical features: Acute: dyspnea, cough; chronic: progressive inflammation and fibrosis leading to restrictive lung disease
Sarcoidosis	• ETI: Unknown • Epidemiology: Black females • Pathology: Development of diffuse noncaseating granulomas • Clinical features: Restrictive lung disease, hilar lymphadenopathy on chest radiograph, erythema nodosum, uveoparotid fever, hypercalcemia • Diagnosis: Increased angiotensin-converting enzyme levels, biopsy

Goodpasture syndrome	• ETI: Antibodies to alveolar and glomerular basement membrane • Pathology: Focal necrosis of alveolar walls, intraalveolar hemorrhage, thickening of septa • Clinical features: Hemoptysis, dyspnea, hematuria, rapidly progressive renal failure
Cryptogenic fibrosing alveolitis	• ETI: Unknown • Pathology: Alveolitis, epithelial cell injury, fibrosis, honeycomb lung • Clinical features: Dyspnea, hypoxia, cor pulmonale

PULMONARY VASCULAR DISEASE

Pulmonary embolism	• Risk factors: Acquired such as trauma; prolonged bed rest; cancer; or congenital such as genetic hypercoagulable state (e.g., factor V Leyden) • Pathology: Ischemia and hypoxia; if large, leads to increased pulmonary artery pressure → decreased cardiac output + acute cor pulmonale • Clinical features: Ranges from asymptomatic to sudden death
Pulmonary hypertension	• ETI: Primary is unknown but may be related to mutation of bone morphogenetic protein receptor type 2 (BMPR2); secondary cause: chronic obstructive pulmonary disease, chronic hypoxia, recurrent emboli, left-to-right cardiac shunt (Eisenmenger complex) • Pathology: Increased pulmonary vascular tone, increased right heart strain, right ventricular hypertrophy (RVH) • Clinical features: Chest pain, dyspnea, cyanosis, fatigue, syncope

PNEUMONIA AND TUBERCULOSIS (FIG. IV-4)

Lobar pneumonia	• ETI: *Streptococcus pneumoniae* infection • Pathology: Intraalveolar exudate → affects adjacent lung units through pores of Kohn → lobar consolidation
Bronchopneumonia	• ETI: *Staphylococcus aureus, Klebsiella* sp., *Streptococcus pyogenes* • Pathology: Infiltrate moves from bronchioles → alveoli → patchy distribution
Interstitial pneumonia	• ETI: Viruses, *Mycoplasma pneumoniae, Legionella pneumophila* • Pathology: Diffuse patchy inflammation in alveolar walls
Lung abscess	• ETI: Anaerobes secondary to aspiration, *S. aureus, Klebsiella, Pseudomonas* • Clinical features: Currant jelly foul sputum, high fever

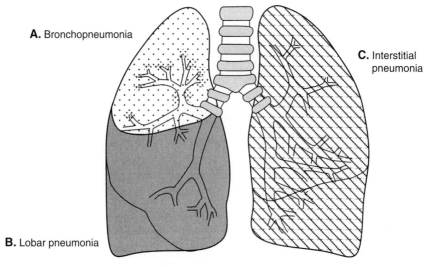

A. Bronchopneumonia

C. Interstitial pneumonia

B. Lobar pneumonia

● **Figure IV-4** Main forms of acute pneumonia. (**A**) Bronchopneumonia. (**B**) Lobar pneumonia. (**C**) Interstitial pneumonia.

Tuberculosis	• Primary
	○ Pathology: Formation of Ghon complex (parenchymal lesion + hilar lymphadenopathy) → usually resolves
	○ Clinical features: Usually asymptomatic, solitary nodule on chest radiograph
	• Secondary
	○ Pathology: Reactivation leading to caseous necrosis, formation of cavitations, fibrosis, and calcification; very rarely spreads hematogenously and lymphatically as miliary tuberculosis and diffuse granulomas in distal organs
	○ Clinical features: Fevers, night sweats, hemoptysis, chronic cough, pleuritic chest pain

LUNG CANCER

Bronchogenic carcinoma	• Squamous cell carcinoma: Central or hilar mass; may result in cavitation; may cause paraneoplastic syndrome (increased parathyroid hormone related polypeptide (PTHrP) leading to hypercalcemia)
	• Adenocarcinoma: Peripheral; develops on areas of previous injury; less related to smoking
	• Bronchioloalveolar carcinoma: Peripheral; grows along bronchioles and alveoli; less related to smoking
	• Large cell carcinoma: Peripheral; undifferentiated has a poor prognosis
	• Small cell carcinoma: Central; undifferentiated and highly aggressive with early metastasis has a poor prognosis; may cause paraneoplastic syndrome (increased adrenocorticotropic hormone or antidiuretic hormone)

Clinical manifestations of lung cancer	• Cough, hemoptysis, pleuritic chest pain, recurrent pneumonia

- Cough, hemoptysis, pleuritic chest pain, recurrent pneumonia
- Virchow node (supraclavicular node)
- Pancoast tumor (apical tumor) leading to injury to cervical sympathetic fibers and Horner's syndrome (ptosis, miosis, hemianhydrosis)
- Superior vena cava (SVC) syndrome: Compression of SVC, increased jugular venous distention, facial swelling, cyanosis
- Hoarseness: Compression of superior laryngeal nerve
- Paraneoplastic syndromes
- Metastasis: Brain, liver, bones

Topic **5**

Gastrointestinal System

Must Knows

- Gastroesophageal diseases
- Diseases of the small and large intestine
- Diseases of the liver, gallbladder, and pancreas

GASTROESOPHAGEAL DISEASES

Achalasia	• ETI: Idiopathic, secondary to Chagas disease • Pathology: Derangement of innervation to myenteric plexus, aperistalsis and incomplete relaxation of lower esophageal sphincter and increased tone leads to dilation of lower esophagus, ulceration, and fibrotic thickening • Clinical features: Difficulty swallowing, regurgitation • Diagnosis: Barium swallow shows "bird beak"
Esophageal varices	• Pathology: Portal hypertension, diversion of blood to esophageal veins, dilated tortuous vessels • Clinical features: Rupture leads to massive hematemesis
Mallory-Weiss syndrome	• Pathology: Longitudinal tears in esophageal mucosa secondary to severe emesis • Clinical features: Severe pain

Barrett esophagus	• ETI: Chronic esophagitis
	• Pathology: Metaplasia of distal stratified squamous mucosa to columnar mucosa with goblet cells, increased risk of adenocarcinoma
	• Diagnosis: Red velvety mucosa on esophagogastroduodenoscopy
Esophageal carcinoma	• Risk factors: Increased mucosal exposure to carcinogens (most important is tobacco), achalasia, esophagitis or Barrett esophagus, family history
	• Pathology: Early local spread and metastasis
Gastritis	• Chronic: Autoimmune, *H. pylori* infection
	• Acute: Excess nonsteroidal anti-inflammatory agent use, alcohol, tobacco, stress, ischemia or trauma
	• Pathology: Mucosal inflammation leading to disruption of mucous layer, decreased HCO_3, decreased mucosal blood flow, and development of erosions
	• Clinical features: Epigastric pain, nausea and vomiting, hematemesis, melena, anemia
Peptic ulcer disease	• Ulcer: Breach through muscularis mucosa to submucosa or deeper
	• Erosion: Loss of superficial epithelium of mucosa
	• **Gastric ulcer:** From decreased defenses against gastric acid; pain increased with meals
	• **Duodenal ulcer:** From increased offenses (increased gastric acid secretion); leads to Brunner's gland hypertrophy; pain decreased with meals
	• Clinical features: Nausea and vomiting, epigastric pain, hematemesis, melena, anemia, perforation leading to peritonitis
Stress ulcers	• Curling's ulcers: Caused by extensive burns
	• Cushing's ulcers: Caused by central nervous system injury
Gastric adenocarcinoma	• ETI: *H. pylori,* nitrosamines, pernicious anemia, alcohol, smoking
	• Pathology: Often around lesser curvature in two patterns:
	○ Intestinal variant: Gastric mucous cells with metaplasia in setting of chronic gastritis leading to fungating or exophytic mass
	○ Diffuse: Occurs de novo from poorly differentiated mucous cell; leads to infiltration of stomach walls with fibrotic change giving the stomach a leather bottle appearance (linitis plastica)
	• Clinical features: Early metastasis to Virchow node (supraclavicular lymph node), early satiation, anemia

DISEASES OF THE SMALL AND LARGE INTESTINE

Celiac disease	• ETI: Sensitivity to gluten (wheat, oats, barley, rye) resulting in an abnormal T-cell reaction • Pathology: T-cell reaction to gliadin leading to mucosal inflammation and villous atrophy • Clinical features: Chronic diarrhea, failure to thrive, weakness, rash of dermatitis herpetiformis (pruritic erythematous papulovesicular lesions) • Diagnosis: Intestinal biopsy, anti-gliadin and anti-endomysial antibodies
Intussusception	• Epidemiology: Infants and young children • ETI: Hypertrophy of Peyer patches secondary to infection, Meckel diverticulum • Pathology: Telescoping of proximal bowel into distal bowel leading to obstruction • Clinical features: Abdominal pain, sausage-like mass, rectal bleeding (Currant jelly stool)
Volvulus (Fig. IV-5)	• Epidemiology: Usually elderly individuals (sigmoid colon) • Pathology: Twisting of gut around its mesenteric blood supply leading to ischemia • Clinical features: Acute abdominal pain, perforation, peritoneal signs

Inflammatory bowel disease	• Crohn's disease
	  ○ ETI: Autoimmune
	  ○ Pathology: Transmural inflammation of any part of GI tract usually with skip lesions leading to thickening and fibrosis, linear mucosal ulcerations, mucosal edema, granuloma formation
	  ○ Clinical features: Abdominal pain, diarrhea, obstruction from strictures, fistulas
	
	• Ulcerative colitis
	  ○ ETI: Autoimmune
	  ○ Pathology: Mucosal inflammation of colon in retrograde pattern starting at the rectum leading to crypt abscesses and pseudopolyps
	  ○ Clinical features: Abdominal pain, bloody diarrhea, toxic megacolon, increased risk of colon cancer

Pseudomembranous colitis	• ETI: *Clostridium difficile* that may colonize after extended use of broad-spectrum antibiotics • Clinical features: Fever, abdominal pain, bloody diarrhea

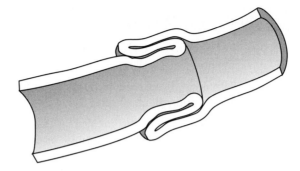

A. Intussusception

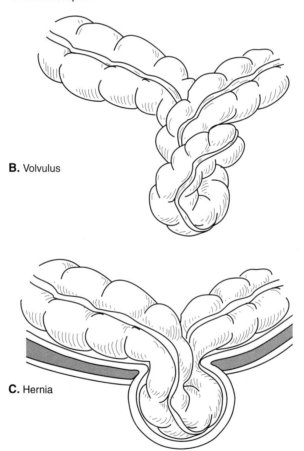

B. Volvulus

C. Hernia

● **Figure IV-5** Intestinal obstructions. (**A**) Intussusception. (**B**) Volvulus. (**C**) Hernia.

Diverticulosis	• ETI: Abnormal colonic intraluminal pressure (chronic constipation)
	• Pathology: Focal areas of weakness exist in the muscular wall where vasarecta penetrates the inner circular muscle adjacent to taeniae. When abnormal pressures develop, these areas become potential herniation sites.

- Clinical features: Asymptomatic or vague abdominal discomfort. If diverticulum becomes colonized with bacteria, fever, pain, perforation, and peritonitis occur.

Appendicitis

- ETI: Lymphoid hyperplasia, fecalith
- Pathology: Blockage of lymphatic drainage, blockage of venous drainage, blockage of arterial supply, bacterial overgrowth, and perforation
- Clinical features: Fever, periumbilical pain that migrates to McBurney point; nausea and vomiting; Rovsing's, psoas, or obturator sign;, rebound tenderness

Angiodysplasia

- Pathology: Tortuous dilations of veins in mucosa or submucosa, usually in the cecum and right colon induced by wall stresses over decades; leads to lower GI bleeding

Ischemic colitis

- ETI: Thrombus, embolus, cardiac failure, shock, excess vasopressors
- Pathology: Ischemia leading to edema and hemorrhage, necrosis, and ulceration
- Clinical features: Acute abdominal pain, bloody diarrhea, abdominal distension, peritoneal signs

Familial polyposis coli

- ETI: Autosomal dominant; defect in *APC* gene
- Pathology: Diffuse development of adenomatous polyps with 100% risk of developing colon cancer

Adenocarcinoma of colon

- ETI: Unknown in 80% of cases. May be associated with mutations of APC or mismatch repair genes such as *MLH1, MSH2, MSH6,* and *PMS2* (typically mutated in hereditary non-polyposis colon cancer [HNPCC]). TP53 plays an important role.
- Pathology: Develops first as adenomatous polyps
  - Tubular adenomas: Small, pedunculated; decreased risk of malignancy
  - Tubulovillous adenomas: Small; pedunculated with villi; intermediate risk of malignancy
  - Villous adenomas: Larger; sessile; large number of villi; increased risk of malignancy
  - Over time, polyps develop to carcinoma and metastasis
- Clinical features: Cecal or right sided: fatigue, weakness, anemia; Left side: Decreased diameter of stool, frank blood, crampy lower left quadrant pain

DISEASES OF THE LIVER AND GALLBLADDER

Hyperbilirubinemia

- Gilbert syndrome
  - Pathology: Deficiency of UDP-glucuronyl transferase → increased unconjugated bilirubin
  - Clinical features: Usually asymptomatic

- Crigler-Najjar syndrome type 1
  - Pathology: Absent UDP-glucuronyl transferase leading to increased unconjugated bilirubin severe jaundice, and kernicterus
  - Clinical features: Death in infancy
- Dubin-Johnson syndrome
  - Pathology: Defective bilirubin transport leading to increased conjugated bilirubin and dark liver
- Rotor syndrome
  - Pathology: Similar to Dubin-Johnson but without formation of dark liver

Hepatitis	- ETI: HAV, HBV, HCV, HEV, alcoholism, autoimmune, drug induced - Pathology: Inflammation, necrosis, repair and fibrosis, cirrhosis - Clinical features: Fever, right upper quadrant (RUQ) pain, jaundice, diarrhea, hepatomegaly - Diagnosis: Serologic confirmation of viral infection
Alcoholic liver disease	- Epidemiology: Most common cause of liver disease in the United States - Pathology: Excess alcohol leads to steatosis (reversible), steatonecrosis (fatty change with neutrophilic infiltrate and intracytoplasmic eosinophilic hyaline inclusions = Mallory bodies) and micronodular cirrhosis - Clinical features: Cirrhosis (see below)
Clinical findings of cirrhosis (Fig. IV-6)	- Cardiovascular: Hypoalbuminemia, ascites and anasarca, coagulopathy secondary to deficient clotting factors - GI: Portal hypertension, esophageal varices, hemorrhoids, caput medusae, splenomegaly - Skin: Jaundice, scleral icterus, spider nevi - Endocrine: Increased estrogen, palmar erythema, gynecomastia, testicular atrophy - Central nervous system: Encephalopathy, asterixis
Hemochromatosis	- ETI: Primary (autosomal recessive [AR]), secondary to multiple transfusions (e.g., thalassemia major) - Pathology: Increased iron levels, deposition in multiple organs - Clinical features: Bronze diabetes, micronodular cirrhosis, decreased TIBC, increased ferritin
Wilson's disease	- ETI: AR - Pathology: Decreased ability to excrete copper, accumulation of copper in organs - Clinical features: Hepatolenticular degeneration (cirrhosis, degeneration of basal ganglia, asterixis, chorea, dementia), decreased ceruloplasmin levels, Kayser-Fleischer rings on the cornea

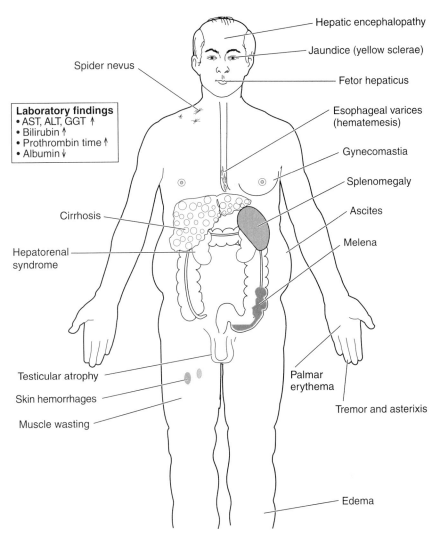

● **Figure IV-6** Clinical manifestations of cirrhosis. ALT = alanine aminotransferase; AST = aspartate aminotransferase; GGT = γ-glutamyl transferase.

Reye syndrome	• ETI: Viral syndrome and aspirin
	• Pathology: Microvesicular fatty change and encephalopathy
	• Clinical features: Mental status change, coma, death
Hepatocellular carcinoma	• Risk factors: HBV, HCV, alcoholic cirrhosis, hemochromatosis, Wilson's disease
	• Clinical features: Increased AFP, hematogenous metastasis
Cholelithiasis and cholecystitis	• Risk factors: Obesity, female gender, fertile, hemolysis, Crohn disease
	• Pathology: Precipitation of cholesterol or bilirubin
	• Clinical features: RUQ pain secondary to biliary colic, obstructive jaundice, ascending cholangitis (fever, jaundice, and RUQ pain), acute pancreatitis

Pancreatitis	• ETI: Gallstones, alcohol, drugs (steroids, didanosine, zidovudine, thiazide diuretics), hyperlipidemia, hypercalcemia, mumps, scorpion toxin • Pathology: Activation of pancreatic enzymes, leakage into abdomen, fat necrosis, formation pseudocyst, abscess • Clinical features: Severe abdominal pain, fever, prostration, Grey Turner sign (ecchymoses of flank), and Cullen sign (periumbilical ecchymoses) • Diagnosis: Increased serum amylase and lipase
Pancreatic adenocarcinoma	• Pathology: Adenocarcinoma arising at pancreatic head • Clinical features: Abdominal pain, jaundice, weight loss, Trousseau's syndrome (migratory thrombophlebitis), very aggressive, leads to death

Topic **6**

Genitourinary System and Diseases of the Breast

Must Knows

● Diseases of the kidney and urinary tract

● Diseases of the penis, testes, and prostate

● Diseases of the vagina, uterus, and ovary

Diseases of the breast

DISEASES OF THE KIDNEY AND URINARY TRACT

Nephritic syndrome	• Hypertension • Oliguria • Azotemia • Hematuria
Poststreptococcal glomerulonephritis (Fig. IV-7)	• ETI: Occurs after infection with group A β-hemolytic streptococci

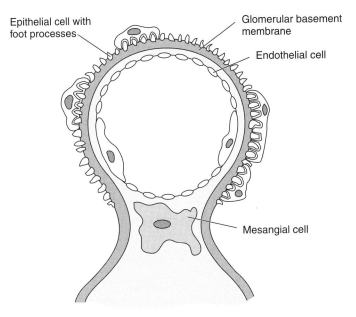

Epithelial cell with foot processes

Glomerular basement membrane

Endothelial cell

Mesangial cell

A. Normal glomerulus

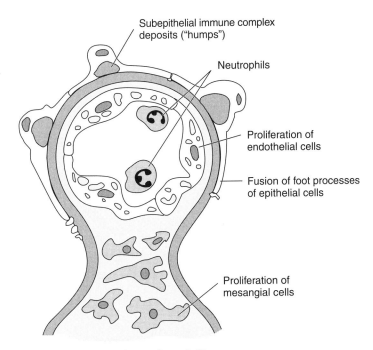

Subepithelial immune complex deposits ("humps")

Neutrophils

Proliferation of endothelial cells

Fusion of foot processes of epithelial cells

Proliferation of mesangial cells

B. Acute poststreptococcal glomerulonephritis

● **Figure IV-7** (**A**) A normal glomerulus. (**B**) The glomerulus in acute poststreptococcal glomerulonephritis.

- Pathology: Immune complex deposition on glomerular basement membrane; subepithelial humps against basement membrane on electron microscopy (EM) and lumpy bumpy on immunofluorescence (IF)
- Clinical features: Fever; abrupt oliguria; children usually recover

Rapidly progressive glomerulonephritis (Fig. IV-8)	• ETI: Defined as nephritic syndrome with rapid progression to failure • Types: I: Goodpasture's (linear pattern on IF); II: Systemic lupus erythematosus (SLE), post-infectious, Henoch-Schönlein; III: Wegener granulomatosis, polyarteritis nodosa • Pathology: Formation of crescents; eventually, sclerosis and obliteration of glomeruli • Clinical features: Unrelenting course leading to long-term dialysis and transplantation
IgA nephropathy (Berger disease)	• Epidemiology: Most common cause of recurrent hematuria; related to upper respiratory infection • Pathology: IgA deposition in mesangium leading to complement activation • Clinical features: Recurrent hematuria after infection

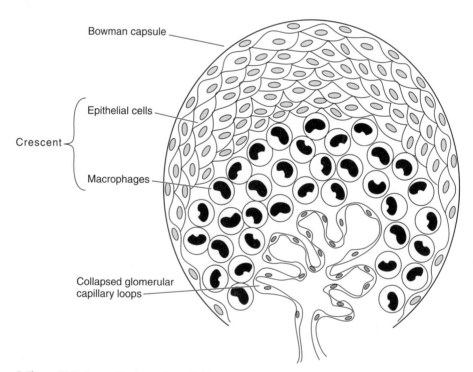

Bowman capsule

Epithelial cells

Crescent

Macrophages

Collapsed glomerular capillary loops

● **Figure IV-8** Crescentic glomerulonephritis.

Nephrotic syndrome	• Proteinuria > 3.5g/d
	• Hypoalbuminemia
	• Edema
	• Hyperlipidemia
Minimal change disease (lipoid nephrosis)	• Epidemiology: Children
	• Pathology: Epithelial cell feet effacement on EM
	• Clinical features: Responds well to steroids
Focal segmental glomerulosclerosis	• ETI: Idiopathic, heroin use, HIV
	• Pathology: Similar to minimal change disease, but in adults and related to hypertension
	• Clinical features: Hematuria, proteinuria, hypertension, poorly responds to steroids
Membranous glomerulonephritis	• ETI: Infection, drugs, cancer, SLE
	• Pathology: Chronic immune complex nephritis; granular pattern on IF
	• Clinical features: Slowly progresses; responds poorly to steroids
Membranoproliferative glomerulonephritis	• Pathology: Mesangial proliferation; thickening of basement membrane with "tram track" appearance on EM
	• Types I: Slowly progressive; II: more aggressive and has C_3 nephritic factor causing hypocomplementemia
Diabetic nephropathy	• Pathology: Thickening of basement membrane or nodular dilatation of mesangial areas (Kimmelstiel-Wilson disease)
Systemic lupus erythematosus (SLE)	• Five types; type IV is most severe (diffuse proliferative form); includes mesangial proliferation and "wire loops"
Acute tubular necrosis	• ETI: Ischemia, sepsis, rhabdomyolysis, nephrotoxicity (antibiotics, contrast dyes)
	• Pathology: Tubular necrosis with tubulorrhexis and protein casts on urinalysis
	• Clinical features: Three phases:
	○ Prodromal phase (decreased urine output, increased blood urea nitrogen)
	○ Oliguric phase (oliguria, hypervolemia, uremia)
	○ Postoliguric phase (steady increased urine o/p)
Interstitial nephritis	• ETI: Methicillin, nonsteroidal anti-inflammatory agents, diuretics
	• Pathology: Hypersensitivity reaction
	• Clinical features: Fever, eosinophilia, skin rash, hematuria, pyuria

Nephrolithiasis	• Calcium stones (most common): Hypercalciuria secondary to hypercalcemia; radiopaque
	• Triple phosphate (ammonium magnesium phosphate): Related to *Proteus* sp.; staghorn calculi, radiopaque
	• Uric acid: Hyperuricemia secondary to gout or myeloproliferative disorders; radiolucent
	• Cystine (least common): Secondary to cystinuria; radiolucent
Urinary tract infection	• Epidemiology: Sexually active women, elderly individuals, urinary catheters
	• ETI: *Escherichia coli, Staphylococcus saprophyticus, Proteus* sp.
	• Clinical features: Dysuria, frequency, hematuria, pyuria
Pyelonephritis	• ETI: Ascending urinary tract infection (UTI); uncommonly secondary to hematogenous seeding
	• Clinical features: Same as for UTI plus fever or chills, nausea or vomiting, back pain, costovertebral angle tenderness, papillary necrosis if untreated
Uremia	• Clinical features: Anorexia, nausea, vomiting, mental status change, bleeding disorder, uremic frost, uremic fetor, fibrinous pericarditis, pleuritis, metabolic acidosis
Adult polycystic kidney disease	• ETI: Autosomal dominant; mutation of *PKD1* (90%) or *PKD2* (10%)
	• Pathology: Formation of bilateral masses of fluid filled cysts; compression of vasculature; ischemic atrophy; renal failure
	• Clinical features: Flank pain, intermittent gross hematuria, hypertension with increased incidence of berry aneurysms, renal failure, death
Renal cell carcinoma	• ETI: Unknown, von Hippel-Lindau (VHL) gene deletion found in more than 90%
	• Pathology: Clear lipid-laden cells; aggressive spread up inferior vena cava + hematogenous metastases
	• Clinical features: Painless hematuria, chronic fever, dull flank pain, polycythemia secondary to increased erythropoietin (EPO), paraneoplastic syndromes
Wilms tumor	• Epidemiology: Third most common cancer in children under age 10 years
	• ETI: autosomal dominant; deletion of *WT1* (tumor suppressor gene on chromosome 11)
Transitional cell carcinoma	• ETI: Smoking, chronic cystitis, schistosomiasis, β-naphthylamine
	• Clinical features: Painless hematuria

DISEASES OF THE PENIS, TESTES, AND PROSTATE

Abnormalities of the penis	• Hypospadias: Opening of the urethra on the ventral surface of the penis • Epispadias: Opening of the urethra on the dorsal side of the penis; less common than hypospadias • Phimosis: Constriction of the foreskin that occurs as a consequence of repeated balanitis of the glans penis; results in difficulty or inability to retract foreskin; may cause balanitis (an inflammation of the glans penis)

Neoplasms of the penis	• Erythroplasia de Queyrat
	  ○ Epidemiology: Uncircumcised middle-aged men
	  ○ Pathology: Carcinoma in situ that progresses to carcinoma in 10%
	  ○ Clinical features: Erythematous plaque involving the glans penis
	• Carcinoma
	  ○ Epidemiology: More common in uncircumcised men and outside the United States
	  ○ Pathology: Usually squamous cell carcinoma; may be associated with HPV 16 and 18

Testicular diseases	• Torsion: Twisting of the testicle around the testicular artery resulting in strangulation. Usually caused by trauma and is associated with an accessory epididymis. It is a medical emergency. • Hydrocele: Fluid in the tunica vaginalis. Often caused by communication with the peritoneal cavity through a patent processus vaginalis. • Varicocele: Defective valves prohibit normal draining of the pampiniform plexus resulting in abnormal dilation. Morphologically resembles a bag of worms. Occurs on the left side more than the right. • Cryptorchism: Failure of the testis to descend down the inguinal canal into the scrotum. Even if corrected with surgery, the testicle still has an increased chance of seminoma. Treatment is orchiectomy.
Testicular infections	• Mumps: Caused by a paramyxovirus that results in orchitis and parotitis. May result in sterility. • Epididymitis: Infection by *Neisseria gonorrhoeae* or *Chlamydia trachomata*

Germ cell testicular tumors	• Seminoma
	  ○ Epidemiology: Men age 25 to 45 years; more common in men with cryptorchidism
	  ○ Pathology: Analogous to dysgerminoma of the ovary
	  ○ Clinical features: Painless enlargement of the testis
	  ○ Diagnosis: No serologic markers

- Treatment: Cured by surgery and, if needed, radiotherapy in more than 90% of cases
  - Embryonal carcinoma
    - Epidemiology: Adults age 20 to 40 years
    - Pathology: More aggressive than seminoma
    - Treatment: Surgery and chemotherapy cure rate in more than 90% of cases
  - Yolk sac tumor (endodermal sinus tumor)
    - Epidemiology: Infancy and early childhood
    - Diagnosis: α-Fetoprotein (AFP) increased in serum; on microscopy, endodermal sinuses appear as primitive glomeruli
    - Treatment: Surgery curative in 99% if done before age 4 years
  - Teratoma
    - Pathology: Germ cell tumor consisting of all three germ cell lines. In males, is always considered malignant (unlike females, in which they are always benign).
  - Choriocarcinoma
    - Pathology: Highly malignant and consists of both cytotrophoblasts and syncytiotrophoblasts. Usually found as part of a mixed cell tumor. It widely metastasizes early.
    - Diagnosis: Human chorionic gonadotrophin
  - Nonseminomatous germ cell tumors (NSGCT)
    - 60% of all germ cell neoplasms in adults; contain embryonal carcinoma, choriocarcinoma, yolk sac tumor, and teratoma elements
    - Diagnosis: hCG and AFP in serum
    - Treatment: Surgery and chemotherapy curative in more than 90% of cases

Sex cord stromal tumors	- Leydig tumor
	  - Pathology: Rare steroid producing a benign tumor
	  - Clinical features: Testicular mass, gynecomastia, precocious puberty
	  - Diagnosis: Microscopy shows polygonal cells with abundant eosinophilic cytoplasm. Intracytoplasmic crystalloids called Reinke crystals are present.
	- Sertoli tumor
	  - Pathology: Rare benign tumor composed of Sertoli cells

Acute prostatitis	- ETI: Gram negatives: *E. coli, Enterococcus, S. aureus* - Pathology: Infection usually spreads contiguously from bladder or urethra - Clinical features: Fever; chills; dysuria; large, tender, boggy prostate

Benign prostatic hyperplasia	• Epidemiology: 90% of men by time they are 70 years old
	• ETI: Dihydrotestosterone (DHT)
	• Pathology: DHT promotes hyperplasia of prostatic tissue leading to enlargement; compression of the prostatic urethra; urinary hesitancy, frequency, nocturia; and urinary retention with stasis and increased susceptibility to UTIs
Prostatic adenocarcinoma	• Epidemiology: Most common cancer in men
	• Pathology: Usually develops in the peripheral parts of the prostate
	• Hematogenous mets to vertebra causing osteoblastic lesions
	• Diagnosis: Needle biopsy and elevated serum prostate-specific antigen (PSA)
	• Treatment: Surgical resection, radiotherapy, hormonal therapy, orchiectomy

DISEASES OF THE VAGINA, UTERUS, AND OVARY

Vulvar intraepithelial neoplasia (VuIN)	• ETI: Lichen sclerosis, HPV 16 or 18
	• Pathology: Carcinoma in situ that presents as raised lesions. May progress to invasive vulvar carcinoma if not treated.
Paget disease	• Pathology: Anaplastic mucin positive tumor cells that occupy the epidermis
	• Clinical features: Red and sharply demarcated; pruritic
Cervical intraepithelial neoplasia (CIN)	• Epidemiology: Risk factors include early sexual intercourse, multiple partners
	• ETI: HPV 16 and 18
	• Pathology:
	○ CIN I: Superficial cellular atypia with epithelial maturation
	○ CIN II: Atypia spreads deeper towards the basal layer
	○ CIN III (CIS): Atypia occupies all layers; cells lack maturation
	• Clinical features: CIN may progress to carcinoma if not treated. Carcinoma may present as cervical bleeding, cervical ulceration, or fungating mass.
	• Diagnosis: Pap smears
Condyloma acuminatum	• ETI: HPV 6 and 11
	• Clinical features: Genital warts in the perineal area
Pelvic inflammatory disease (PID)	• ETI: *C. trachomatis, N. gonorrhea,* or postpartum (especially with cesarean section)
	• Epidemiology: Risk factors include multiple sexual partners, history of STD

- Clinical features: Triad includes fever, chills, cervical motion tenderness, and abdominal pain; other clinical features include peritonitis, salpingitis, tuboovarian abscess and sequelae of ectopic pregnancy and infertility

Dysfunctional uterine bleeding	<ul><li>Pathology: Irregular menstrual bleeding without anatomic lesions of the uterus; caused by chronic unopposed estrogen stimulation</li><li>Clinical features: Menorrhagia or metrorrhagia</li><li>*Postmenopausal bleeding is cancer until proven otherwise*</li></ul>
Amenorrhea	<ul><li>Most likely caused by pregnancy</li></ul>
Endometriosis	<ul><li>ETI: 10% to 15% of women of reproductive age</li><li>Pathology: Ectopic endometrial tissue most commonly on ovaries (causing chocolate cysts), pelvic peritoneum, and uterosacral ligaments</li><li>Clinical features: Dysmenorrhea, dyspareunia, infertility, pelvic pain</li><li>Diagnosis: Direct visualization by laparoscopy</li></ul>
Adenomyosis	<ul><li>Pathology: Extension of the endometrium into the myometrium</li><li>Clinical features: Dysmenorrhea, menorrhagia, boggy uterus</li></ul>
Fibroids	<ul><li>Epidemiology: 20% to 30% of U.S. women; risk factors: black, obese, perimenopausal</li><li>Pathology: Benign local proliferation of uterine smooth muscle that is estrogen sensitive. There are four different types: intramural, submucosal, subserosal, and parasitic.</li><li>Clinical features: Asymptomatic (> 50%), pain, abnormal menstruation, infertility</li></ul>
Endometrial hyperplasia	<ul><li>Pathology: Abnormal proliferation of endometrial glands in response to excess estrogen stimulation. May develop into endometrial carcinoma.</li><li>Clinical features: Postmenopausal bleeding</li><li>Diagnosis: Endometrial biopsy looking for cellular atypia</li></ul>
Endometrial carcinoma	<ul><li>Epidemiology: Risk factors include early menarche, late menopause, nulliparity, obesity, unopposed estrogen, loss of *PTEN* tumor suppressor gene</li><li>Pathology: May develop as consequence of endometrial hyperplasia</li><li>Clinical features: Postmenopausal bleeding</li><li>Diagnosis: Endometrial biopsy</li></ul>
Ovarian cysts	<ul><li>Follicular cysts</li><ul><li>Epithelial cysts are common and non-neoplastic; grow to large sizes and cause abdominal pain, which is acute if they rupture</li></ul></ul>

- Polycystic ovarian syndrome
  - ○ Epidemiology: Young women
  - ○ Pathology: Increased luteinizing hormone and follicle-stimulating hormone stimulating adrenal androgen production and development of ovarian follicles without ovulation
  - ○ Clinical features: Amenorrhea, infertility, obesity, hirsutism

Epithelial ovarian tumors	- Epidemiology: Women older than age 30 years - Serous cystadenocarcinoma: Malignant; most common; may be bilateral - Mucinous cystadenocarcinoma: Malignant; may seed peritoneum as pseudomyxoma peritonei - Endometrioid carcinoma: Malignant; microscopically similar to endometrium - Brenner tumor: Rare; benign; epithelial cells resemble transitional epithelium
Ovarian germ cell tumors	- Epidemiology: Women and girls younger than age 30 years - Dysgerminoma: Malignant; homologous to testicular seminoma - Yolk sac tumor (endodermal sinus tumor): Homologous to yolk sac tumor of testicle; secretes AFP - Teratoma: Benign tumor (dermoid cyst) - Immature teratoma: Malignant because it contains immature neural tissue that may metastasize - Choriocarcinoma: Malignant; secretes hCG; early metastasis
Ovarian sex cord stromal tumors	- Granulosa cell tumor: Secretes estrogen; low-grade malignancy; may causes precocious puberty; Call-Exner bodies on microscopy - Sertoli-Leydig cell tumor: Secretes androgens; causes virilization

DISEASES OF THE BREAST

Inflammation	- Acute mastitis: A bacterial infection of the breast secondary to the development of fissures and cracks in the nipple during breastfeeding. Clinical features include the classic signs of inflammation: dolar, rubor, calor, and tumor. - Fat necrosis: Occurs secondary to trauma of the breast; results in fibrosis, which may be mistaken for a mass

Fibrocystic breast disease	- Epidemiology: Common in women age 20 to 40 years
	- Pathology: Formation of cysts and stromal fibrosis as an irregular response to hormonal stimuli. Three patterns:
	  ○ Simple fibrocystic changes: Fibrotic changes with epithelial cell hyperplasia; common and not associated with risk of neoplasm
	  ○ Proliferative fibrocystic change: Epithelial cell hyperplasia; increases risk of invasive carcinoma. If hyperplastic cells

show signs of atypia, risk of invasive carcinoma is considerably increased.

- ○ Sclerosing adenosis: Intralobular fibrosis and proliferation of ductal epithelium. The pattern suggests increased risk of neoplasia.

Breast tumors	• Fibroadenoma: Most common tumor of the breast
	  ○ Epidemiology: Women age younger than age 30 years
	  ○ Pathology: Benign proliferation of stroma and ducts
	  ○ Clinical features: Large, freely movable mass
	• Intraductal papilloma
	  ○ Pathology: Benign papillary growth in a lactiferous duct; increased risk of invasive carcinoma
	  ○ Clinical features: Bloody serous discharge from nipple
	• Phyllodes tumor
	  ○ Pathology: Massive variant of a fibroadenoma; usually benign but has potential for malignant transformation

Breast carcinomas	• Epidemiology: Affects one in 10 women. Risk factors include early age of menarche, late age of menopause, nulliparity, obesity, family history, proliferative atypical fibrocystic disease
	• ETI: Genetic components (*BRCA1* and *BRCA2*, *TP53*), excess circulating estrogen
	• Pathology: According to type of carcinoma:
	  ○ Ductal carcinoma in situ: Usually nonpalpable and seen as irregular calcifications on mammogram. It requires excision to prevent development of invasive carcinoma.
	  ○ Invasive ductal carcinoma: Most common carcinoma of the breast. Tumor cells are encased in dense fibrous tissue.
	  ○ Invasive lobular carcinoma: May be bilateral. "Indian file" cells on microscopy.
	  ○ Paget disease of the breast: Underlying ductal carcinoma that presents with dermatitis or macular rash over nipple and areola. On microscopy, Paget cells appear large and surrounded with clear area.
	  ○ Inflammatory carcinoma: Classic symptoms of inflammation, early lymphatic involvement with rapid metastasis. Poor prognosis
	• Clinical features: Fixed, irregular, immovable mass; nipple retraction; nipple discharge; dimpling on the surface of the breast. Note that all women over age 50 years should have annual mammograms.
	• Treatment: Modified radical mastectomy or lumpectomy with or without radiation. If estrogen receptor positive, tamoxifen or raloxifene are added.

Topic **7**

Rheumatology and the Musculoskeletal System

Must Knows

- Arthropathies and connective tissue disorders
- Muscle diseases
- Metabolic bone diseases
- Nonneoplastic bone diseases
- Bone tumors

ARTHROPATHIES AND CONNECTIVE TISSUE DISORDERS

Rheumatoid arthritis (RA)	• ETI: Autoimmune (HLA-DR1,4) • Pathology: Acute inflammatory response; activation of neutrophils, lymphocytes, plasma cells; proliferation and hypertrophy of synovial lining with revascularization; panis formation (granulation tissue); destruction of bone and cartilage; fibrosis and calcification; ankylosis • Clinical features: Symmetric polyarticular arthritis worse in the morning; gelling; involvement of proximal interphalangeal (PIP) joints; swan neck or boutonnière deformity; ulnar deviation; rheumatoid nodules over extensor surfaces; constitutional symptoms • Systemic features: Pleuritis, pericarditis, uveitis, pulmonary fibrosis, anemia of chronic disease, vasculitis • Felty syndrome: RA, splenomegaly, and neutropenia • Still disease: Juvenile RA, acute fever, generalized lymphadenopathy, and hepatosplenomegaly
Osteoarthritis (degenerative joint disease [DJD])	• ETI: Usually of unknown etiology and called DJD; secondary to joint trauma, hemochromatosis, hemophilia, Wilson's disease, alkaptonuria • Pathology: Slow increase of joint H_2O, decreased proteoglycans and weakening of collagen network, decreased tensile strength and resilience, increased repair response of deeper chondrocytes

by increased secretion of collagen and proteoglycans, eventual exhaustion, increased secretion of interleukin-1 (IL-1) increased production of proteolytic enzymes by surrounding chondrocytes, and further degeneration

- Structural changes: Fibrillation or splitting of articular surface, eburnation and formation of joint mice, subchondral sclerosis, osteophyte formation
- Clinical features: Joint stiffness and crepitus in weight-bearing joints (e.g., hips, knees); joint fusion does not occur
- Heberden nodes: Osteophytes on distal interphalangeal joints
- Bouchard nodes: Osteophytes on proximal interphalangeal joints

Gout	• ETI: Hyperuricemia secondary to abnormal purine metabolism, decreased renal excretion, increased nucleic acid turnover secondary to neoplastic process, Lesch-Nyhan syndrome • Pathology: Uric acid precipitation in joints, complement activation, activation of neutrophils, release of proteases and inflammatory mediators, tissue injury and inflammation • Clinical features: Podagra (metatarsophalangeal joint [MTP]), tophaceous deposits (ear, Achilles), urolithiasis, subcutaneous nodules (tophi) • Diagnosis: Needle-shaped, negatively birefringent crystals in joint fluid or tophi
Pseudogout	• Pathology: Deposition of calcium pyrophosphate dehydrate crystals; inflammation • Clinical features: Monoarticular attacks in the knee, wrist, shoulder, and ankle • Diagnosis: Positively birefringent crystals

Seronegative arthritis	• Common features:
	  ◦ Inflammatory axial arthritis, sacroiliitis, spondylitis
	  ◦ Peripheral asymmetric oligoarthritis
	  ◦ Enthesitis
	  ◦ HLA-B27
	
	• **Ankylosing spondylitis**
	  ◦ Pathology: Erosive changes leading to fibrous ankylosis; starts at sacroiliac joint and ascends
	  ◦ Clinical features: Inflammatory back pain, immobility, morning stiffness
	  ◦ Diagnosis: Bamboo spine on radiograph
	
	• **Reiter syndrome**
	  ◦ Pathology: Acute inflammatory arthritis occurring 1 to 4 weeks after infection (*Chlamydia trachomatis, Yersinia enterocolitica, Campylobacter jejuni*)
	  ◦ Clinical features: Uveitis, urethritis, arthritis

- **Psoriatic arthritis**
  - Clinical features: Nail pitting, distal interphalangeal (DIP) joint involvement, exacerbated during outbreaks of psoriasis

Systemic lupus erythematosus (SLE)	• Epidemiology: F:M=7:1. Most often affects black women
	• ETI: Autoimmune; associated with HLA-DR2, 3; drug induced
	  ○ Pathology: Immune complex–mediated lesions causing:
	    Head/neck: Malar rash, discoid rash, oral ulcers
	  ○ Cardiovascular: Libman-Sacks endocarditis (nonbacterial verrucous), pericarditis, Raynaud phenomenon, vasculitis
	  ○ Respiratory: Diffuse interstitial pulmonary fibrosis, pleuritis
	  ○ Renal: Glomerulonephritis
	  ○ Musculoskeletal: Arthralgia and arthritis
	  ○ Skin: Photosensitivity
	  ○ Neurological: Cognitive dysfunction, psychosis
	• Diagnosis: Anti-dsDNA antibody, anti-Sm antibody
	• Treatment: Steroids and immunosuppression

Sjögren syndrome	• ETI: Autoimmune • Clinical features: Conjunctivitis, xerophthalmia, xerostomia (keratoconjunctivitis sicca) • Diagnosis: AntiRo (SS-A) antibody

Scleroderma	• Pathology: Diffuse fibrotic changes causing loss of normal function:
	  ○ Skin: increased dermal collagen, epidermal atrophy, loss of adnexa lead to tightening of skin (especially face), sclerodactyly, and autoamputation of digits
	  ○ Musculoskeletal: Myositis, synovitis, arthralgias
	  ○ Gastrointestinal: Atrophy or fibrosis of submucosa and muscularis leading to esophageal dysmotility and constipation
	  ○ Respiratory: Interstitial fibrosis, pulmonary hypertension, cor pulmonale
	  ○ Renal: Renal failure leading to hypertensive crisis
	• Diagnosis: Anti Scl-70 antibody

CREST syndrome	• Variant of scleroderma • Calcinosis, Raynaud syndrome, esophageal dysmotility, sclerodactyly, telangiectasia • Diagnosis: Anticentromere antibody
Carpal tunnel syndrome	• ETI: Repetitive hand trauma, acromegaly, pregnancy • Pathology: Entrapment of median nerve in carpal tunnel

- Clinical features: Paresthesias in lateral 3.5 fingers, wasting of thenar eminence, difficulty in apposition of thumb, positive Tinel sign and Phalen test

Lyme disease	• ETI: *Borrelia burgdorferi* (vector is *Ixodes* tick) • Stage I (3 days to 4 weeks): Erythema migrans plus diffuse arthralgia or myalgia • Stage II (weeks to months): Bell's palsy, meningoencephalitis, peripheral neuropathy, heart block, peri- or myocarditis • Stage III: Demyelinating encephalopathy, episodic oligoarthritis

MUSCLE DISEASES

Myasthenia gravis	• ETI: Autoimmune disease of young women or older men • Pathology: Antibodies against postsynaptic neuromuscular acetylcholine receptors. May be associated with thymoma in young women. • Clinical features: Muscle weakness that progresses with exertion and throughout the day that is relieved with rest, diplopia. Improved with edrophonium.
Lambert-Eaton syndrome	• ETI: Paraneoplastic syndrome; most often with small cell carcinoma of the lung • Pathology: Antibodies against presynaptic calcium conduction channels in axons • Clinical features: Weakness that improves with repeated exertion
Myotonic dystrophy	• ETI: Autosomal dominant; trinucleotide repeat • Pathology: Defective myotonin protein kinase • Clinical features: Inability to relax muscles after contraction
Duchenne muscular dystrophy	• ETI: X-linked recessive; mutation of dystrophin gene • Pathology: Production of defective dystrophin protein leading to muscle cell death and fibrofatty replacement ("pseudohypertrophy") • Clinical features: Weakness, pseudohypertrophy of calves, Gower maneuver, eventual death
Dermatomyositis or polymyositis	• Clinical features: Symmetric proximal muscle weakness, dysphagia, Gottron papules (erythematous lesions over metacarpophalangeal [MCP] and PIP joints), heliotrope rash, elevated creatine kinase (CK), abnormal electromyogram (EMG)
Fibromyalgia	• ETI: Unknown • Clinical features: Pain along specific trigger points, sleep disturbance, depression

| **Polymyalgia rheumatica** | • Epidemiology: Elderly individuals; 20% have concurrent temporal arteritis
• ETI: Autoimmune, associated with HLA-DR4
• Clinical features: Pain, stiffness, tenderness in shoulder girdle, hip, neck |

METABOLIC BONE DISEASES

Osteoporosis	• Pathology: Increased osteoclast activation, increased bone resorption, fractures • Clinical features: Initially asymptomatic, decreased bone density on radiograph, pathologic fractures
Rickets and osteomalacia	• ETI: Vitamin D deficiency • Pathology: Defective mineralization of bone with increased osteoid • Clinical features: Soft bones, bowed legs

NONNEOPLASTIC BONE DISEASES

Osteomyelitis	• ETI: *S. aureus* (most common), *Salmonella* sp. (sickle cell anemia), *Pseudomonas* sp. (IVDA), *E. coli* + *S. pyogenes* (neonates) • Pathology: Subperiosteal inflammation that leads to eventual necrosis • Clinical features: Fever, leukocytosis, increased erythrocyte sedimentation rate (ESR), local swelling and pain
Pott disease	• Tuberculous osteomyelitis of vertebrae; bone destruction; deformity and collapse, and extension to adjacent soft tissue and formation of "cold" abscess in psoas muscle

Paget disease of bone	• Pathology: Three phases:
	  ○ Osteolytic: Extensive osteoclastic activity with replacement of marrow with vascular connective tissue
	  ○ Mixed: Superimposed osteoblastic activity
	  ○ Osteosclerotic: Irregular bone deposition in a jigsaw puzzle pattern
	• Clinical features: Usually asymptomatic, increased serum alkaline phosphatase, back pain, enlargement of head, visual disturbances and deafness (decreased diameter of skull foramina), warmth of overlying skin, high-output cardiac failure caused by hypervascularity of bone marrow

Legg-Calvé-Perthes disease	• Epidemiology: Boys age 4 to 9 years • Pathology: Aseptic avascular necrosis in femoral head • Clinical features: Hip pain, normal ESR and leukocytes

Slipped capital femoral epiphysis (SCFE)	• Epidemiology: Obese male adolescents • Clinical features: Dull aching hip or knee pain made worse with movement
Osteogenesis imperfecta	• ETI: Autosomal dominant; mutation of collagen I genes • Pathology: Abnormal synthesis of collagen, defective bones, fractures • Clinical features: Multiple fractures, blue sclera, hearing loss
Achondroplasia	• ETI: Autosomal dominant; mutation of fibroblast growth factor III receptor gene • Pathology: Abnormal cartilage in developing growth plate, short stature

BONE TUMORS

Osteochondroma, also known as exostosis (benign)	• Epidemiology: Younger than age 25 years; males:females = 3:1; most common benign bone tumor • Clinical features: Tubular bones, most often distal femur and proximal tibia
Giant cell tumor (benign, but may recur)	• Epidemiology: Age 20 to 40 years; females > males • Pathology: Multinucleated giant cells within fibrous stroma • Clinical features: Epiphysis of distal femur and proximal tibia; soap bubble appearance on radiograph • Treatment: Surgery (extensive curettage or resection); 10% to 20% recur
Osteosarcoma (malignant)	• Epidemiology: Age 10 to 20 years; males > females • Clinical features: Metaphysis of long bones; 60% are around the knee joint. On radiograph, bone spicules are visible with sunburst pattern, Codman triangle (periosteal elevation). Early hematogenous metastases. • Treatment: Surgery and chemotherapy results in 65% long-term survival.
Ewing sarcoma (malignant)	• Epidemiology: Children; more common in boys • Pathology: Small blue cell tumor, equivalent to primitive neuroectodermal tumor (PNET). Related to translocation t(11;22) of the *EWS* gene and formation of the *EWS-FLI1* fusion gene; found in 85% of all EWS-PNET. • Clinical features: Diaphysis of long bones, pelvis, ribs, early metastases • Treatment: Surgery and chemotherapy results in 50% long-term cure

Topic **8**

Dermatology

Must **Knows**

- Terminology
- Common dermatoses
- Bullous diseases
- Disorders of pigmentation
- Benign and premalignant epithelial lesions
- Malignant epithelial lesions
- The phakomatoses

TERMINOLOGY

Macule	Flat discoloration < 1 cm in diameter
Papule	Elevated lesion < 1 cm in diameter
Plaque	Elevated skin lesion > 1 cm in diameter
Vesicle	Fluid containing lesion < 0.5 cm
Bulla	Fluid containing lesion > 0.5 cm
Petechiae	Flat, small, nonblanching, red-purple lesion caused by hemorrhage
Purpura	Flat, large, nonblanching, red-purple lesion caused by large area of hemorrhage
Hyperkeratosis	Increased thickness of stratum corneum
Parakeratosis	Hyperkeratosis with retention of nuclei in stratum corneum
Lichenification	Thickened rough skin from repeated scratching
Excoriation	A traumatic lesion to the epidermis, usually by scratching
Acanthosis	Thickening of epidermis
Spongiosis	Epidermal edema resulting in widened intercellular space

Acantholysis	Separation of epidermal cells by extracellular fluid
Folliculitis	Infection of hair follicle
Furuncle	Infection of hair follicle and surrounding deep tissue
Carbuncle	Multiple connected furuncles resulting in an abscess

DERMATOSES

Urticaria	• Pathology: Localized mast cell degranulation secondary to antigen-induced release; increased dermal microvascular permeability; edematous plaques called wheals
Eczema	• ETI: Contact, atopic, drug induced, photo induced • Pathology: Antigens are processed by epidermal Langerhans cells; T-cell sensitization; reexposure; CD4+ T cell activation; cytokine release; inflammation • Clinical features: Red, papulovesicular, oozing, crusted lesions; raised scaling plaques; spongiosis on microscopy
Psoriasis	• ETI: Possibly autoimmune • Pathology: Chronic inflammation; acanthosis, parakeratosis, and development of Munro microabscesses (neutrophilic abscess) • Clinical features: Silvery-white scaly plaques over extensor surfaces, pitting of nails, Auspitz sign (pinpoint bleeding of plaque when lifted), Koebner phenomenon (lesions appear at points of chronic irritation); may also be associated with arthritis
Lichen planus	• ETI: Associated with hepatitis C virus (HCV) • Pathology: Hyperkeratosis and mononuclear infiltrate in dermis • Clinical features: Four Ps: pruritic, purple, polygonal papules

DISORDERS OF PIGMENTATION

Vitiligo	• ETI: Unknown; may be autoimmune or associated with Graves' disease • Pathology: Loss of melanocytes • Clinical features: Sharply demarcated depigmented patches

Albinism	• Ocular albinism: Lack of melanin limited to the eyes
	• Oculocutaneous albinism
	  ○ Pathology: Ingrown error of metabolism secondary to defective *tyrosinase*
	  ○ Clinical features: Unpigmented skin, hair, eyes; predisposes to actinic keratosis, squamous cell carcinoma, malignant melanoma

Nevus	• Nevocellular nevus: Benign tumor derived from melanocytes • Dysplastic nevus: Disorderly proliferation of melanocytes resulting in atypical irregularly pigmented lesion; may progress to malignant melanoma
Erythema nodosum	• ETI: Unknown but may be related to infections (e.g., *Mycoplasma, fungi*), inflammatory bowel disease, sarcoidosis, rheumatic fever • Pathology: Inflammation of subcutaneous tissue in the extremities (usually the legs) • Clinical features: Tender red nodules occurring on lower legs
Capillary hemangioma	• Pathology: Red macules or papules or plaques that consist of blood-filled capillaries • Clinical features: Port-wine stain of face or neck; strawberry hemangioma is raised; cherry angioma is a dome-shaped papule
Granuloma pyogenicum	• Vascular pedunculated lesion
Acanthosis nigricans	• ETI: Associated with diabetes and underlying malignancy • Clinical features: Dark intertriginous areas
Xanthoma	• ETI: Hypercholesterolemia • Clinical features: Yellow plaques and papules over tendon surfaces and eyelids (xanthelasma) • Diagnosis: Patient must be worked up for hypercholesterolemia

BULLOUS DISEASES

Pemphigus vulgaris	• ETI: Autoimmune type II hypersensitivity reaction • Pathology: IgG autoantibodies against the desmosome; acantholysis of epidermis; intraepidermal bullae • Clinical features: Intraepidermal vesicles; lesions begin on oral mucosa followed and then erupt over skin; fatal unless treated • Treatment: Steroids
Bullous pemphigoid	• ETI: Autoimmune type II hypersensitivity reaction • Pathology: IgG autoantibodies against the hemidesmosome; separation between the basal cell layer and lamina lucida; subepidermal bullae • Clinical features: Subepidermal vesicles; similar to pemphigus vulgaris but not as extensive with sparing of mucous membranes
Dermatitis herpetiformis	• Epidemiology: Associated with celiac sprue • ETI: Autoimmune • Pathology: Deposits of IgA on tips of dermal papillae; development of neutrophilic infiltrate; microabscess formation; separation of dermis and epidermis; subepidermal bullae

	• Clinical features: Pruritic grouped vesicles that are typically bilateral and symmetric
	• Treatment: Gluten-free diet
Erythema multiforme	• ETI: Unknown but may be a hypersensitivity reaction in response to certain infections or drugs, malignancy, or collagen vascular disease
	• Pathology: Lymphocytic infiltrate; dermal edema; margination of lymphocytes along dermoepidermal junction; subepidermal bullae
	• Clinical features: Diffuse erythematous target lesions of various shapes, vesicles, and bullae seen on dorsum of hands, palms, soles
Stevens-Johnson syndrome	• Similar to erythema multiforme with prodrome of 1 to 14 days of fever, arthralgia, and myalgia followed by sudden onset of high fever and bullae that may include the respiratory system and gastrointestinal (GI) tract
Toxic epidermal necrolysis	• ETI: Sulfa drugs, anticonvulsants, nonsteroidal anti-inflammatory drugs
	• Pathology: Deadly variant of erythema multiforme with mortality approaching 30%
	• Clinical features: Morbilliform rash that develops into bullae; lesions start on face and descend; other features include elevated liver enzymes, renal failure, electrolyte imbalance, sepsis, shock

BENIGN SKIN LESIONS

Seborrheic keratosis	• Epidemiology: Elderly individuals
	• Clinical features: Round, flat, tan to dark brown, coinlike lesions that occur on head, trunk, and extremities; appear stuck to skin surface
Verrucae (warts)	• ETI: HPV 1 to 4
	• Pathology: HPV infection; papillomatous epidermal hyperplasia and koilocytosis from cytoplasmic vacuolization
	• Clinical features: Verruca vulgaris (hand wart); verruca plana (flat wart)
Keloid	• Epidemiology: Blacks
	• ETI: Trauma to skin
	• Pathology: Abnormal regeneration of connective tissues after trauma
	• Clinical features: Dark, large, raised, irregularly shaped lesions

MALIGNANT SKIN TUMORS

Carcinoma in situ
- ETI: Excessive exposure to sunlight
- Pathology: Epidermal dysplastic changes with accumulation of keratin
- Clinical features: < 1 cm tan-brown, red sandpaper-like lesions; considered premalignant and may progress to squamous cell carcinoma

Actinic keratosis
- ETI: Sun exposure
- Pathology: Intraepithelial neoplasia involving one half of the epithelium; may progress to invasive squamous cell carcinoma

Malignant melanoma
- Epidemiology: Fair-skinned individuals with excessive sunlight exposure
- Pathology: Radial phase of growth (no metastasis); vertical phase (chance of metastasis proportional to depth of invasion)
- Clinical features: Remember A-B-C-D-E: Asymmetric, borders (irregular), color (multicolor), diameter (> 6 mm), elevation (raised)

Basal cell carcinoma
- Epidemiology: Most common skin tumor
- Pathology: Locally aggressive; may cause ulceration and bleeding; microscopy shows palisading nuclei
- Clinical features: Usually on head and neck

Squamous cell carcinoma
- Pathology: Locally invasive; may be preceded by actinic keratosis
- Clinical features: Appears on sun-exposed areas (lower lip, ears, nose)

Kaposi sarcoma
- Epidemiology: AIDS
- ETI: HHV-8
- Clinical features: Red/purple plaques and nodules on skin and mucosa; may affect epithelial lining of lungs, GI tract

PHAKOMATOSES

Neurofibromatosis
- Neurofibromatosis 1 (NF1)
  - ETI: Autosomal dominant mutation of *NF1* on chromosome 17q
  - Pathology: Café-au-lait spots, neurofibromas, axillary or inguinal freckling, Lisch nodules (pigmented iris hamartomas), kyphoscoliosis
- Neurofibromatosis 2 (NF2)
  - ETI: Autosomal dominant mutation of *NF2* on chromosome 22
  - Pathology: Bilateral acoustic neuromas and café-au-lait spots but no other features of NF1

Tuberous sclerosis	• Ash-leaf hypopigmented lesions on trunk and extremities; small, red sebaceous adenomas on face; shagreen patch (rough papule in lumbosacral region); seizures; mental retardation
Sturge-Weber syndrome	• Port-wine stain on face in cranial nerve V distribution; multiple meningeal hemangiomas; seizures; mental retardation

Topic **9**

Endocrine System

Must **Knows**

- Pituitary lesions
- Thyroid and parathyroid lesions
- Adrenal lesions
- Diabetes
- Multiple endocrine neoplasia syndromes

PITUITARY LESIONS

Pituitary adenomas	• Epidemiology: Order of frequency is prolactinoma, growth hormone (GH) adenoma, corticotroph
	• Prolactinoma
	○ Clinical features: Amenorrhea, galactorrhea, decreased libido; the largest of the pituitary adenomas and may cause mass effects resulting in headaches and bitemporal hemianopsia
	○ Diagnosis: Pregnancy, hypothyroidism, hypothalamic lesions, antipsychotic medications
	○ Treatment: bromocriptine
	• GH adenomas
	○ Clinical features: Gigantism (before epiphyseal closure), acromegaly (after closure), glucose intolerance, proximal muscle weakness, hypertension
	• Corticotroph adenomas
	○ Clinical features: Cushing disease (Cushing syndrome caused by excess adrenocorticotropic hormone [ACTH]); hyperpigmentation from excess ACTH

Hypopituitarism	• Clinical features: Amenorrhea, decreased libido, genital atrophy, impotence, loss of pubic and axillary hair, hypoadrenalism, hypothyroidism
	• Sheehan syndrome (postpartum anterior pituitary necrosis)
	○ Pathology: During pregnancy, the anterior pituitary hypertrophies while providing adequate prolactin, but blood supply does not increase. If the mother becomes hypotensive during delivery, the enlarged gland is susceptible to necrosis.
	• Empty sella syndrome
	○ Pathology: Defect in diaphragm sellae; chronic herniation of subarachnoid mater and cerebrospinal fluid; expansion of the sella turcica and compression of the pituitary
Diabetes insipidus	• ETI: Head trauma, neoplasm
	• Clinical features: Polyuria, polydipsia, hypernatremia
	• Diagnosis: Response to DDAVP (1-desamino[8-D-arginine] vasopressin) administration

THYROID AND PARATHYROID LESIONS

Hyperthyroidism	• ETI: Graves' disease, exogenous ingestion, hyperfunctional thyroid, adenoma
	• Clinical features according to system:
	○ General: Heat intolerance, increased appetite, weight loss
	○ Face: Exophthalmos (only in Graves' disease)
	○ Neck: Palpable nodule (adenoma), diffuse enlargement (Graves' disease), dysphagia
	○ Cardiovascular: Palpitation, atrial fibrillation
	○ Gastrointestinal: Diarrhea
	○ Extremities: Pretibial myxedema (Graves' disease)
	○ Neurological: Increased sympathetic outflow (eyelid lag, tremor), irritability, insomnia
	• Diagnosis: Serum thyroid-stimulating hormone (TSH) level, free T_4 levels, iodine uptake
	• Treatment: Propylthiouracil, methimazole; propranolol and iodine for thyroid storm; permanent treatment requires surgery or radioactive iodine
Hypothyroidism	• ETI: Hashimoto disease (women ages 30 to 50 years), iatrogenic (surgery, radiation therapy), iodine deficiency (worldwide; not United States), Li^{2+} therapy for bipolar
	• Clinical features according to system:
	○ General: Cold intolerance, fatigue
	○ Face: Myxedema of the face (puffiness of face and eyelids)
	○ Neck: Diffuse enlargement, dysphagia

- ◦ Cardiovascular: Bradycardia
- ◦ Gastrointestinal: Constipation
- ◦ Extremities: Carpal tunnel syndrome, coarse hair
- ◦ Neurological: Delayed reflexes; may mimic depression
- Diagnosis: Serum TSH
- Treatment: Levothyroxine

Graves' disease	• Epidemiology: Women, HLA-DR3 • ETI: Thyroid-stimulating immunoglobulins (TSIs) • Pathology: Chronic stimulation of thyroid by TSI; diffuse hypertrophy and hyperplasia of thyroid follicles; increased production of T_3/T_4 • Clinical features: Hyperthyroidism, exophthalmos, pretibial myxedema • Diagnosis: TSI, decreased TSH, increased free T_4, increased iodine uptake

Thyroiditis	• **Hashimoto thyroiditis**
	  ◦ ETI: Autoimmune; females more often than males
	  ◦ Pathology: Lymphocytic infiltrate; atrophy of follicles, Hürthle cells
	  ◦ Clinical features: Painless enlargement of thyroid with hypothyroidism; may also have transient periods of hyperthyroidism
	  ◦ Diagnosis: Decreased T_3/T_4, increased TSH, antithyroid peroxidase AB, antithyroglobulin AB
	• Subacute (de Quervain) thyroiditis
	  ◦ ETI: Viral infections such as upper respiratory tract infections, coxsackie
	  ◦ Clinical features: Flulike symptoms, neck pain, and thyroid tenderness; self-limited
	• Riedel thyroiditis
	  ◦ Pathology: Extensive fibrosis of thyroid gland
	  ◦ Clinical features: Hard thyroid that may mimic carcinoma

Neoplasms	• Solitary nodules are more likely neoplastic than multiple nodules • Hot nodules (take up iodine on imaging) are most likely benign
Carcinomas	• Papillary carcinoma: Most common; ground-glass or orphan Annie nuclei; psammoma bodies; prognosis is good • Follicular carcinoma: Frequently presents as cold solitary nodules; not as good prognosis as papillary carcinoma • Medullary carcinoma: Neuroendocrine neoplasms that develop from parafollicular C cells and produce calcitonin; amyloid deposits on biopsy; associated with MEN2A and MEN2B

- Anaplastic carcinoma: Occurs in elderly patients in areas of endemic goiter; Pleomorphic cells, spindle cells, and small anaplastic cells on biopsy; very poor prognosis; one of the most aggressive cancers with death in less than 1 year

Hyperparathyroidism	• Primary hyperparathyroidism
	  ○ ETI: Parathyroid adenoma, parathyroid hyperplasia, bronchogenic squamous cell carcinoma, or renal cell carcinoma (release PTHrP)
	  ○ Clinical features: Hypercalcemia, increased alkaline phosphatase, decreased phosphate
	• Secondary hyperparathyroidism
	  ○ ETI: Renal failure; decreased synthesis of active vitamin D; decreased serum Ca^{2+}; increased parathyroid hormone (PTH)
	  ○ Clinical features: Hypercalcemia, renal failure

Hypoparathyroidism	• ETI: Iatrogenic secondary to excision during thyroidectomy (most common), DiGeorge syndrome • Clinical features: Hypocalcemia

Clinical findings of hypercalcemia	• Painful bones, renal stones, abdominal groans, psychic moans
	• GI: Constipation, dyspepsia, pancreatitis
	• Musculoskeletal:
	  ○ Osteitis fibrosa cystica: Hemorrhage and cystic changes in bone secondary to overactive osteoclastic bone resorption
	  ○ Brown tumors (masses caused by fibrous replacement of resorbed bone)
	• Genitourinary: Nephrolithiasis, polyuria, and polydipsia
	• Neurological: Lethargy, depression, weakness, hypotonia

Clinical findings of hypocalcemia	• Gastrointestinal: Diarrhea • Neurological: Spasms; positive Chvostek's and Trousseau's signs

ADRENAL LESIONS

Hyperadrenalism	• Exogenous steroid hormones (most common) • Cushing disease (pituitary tumor) • Adrenal neoplasm (adenoma more common than carcinoma) • Ectopic production (small cell lung carcinoma)
Diagnosis of hyperadrenalism	• 24-hour urinary cortisol • Dexamethasone suppression test: Administration of dexamethasone will cause suppression of ACTH from pituitary leading to decreased cortisol production. In contrast, hyperadrenalism from exogenous, neoplasm, or ectopic source will not be affected.

Clinical findings of Cushing syndrome	• General: Weight gain, truncal obesity, moon facies, buffalo hump, hirsutism
	• Cardiovascular: Hypertension (HTN)
	• Musculoskeletal: Proximal muscle limb weakness, osteoporosis
	• Dermatological: Thin skin, abdominal striae, acne
	• Genitourinary: Amenorrhea, impotence
	• Endocrine: Hyperglycemia, glucosuria, polydipsia
	• Neurological: Behavioral changes, psychosis
Adrenal insufficiency	• Congenital adrenal hyperplasia: 21-hydroxylase deficiency: Hyponatremia, hyperkalemia, virilization (females), precocious puberty (males)
	• 11-hydroxylase deficiency: Hypernatremia, hypokalemia, HTN
	• Addison disease: Autoimmune adrenalitis, infection (tuberculosis, histoplasma, coccidioides)
Clinical findings of adrenal insufficiency	• Fatigue, weight loss, hypotension, anorexia, nausea, vomiting, diarrhea, hyperpigmentation (only in primary adrenal insufficiency), hyponatremia and hyperkalemia (except for 11-hydroxylase deficiency)
Acute adrenal crisis	• ETI: Precipitated by physiologic stress during chronic insufficiency or failure to conduct a steroid taper in a patient who has been taking steroids for long periods. Also may be caused by Waterhouse-Friderichsen syndrome, which is necrosis of the adrenal glands secondary to N. *meningitides* infection or pituitary apoplexy.
	• Clinical features: Intractable vomiting, abdominal pain, hypotension, loss of consciousness, death
Neoplasms	• Adrenal gland is a common site for metastasis, but primary tumors are uncommon
Hyperaldosteronism	• Primary aldosteronism (Conn syndrome)
	○ ETI: Excessive production of mineralocorticoids secondary to functional adenoma
	○ Clinical features: Hypertension, hypernatremia, hypokalemic metabolic alkalosis, decreased serum renin
	• Secondary aldosteronism
	○ ETI: Congestive heart failure, renal vascular disease
	○ Clinical features: Same as above, but renin levels are elevated
Pheochromocytoma	• Epidemiology: 10% malignant, 10% bilateral, 30% familial
	• Clinical features: HTN, palpations, headaches, diaphoresis, tremors
	• Diagnosis: Increased urinary catecholamines

Neuroblastoma	• Epidemiology: Children younger than age 5 years • Pathology: Malignant tumor; produces catecholamines • Clinical features: Large abdominal mass, HTN • Diagnosis: Increased urinary catecholamines, palpable mass in abdomen, computed tomography scan

DIABETES MELLITUS

Clinical findings of diabetes mellitus (DM)	• Eye: Diabetic retinopathy, cataracts • Cardiovascular: Coronary artery disease, increased risk of myocardial infarction • Gastrointestinal: Gastroparesis, nausea, vomiting, abdominal pain, polydipsia • Genitourinary: Impotence, diabetic nephropathy (Kimmelstiel-Wilson disease), polyuria • Extremities: Peripheral vascular disease, diabetic foot ulcers • Neurological: Peripheral neuropathy
Type 1	• Epidemiology: Onset at or before adolescence • ETI: Autoimmune destruction of pancreatic islets secondary to a combination of genetic predisposition and environmental factors • Pathology: Destruction of pancreatic islets leads to an absolute deficiency of insulin; inability for glucose to enter cells; "starvation in the midst of plenty"; initiation of gluconeogenesis, lipolysis, ketogenesis, ketoacidosis, dehydration, and mental status changes
Type 2	• Epidemiology: Middle age; associated with obesity • ETI: Peripheral insulin resistance • Pathology: Relative deficiency of insulin leads to difficulty for glucose to enter cells; usually does not lead to ketoacidosis; instead, hyperosmolar coma is more common
Other secondary causes of DM	• Hereditary hemochromatosis (bronze diabetes) • Pancreatitis

MULTIPLE ENDOCRINE NEOPLASIA (MEN)

MEN1	• Pituitary, parathyroid, pancreatoma (Zollinger-Ellison, hyperinsulinism)
MEN2A	• Pheochromocytoma, medullary carcinoma, hyperparathyroidism
MEN2B	• Pheochromocytoma, medullary carcinoma, mucocutaneous neuromas (especially gastrointestinal tract)

Topic **10**

Nervous System

Must Knows

- Different types of herniations, hydrocephalus, and hematomas
- Disorders of circulation
- Degenerative diseases
- Demyelinating diseases
- Neoplasia

Herniation	<ul><li>Common ETI includes trauma or mass effects</li><li>Transtentorial (uncinate)<ul><li>Pathology: Compression of medial temporal lobe leads to herniation of tentorium cerebelli, compromise of posterior cerebral artery, and ischemia</li><li>Clinical features: Compression of cranial nerve (CN) III causes pupillary dilation and occulomotor palsy</li></ul></li><li>Subfalcine<ul><li>Pathology: Asymmetric expansion of cerebral hemisphere leads to displacement of cingulated gyrus under falyx cerebri and compromise of anterior cerebral artery branches</li></ul></li><li>Tonsillar<ul><li>ETI: Displacement of cerebellar tonsils through foramen magnum leads to brain stem compression</li><li>Clinical features: Decreased respiratory rate and compromise of the basilar arteries causing median and paramedian ischemia and infarction</li></ul></li></ul>
Hydrocephalus	<ul><li>Communicating: Enlargement of entire ventricular system secondary to an obstruction outside the system, usually in the subarachnoid space or arachnoid granulations</li><li>Noncommunicating: Local enlargement of one or more ventricles secondary to obstruction within the ventricular system</li><li>Hydrocephalus ex vacuo: Dilation of the ventricles secondary to atrophy of parenchyma</li></ul>

Hematoma	• Epidural hematoma
	○ ETI: Often from trauma to the temporoparietal area
	○ Pathology: Damage to middle meningeal artery leads to hemorrhage of blood into the epidural space, separation of dura from the calvarium, mass effects, increased intracranial pressure (ICP), ischemia, herniation, and death
	○ Clinical features: Lucid intervals, unconsciousness
	• Subdural hematoma
	○ ETI: Falls, assaults
	○ Pathology: Impact causes shearing effect on bridging veins in the subdural space leads to hemorrhage; may stop, continue to enlarge, or be reabsorbed
	○ Clinical features: Headache, seizures, mental status changes, motor weakness

DISORDERS OF CIRCULATION

Ischemia and infarction	• Ischemia: May be global from decreased perfusion causing watershed infarcts and laminar necrosis (caused by decreased perfusion pressure to deep cortical structures); may be regional from atherosclerosis
	• Infarction: Embolization leads to abrupt infarct, necrosis of ischemic region and vessels. and thrombosis; occurs gradually
Cerebral hemorrhage	• Intracerebral hemorrhage
	○ ETI: Most commonly hypertension
	○ Pathology: Hypertension leading to lipohyalinosis of vessel walls, weakening, Charcot-Bouchard aneurysms (fusiform shaped aneurysms located at vessel trunk), and rupture
	○ Clinical features: Most often occurs in basal ganglia and thalamus
	• Subarachnoid hemorrhage
	○ ETI: Two thirds from rupture of preexisting aneurysm; 10% from arteriovenous malformation and trauma
	○ Clinical features: Sudden onset; "worst headache in life"
Berry aneurysms	• Pathology: Saccular aneurysms that occur at branch points; lead to rupture as subarachnoid, intracerebral, or intraventricular hemorrhages
	• Clinical features: Sudden severe headache, mental status changes, death

DEGENERATIVE DISEASES

Alzheimer's disease	• Epidemiology: Most common cause of dementia in elderly individuals

- ETI: Abnormal amyloid protein (chromosome 21), loss of choline acetyltransferase, apoprotein E-ϵ_4
  - Pathology: Deposits of amyloid β-protein form neuronal plaques
  - Neurofibrillary tangles from microtubules and neurofilaments
  - Granulovacuolar degeneration in pyramidal cells of hippocampus
  - Global cerebral atrophy with dilated ventricles
- Clinical features: Gradual dementia, behavioral changes, aphasia
- Treatment: Acetylcholinesterase inhibitors

Pick disease	• Epidemiology: More frequent in women • Pathology: Cortical atrophy in frontal and temporal lobes; Pick bodies seen in neurons (round intracytoplasmic inclusion bodies) • Clinical features: Similar to Alzheimer's disease
Parkinson's disease	• Epidemiology: Frequency is 2% of American population • Pathology: Loss of dopaminergic neurons in the basal ganglia (specifically the substantia nigra); morphologic changes include depigmentation of the substantia nigra and locus ceruleus and development of Lewy bodies (eosinophilic intracytoplasmic inclusion bodies) • Clinical features: Masklike facies, pill rolling tremor, cog wheel rigidity, shuffling gait, bradykinesia • Treatment: Levodopa and carbidopa, amantadine
Huntington's disease	• ETI: Autosomal dominant; caused by trinucleotide expansion on chromosome 4 • Pathology: Atrophy of caudate nucleus, putamen, and frontal cortex leads to choreiform movements and behavioral changes • Clinical features: Chorea, athetosis, aggressive and disinhibited behavior, dementia, and death
Amyotrophic lateral sclerosis	• Pathology: Degeneration of upper (ventral motor neurons) and lower motor neurons • Clinical features: Lower motor neuron signs (atrophy, fasciculations, weakness) and upper motor neuron signs (hyperreflexia, spasticity) leading to respiratory failure and death
Multi-infarct dementia	• Epidemiology: Second most common cause of dementia • Pathology: Diffuse cerebral atherosclerosis • Clinical features: Acute stepwise progression of deficits and decreased neurologic function

DEMYELINATING DISEASES

Multiple sclerosis (MS)	• Epidemiology: Female:male = 2:1; mean age at diagnosis is 30 years; more common in colder climates, with increased incidence with increased distance from equator • ETI: Autoimmune associated with HLA-DR2 • Pathology: T cells attack central nervous system (CNS) myelin; leads to plaque development, gliosis, and dysfunction of denuded axons • Clinical features: Onset in the third to fourth decade of life, blurred vision, double vision, internuclear ophthalmoplegia, vertigo, weakness in one or both legs, numbness in extremities; clinical features may follow a chronic relapsing and remitting course • Diagnosis: Oligoclonal bands in cerebrospinal fluid (CSF), magnetic resonance imaging of plagues
Guillain-Barré syndrome	• ETI: Autoimmune, after infectious (viral upper respiratory tract infection, *Campylobacter jejuni*) • Pathology: Acute ascending inflammatory demyelinating peripheral neuropathy • Clinical features: Ascending muscle weakness and paralysis leading to respiratory paralysis and death • Diagnosis: Albuminocytologic dissociation in CSF (increased protein; no hypercellularity)
Acute disseminated encephalomyelitis (ADEM)	• ETI: Autoimmune and follows infection (mumps, measles, rubella [MMR], varicella) • Pathology: Widespread CNS demyelination similar to MS • Diagnosis: Oligoclonal bands in CSF, MRI

NEOPLASIA

Metastatic tumors	• Most common CNS tumor • Usually seeds in grey-white junction from primary sites: Lung, breast, skin, gastrointestinal tract, kidneys
Glioblastoma multiforme	• Epidemiology: Most common adult primary intracranial tumor; also the most deadly • Pathology: Highly anaplastic astrocytoma with endothelial cell proliferation causing areas of necrosis and hemorrhage; may cross the corpus callosum and become bilateral ("butterfly lesion"); death occurs within 1 year
Oligodendroglioma	• Pathology: Arises in white matter of cerebral hemispheres; slow growth without necrosis; cells have clear halo of cytoplasm resembling "fried eggs" • Clinical features: Seizures, increased ICP; survival is 6 to 10 years

Ependymoma	• Pathology: Most common in fourth ventricle; obstruction; non-communicating hydrocephalus; slow growth; may seed arachnoid space and cause spinal cord tumors; survival is 4 to 5 years after surgery
Medulloblastoma	• Epidemiology: Most common intracranial neuroblastic tumor; occurs in first decade of life • Pathology: Emerges from cerebellum as highly malignant and aggressive; appears as sheets of closely packed cells; may disseminate through CSF; 5-year survival after surgery and chemotherapy is 75%
Meningioma	• Epidemiology: Second most common primary intracranial tumor • Pathology: Originates from arachnoid villi and is slow growing and well circumscribed; occurs in parasagittal areas, cerebral hemisphere convexities, olfactory groove, and lateral wing of sphenoid; appears as whorled pattern of meningothelial cells with psammoma bodies • Clinical features: Seizures, anosmia, visual changes, CN palsies • Treatment: Surgery curative in 96% cases; 4% are malignant
Acoustic neuromas (schwannomas) (Fig. IV-9)	• Epidemiology: Third most common primary intracranial tumor; bilateral in NF2

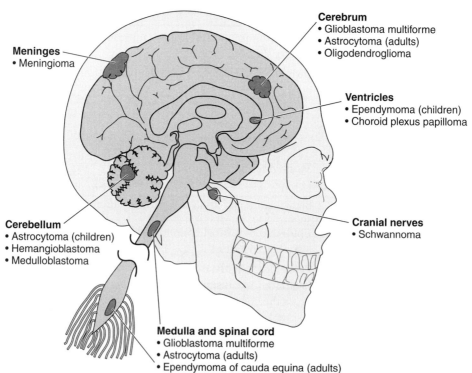

● **Figure IV-9** Anatomic predilection of many brain tumors. All brain tumors are malignant except for meningiomas and schwannomas.

- Pathology: Arises from sheath of CN VIII: unilateral hearing loss and tinnitus, enlargement of meatus and extension into the subarachnoid space and cerebellopontine angle; compression of CN V and VII, brainstem, cerebellum leads to hydrocephalus and tonsillar herniation
- Clinical features: Early as hearing loss, tinnitus, vertigo; late as compromise of brain stem function and death

Microbiology/Immunology

10 Top Tips

Microbiology/Immunology

Topic	Main Focus	USMLE Example
1 Basic Properties of Bacteria and Viruses	Bacteria are classified by morphology, staining, O_2 susceptibility, enzyme reactions; viruses are classified by morphology, tropism, and genome	• A sexually active 16-year-old adolescent presents with acute liver disease. Hepatitis B is suspected. This enveloped virus is defined by a circular dsDNA that requires a viral-coded reverse transcriptase to replicate because viral DNA is synthesized on an RNA template.
2 Microbial Genetics	Bacterial reproduce asexually, but DNA can be transferred (e.g., transformation). Viruses are intracellular parasites with genomes of RNA or DNA.	• A 48-year-old AIDS patient who became infected with a multidrug-resistant strain of *Mycobacterium tuberculosis* is dying because this strain possesses resistant genes against isoniazid, rifamycin, and streptomycin, the standard therapeutic agents.
3 Respiratory Tract Infections	Most upper respiratory tract infections (URIs) are caused by viruses. Bacterial pathogens must be differentiated from normal flora. Tuberculosis (TB) and pneumonias are major lower respiratory infections (LRIs).	• A 10-year-old child who complains of a sore throat is brought to the pediatrician. Although most URIs are caused by viruses (e.g., RSV, adenoviruses, rhinoviruses), the doctor must rule out group A *Streptococcus,* a dangerous pathogen that has potential autoimmune sequelae.
4 Gastrointestinal Infections	Gastroenteritis and nosocomial infections are major disease syndromes.	• On a trip to the Caribbean, a 22-year-old student was incapacitated with diarrhea 12 hours after drinking fresh coconut milk. *Escherichia coli* was isolated that

(Continued)

10 Top Tips

Microbiology/Immunology   *(Continued)*

Topic	Main Focus	USMLE Example
		was found to secrete a heat-labile A-B exotoxin.
5 Urogenital Tract Infections	Fecal contamination and nosocomial infection via catheterization are major causes of urinary tract infections (UTIs).	• Cystitis in a 42-year-old woman who had a hysterectomy 1 week ago is most likely to be attributable to infection with *E. coli* as a result of catheterization during surgery.
6 Central Nervous System, Cardiovascular, Ear, and Eye Infections	Infections of these organs are frequently caused by opportunistic organisms in compromised hosts.	• A 6-month-old infant is rushed to the emergency department with a highly fulminant meningitis. A lumbar puncture is performed to obtain cerebrospinal fluid to test for *Streptococcus pneumoniae*, *Neisseria meningitis,* and *Haemophilus influenzae,* which cause meningitis in this age group.
7 Definition of the Immune System	Each component of the immune systems has evolved specifically to address unique and distinct threats.	• A 17-year-old girl presents with signs of septic shock caused by an enterotoxin-bearing *Staphylococcus aureus* (toxic shock). This condition results when massive amounts of shock-inducing cytokines are released when this superantigen binds to multiple clones of T cells at a site independent of the antigen-specific receptor site.
8 Innate and Humoral Immunity	Innate immunity is nonspecific and does not require host adaptation. Humoral immunity involves antigen-presenting cells (APCs) and T-cell activation of B-cell antibody production.	• A 7-month-old boy presenting with recurrent pyogenic infections was found to have no tonsils, B cells, or lymph node germinal centers in the presence of normal T cells and thymus. Bone marrow studies reveal a developmental defect characterized by the loss of a tyrosine kinase gene during the transition of pre-B to B cells. The child was referred to an experimental gene therapy program.
9 Cell-Mediated Immunity	Cell-directed inflammation and cytotoxic	• A 32 year-old homeless man with a chronic cough and a cavitary lung lesion

(Continued)

10 Top Tips

Microbiology/Immunology   *(Continued)*

Topic	Main Focus	USMLE Example
	killing is used to fight infection.	had sputum positive for *Mycobacterium tuberculosis*. Cell-mediated immunity, which results in granuloma formation, is the principal host defense for TB.
10 **Disorders of the Immune System**	Lesions to distinct components of the immune system result in unique patterns of humoral immunity and cell-mediated immunity disorders.	• A 35-year-old man who was diagnosed with HIV 6 years ago has a CD 4 count of 150 cells/μ and clinical *Pneumocystis carinii*. His sexual partner, who has never tested positive for HIV, lacks an obligatory viral co-receptor, a CXCR 4 chemokine, required for fusion of the virus into the T cell.

Topic **1**

Basic Properties of Bacteria and Viruses

Must Knows

- Bacterial structure
- Basic bacterial characteristics
- Viral organization

BACTERIAL STRUCTURE

Basics	• Prokaryotes; possess no organelles; no membrane-bound nucleus; most reproduce by binary fission
Cell wall	• Gram positive: Approximately 50% peptidoglycan, teichoic and teichuronic acids, polysaccharides
	• Gram negative: Approximately 2% to 10% peptidoglycan, lipoprotein, and an outer phospholipid membrane of lipopolysaccharide (LPS)
	• LPS: Endotoxin; lipid A is the toxic moiety
	• Peptidoglycan: A site of action for antibiotics (e.g., penicillin, cephalosporins)
Virulence factors	• Several pathogens possess capsules (i.e., *Streptococcus pneumoniae*, *Haemophilus influenzae*), which protect from phagocytosis; antibodies against the capsule are protective
	• Glycocalyx slime layer: Facilitates adherence
	• Spores: Resistant to boiling or freezing; killed by autoclaving

BACTERIAL CHARACTERISTICS

Antimicrobial chemotherapy	• Antimetabolites: Sulfonamides, trimethoprim, isoniazid
	• Inhibitors of cell wall biosynthesis: Penicillins, cephalosporins, vancomycin
	• Inhibitors of protein biosynthesis: Streptomycin, tetracycline, erythromycin, clindamycin
	• Inhibitors of nucleic acid synthesis: Quinolones, novobiocin, rifampin

Chemical disinfectants	• Agents are compared with phenol (phenol coefficient), which compares the rate of the minimal sterilizing concentration of phenol to that of a test compound • Examples: Ethylene oxide, an alkylating agent useful for sterilizing hospital instruments; iodine is an oxidizing agent, bactericidal in a 2% KI aqueous solution; alcohol, isopropyl alcohol at 90% to 95%
Bacteria expressing A-B type toxins	• *Corynebacteria diphtheriae, Pseudomonas aeruginosa, Shigella dysenteriae, Vibrio cholerae, Escherichia coli, Campylobacter jejuni, Bordetella pertussis, Clostridium tetani, Clostridium botulinum*
Bacteria expressing single polypeptide toxins	• *Clostridium perfringens* (phospholipase C enzyme), *Escherichia coli* (activates guanylate cyclase), *Salmonella* sp. (activates cyclic AMP), *Staphylococcus aureus* (exfoliative epidermal toxin), *Streptococcus pyogenes* (erythrogenic and pyrogenic toxins)
Distinguishing bacterial species	• Biochemical reactions, susceptibility to O_2, enzyme content, hemolysis, nuclear probe analysis, growth on selective media, cell wall type

VIRAL ORGANIZATION

Basics	• Obligate intracellular parasites • Classified into 21 families based on morphology, DNA content, single or double stranded, +/− sense RNA, transmission, trophism, pathology, and whether enveloped • Inclusion bodies aid in identification of certain viral infections • Virion is the infective unit
DNA viruses	• Contain dsDNA and icosahedral capsules; intranuclear replication • Capsid protein coat is composed of capsomeres; this protein coat determines host specificity, binding to specific host receptors, antigenicity, and protects nucleic acids from host nucleases • DNA virus families: Adenoviruses, hepadnaviruses, herpesviruses, papovaviruses, parvoviruses, poxviruses; the later two replicate in the cytoplasm via ssDNA
RNA viruses	• Possess ssRNA (except for dsRNA reoviruses); are naked or enveloped; can possess a helical or icosahedral capsid • They replicate in the cytoplasm except for orthomyxoviruses and retroviruses, which have both a cytoplasmic and nuclear phase • RNA virus families: Arboviruses, arenaviruses, astroviruses, bunayaviruses, caliciviruses, coronaviruses, filoviruses, flaviviruses, orthomyxoviruses, paramyxoviruses, picornaviruses, reoviruses, retroviruses, rhabdoviruses, togaviruses

Bacteriophage	• Viruses that infect bacteria; contain protein and RNA or DNA
	• Lysogenic phage conversion: A change in bacterial phenotype as a result of limited expression of genes by a temperate prophage; responsible for multiple serological changes in *Salmonella* sp. polysaccharides; also the genetic mechanism by which nontoxigenic strains of *C. diphtheriae* and *C. botulinum* types C and D are converted to toxin-producing strains
Prions	• Infectious proteins devoid of nucleic acid; associated with certain central nervous system (CNS) diseases (e.g., Creutzfeldt-Jakob disease, kuru, bovine spongiform encephalopathy [BSE])
	• Mimic normal host protein but with an altered folding pattern that can change the conformation of its normal counterpart
Viral infection	• Infection triggers secretion of interferons α, β, and γ
	• α and β inhibit viral replication by inducing antiviral proteins in infected cells, which destroy viral mRNA and protect healthy cells
	• γ does so weakly, but is a potent activator of phagocytic cells
Viral vaccines	• Live vaccines use attenuated strains and include measles, mumps, rubella, chickenpox, Sabin polio, yellow fever, and adenovirus
	• Killed vaccines use heat or chemically inactivated viruses and include Salk polio, rabies, influenza, and hepatitis A; hepatitis B virus vaccine uses a recombinant subunit

Topic **2**

Microbial Genetics

Must Knows

● Gene transfer between bacteria

● Bacterial gene expression

● Viral replication process

BACTERIAL GENETICS

Basics	• Most genes are haploid and carried on a single, circular chromosome; specialized genes may be carried on plasmids

- Transposons: Short DNA sequences that cannot replicate; possess insertion sequences and can insert genetic information into other genetic elements; and code for antibiotic resistance and toxins
- Replicons: Circular dsDNA sequences capable of self-replication

Gene transfer (Fig. V-1)

- Results in acquisition of new characteristics; causes serology (antigenic) changes; transfer of toxins to nontoxigenic strains, a major problem in antibiotic resistance
- Conjugation: One-way transfer of DNA plasmids (F pilus) from donor to recipient by physical contact; three plasmid types involved:
  - Fertility cell (F+) transfers a fertility factor to an Hfr donor via a sex pilus, which inserts it into its chromosome, thus transferring the F+ plasmid trait to the F− cell
  - R factors contain genes conferring drug resistance, usually carried on transposons
  - F′ and R′ plasmids are recombinant fertility or resistance plasmids in which limited regions of chromosomal DNA can be replicated and transferred independent of the chromosome

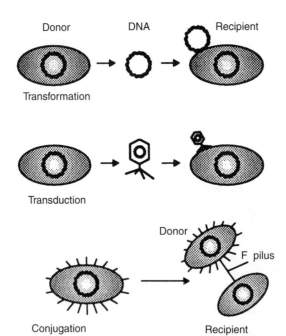

● **Figure V-1** Three major mechanisms of genetic transfer in bacteria. In *transformation,* naked DNA is taken up directly by the recipient cell. During *transduction,* host DNA is transferred attached to viral DNA via bacteriophage. In *conjugation,* donor DNA is transferred via a conjugative plasmid (F pilus) to a recipient cell by physical contact. (Adapted with permission from Atlas RM: *Microbiology: Fundamentals and Application,* 2nd ed. New York, Macmillan, 1988, p. 215.)

- Transduction: Mediated by bacteriophages, occurs when host DNA is packaged in a bacteriophage coat and another bacterium is infected (generalized transduction), no phage genes are transferred

- Transformation: Direct uptake and recombination of naked DNA fragments through the cell wall by competent bacteria

Gene expression	- Transcription: Mediated by RNA polymerase; initiated by binding of σ factor (a subunit of RNA polymerase) to promoter region; involves DNA unwinding, alignment of complementary ribonucleotide bases onto the template from 5′ to 3′
	
	- Translation: Occurs at ribosomes by tRNA-mediated linkage of amino acids to the transcript and assembly of a polypeptide chain
	
	- Negative control: Inhibits transcription by binding of a repressor
	   ○ Example: *lac* operon controls expression of three genes for lactose metabolism via a repressor protein; *trp* operon controls tryptophan synthesis by the binding of a repressor protein to the trp operator, halting tryptophan synthesis when in excess
	
	- Positive control: Transcription initiation in response to binding of an activator protein
	   ○ Example: Expression of the *ara* operon proceeds when arabinose binds to a special protein, forming an activator compound necessary for transcription of the *ara* operon.

VIRAL GENETICS

Viral replication	- Similar for all viruses in a family; has a sequential pattern that includes attachment, penetration, uncoating of the genome, synthesis of early proteins involved in genome replication, synthesis of structural components, assembly, and release - One-step multiplication curves show that viruses have an eclipse period (i.e., time from start of infection to detection of intracellular virus)
DNA viruses	- Transcription is intranuclear by host-cell proteins; DNA-dependent RNA polymerases (except for pox viruses) yields transcripts with polyA tail and methylated cap added before translation; may be followed by posttranscriptional processing; translation is followed by transport of synthesized proteins to the nucleus - Genome replication is semiconservative, performed by a DNA-dependent DNA polymerase after synthesis of early proteins - Assembly occurs in the nucleus (except for pox viruses); if inefficient, leads to formation of inclusion bodies
RNA viruses	- Genome ss or dsRNA, segmented or nonsegmented; it can be positive-sense polarity (if ss) and act as mRNA (picornaviruses and retroviruses); it may be negative-sense polarity and comple-

mentary to mRNA (orthomyxoviruses and paramyxoviruses), or it may be ambisense with messenger- and anti-messenger polarity

- Transcription involves RNA-dependent RNA polymerase for all viruses (except retroviruses; they use host-cell, DNA-dependent RNA polymerase); it involves a virion-associated transcriptase for negative sense viruses; it occurs on cytoplasmic polysomes

- Cytoplasmic genome replication (not retro- or orthomyxoviruses) occurs via a viral-specific replicase (except for retroviruses, which have a reverse transcriptase and replicate in the nucleus, and orthomyxoviruses)

Genetic shifts	• Occurs if similar segments from two different strains of a segmented virus replicate independently from the parent, producing a virus with different antigenicity and infectivity (e.g., influenza A virus epidemics)

Topic **3**

Respiratory Tract Infections

Must **Knows**

- ● Organisms involved
- ● Pathogenic mechanisms

UPPER RESPIRATORY TRACT INFECTIONS

***Streptococcus pyogenes* (group A)**	• Classified into 21 Lancefield groups by differences in cell wall carbohydrates; also classified according to hemolysis of erythrocytes:
	○ α-Hemolysis: Incomplete lysis on blood agar with green pigment surrounding colony
	○ β-Hemolysis: Total lysis and release of hemoglobin; leaves a clear area around the colony
	○ γ-Hemolysis: Absence of lysis
	• Cause cellulitis, pharyngitis, scarlet fever, and rheumatic fever
	• Attach to epithelial surfaces via the lipoteichoic acid portion of fimbriae (pili)

- Secrete three types of erythrogenic exotoxins that require lysogenic phages for production
- Exotoxins cause rash in scarlet fever and are superantigens; also produce two leukocidal hemolysins, streptolysin S (responsible for β hemolysis) and streptolysin O (an O_2 sensitive protein)
- Pathogenicity is aided by (1) M proteins, potent virulence factors found on fimbriae, which interfere with phagocytosis, and (2) an antiphagocytic hyaluronic acid capsule
- Differentiated from normal oral flora and other *Streptococci* sp. by culture, specific antisera, and bacitracin sensitivity; are catalase negative in contrast to *Staphylococci*
- Resistance to penicillin is rare

Haemophilus influenzae

- Colonizes upper respiratory tract, requires hemin (X) and nicotinamide-adenine denucleotide NAD (V) as growth factors; polyribitol phosphate capsule inhibits phagocytosis, aiding colonization
- Anticapsular antibody provides protection from invasive disease; IgA protease facilitates colonization
- Non-encapsulated strains are normal upper respiratory tract flora but can cause sinusitis, bronchitis, and otitis media; the second most common cause of bacterial pneumonia, particularly in individuals with chronic obstructive pulmonary disease
- Vaccination of children reduces the incidence of type B invasive disease and resulting meningitis

LOWER RESPIRATORY TRACT INFECTIONS

Streptococcus pneumoniae

- Normal oropharyngeal flora in 40% to 70% of individuals; they are gram-postive, α hemolytic, lancet-shaped diplococci that possess a group-specific carbohydrate common to all pneumococci; it can precipitate C-reactive protein, a test to determine the extent of an inflammation
- Possess a type specific polysaccharide capsule with more than 80 different T-cell–independent antigenic types
- Disease is identified by culture of lung sputum (not saliva); typing is done by Quellung reaction: a swelling of the capsule in the presence of type specific antiserum; virulence is attributable to the antiphagocytic action of the capsule
- Must be distinguished from nonpathogenic *S. viridans* which is also a gram-positive, α-hemolytic diplococcus. *S. pneumoniae* can be differentiated by its sensitivity to Optochin and bile.
- Pathogenicity is associated with disturbances of normal defense, especially in infants, elderly individuals, those with immunosuppression, and alcoholics
- Vaccine containing about 23 type specific polysaccharides is available

Mycoplasma pneumoniae	• Smallest of the bacteria, lack a cell wall, require cholesterol
	• Attach to mucosal cells by the P1 protein.
	• Causes primary atypical pneumonia, characterized by a severe, hacking cough, and fever, followed by interstitial or broncho-pneumonia; is the most common cause of pneumonia from age 5 to 15 years
	• Culture on special media reveals tiny colonies with "fried egg" appearance; can then be defined by polymerase chain reaction
Legionella pneumophila	• An intracellular parasite; causes a fibrinopurulent pneumonia, acquired by inhalation from environmental sources (usually aquatic or air conditioners); infection peaks from July to October; common in smokers and those with chronic lung disease
	• Stains well only with Dieterle's silver stain
	• Requires cysteine and Fe for growth; often diagnosed by direct fluorescent antibody staining
	• Treatment is with erythromycin
Mycobacterium tuberculosis	• Acid-fast bacillus; cell wall contains mycolic acids; cord factor (trehalose mycolate) is the major virulence factor that disrupts mitochondrial membranes, inhibits neutrophil migration, and is associated with granuloma formation; sulfatides potentiate toxicity and promote intracellular survival by inhibiting phagosome–lysosome fusion and superoxide formation
	• Primary tuberculosis (TB): Organisms reside and replicate in phagocytic cells of the lungs, leading to granuloma formation
	• Secondary TB: Occurs with reinfection or reactivation of primary TB by granuloma erosion
	• Diagnosis by microscopy: red, acid-fast bacteria in sputum, confirmation by the Ziehl-Neelsen stain
	• Skin test with purified protein derivative (PPD) of M. tuberculosis indicates exposure, not necessarily current disease; induration of > 15 mm is considered a positive test result in those with unknown background
	• Isoniazid is given as prophylaxis; treatment may consist of isoniazid, rifampin, pyrazinamide and ethambutol given for 2 months followed by 4 months of isoniazid and rifampin; multidrug-resistant strains are emerging
Bordetella pertussis	• Small gram-negative aerobic bacillus; causes whooping cough
	• Possesses three toxins: Pertussis toxin (A-B type) causes local tissue damage with inflammation; hemagglutinins for attachment to cilia; an undefined cough toxin is active neurologically
	• During the catarrhal stage, the organism is confined to the upper respiratory tract; with the paroxysmal stage, it extends to the lower tract, causing severe cough and breathing difficulties leading to anoxia and vomiting; pneumonia can last 1 to 6 weeks during the convalescent period

	• DTaP (diphtheria, tetanus, and pertussis) vaccine includes acellular pertussis filamentous hemagglutinin and pertussis toxoid; its protective activity wanes
Bacillus anthracis	• Causes pulmonary anthrax; results from spore entry into the lungs
	• Pathogenicity is attributable to an antiphagocytic polypeptide consisting of protective antigen, lethal factor, and edema factor; the latter is a calmodulin-activated adenylate cyclase
	• Infection is characterized by high fever, malaise, cough, myalgias, and hemorrhagic necrosis of lymph nodes. The fatality rate is 50%. A cutaneous form of less severity exists.
Influenza viruses	• Classified into types A, B, and C depending on a nucleocapsid antigen; can undergo gene reassortment because of segmented genome
	• Type A major antigens are hemagglutinin (H) and neuraminidase (N). H antigen undergoes frequent minor mutations yielding antigenic drift. Major antigenic shifts (subtypes) result in epidemics after reassortment between the H-coding RNA segments of animal or human viruses. Greater variation is seen in the A strain than the B strain.
	• N antigen is involved in the release of virions from infected cells. It can undergo antigenic shift, but epidemics do not result.
	• Attenuated vaccine contains 2 types of A and 1 type B strain
	• Secondary bacterial pneumonia is a major complication
Respiratory syncytial viruses	• Are the major cause of serious bronchiolitis and pneumonia in infants
	• Characterized by a syncytial effect (cell fusion) in infected cells

Topic **4**

Gastrointestinal Infections

Must **Knows**

● Basic properties of Enterobacteriaceae

● Mechanisms of exotoxins and endotoxins

● Major bacteria involved

● Major viruses involved

ENTEROBACTERIACEAE

Basics
- Composed of hundreds of species that exchange plasmids and DNA, resulting in new antigens and serologic strains
- Gram-negative rods; cause nosocomial and gastrointestinal (GI) infections
- Differentiated according to genera and species by antisera, biochemical reactions, and growth on selective media
- Do not ferment lactose (except *Escherichia coli*); differentiates them from other bacterial GI pathogens
- Nosocomial infections are common, preceded by events introducing organisms (e.g., catheterization, contaminated IV fluids, or surgery), followed in 1 to 2 days by a triad of chills, fever, and hypotension
- GI infection by *Enterobacteriaceae* sp. must be distinguished from those caused by *Staphylococcus* sp. The latter have a shorter incubation period (6 hours vs. 1 to 2 days) and are treated with different antibiotics.

Virulence factors
- Some species (e.g., *Escherichia coli* and *V. cholerae*) secrete heat labile and heat stable A-B exotoxins transmissible by plasmids
- B subunit binds the Gm_1 ganglioside at the epithelial cell brush border of the small intestine, facilitating entrance of subunit A
- Subunit A of heat labile toxin activates adenylate cyclase, increasing cyclic adenosine monophosphate (cAMP) and triggering hypersecretion of H_2O and Cl^- and inhibiting Na^+ reabsorption; the gut lumen becomes distended with fluid, causing hypermotility and diarrhea
- Heat stable toxin activates guanylate cyclase and increases cyclic guanosine monophosphate (cGMP) in epithelial cells, causing a similar syndrome
- Endotoxic lipopolysaccharide (LPS): In the outer membrane, has a common toxic lipid core causing hypotension, shock, fever, hemorrhage and disseminated intravascular coagulation (DIC); triggers systemic release of cytokines interleukin-1 (IL-1), IL-6, *tumor necrosis factor-α* (*TNF-α*), and interferon-γ to induce the syndrome

BACTERIA INVOLVED

Staphylococcus aureus
- β-Hemolytic, catalase (+) coccus; found in the oropharynx and on skin, spread to food from the nares or cutaneous lesions of food preparers
- Produces heat stable enterotoxins in poorly refrigerated high-protein foods
- Infection involves rapid onset nausea, GI pain, vomiting, diarrhea; symptoms resolve quickly, and no treatment is usually necessary

Salmonella sp.	• Can possess both an endotoxin and exotoxin causing the same symptoms as *E coli* infection • Food poisoning is the most common form of *Salmonella* infection caused mainly by *S. typhimurium* and *S. enteritidis* • Sources include poultry products, human carriers, and exotic pets

Shigella sp.	• Categorized into four groups:
	  ○ *Sh. sonnei:* Most common cause of shigellosis, an acute inflammation of the wall of the large intestine
	  ○ *Sh. flexneri:* Also common in the United States
	  ○ *Sh. dysenteriae:* Infections require antibiotics; secretes a potent heat labile A-B exotoxin causing diarrhea and neurotoxicity
	  ○ *Sh. boydii:* Rarely found in the United States

Escherichia coli	• Four strains cause diarrhea:
	  ○ Enteropathogenic: Infects infants and children; is nontoxigenic and adheres to erythrocytes; damages villi
	  ○ Enterohemorrhagic: Transmitted in undercooked meats with cattle as the main reservoir; dominant serotype is 0157-H7 that secretes *Shigella*-like A-B toxin
	  ○ Enteroinvasive: Causes bloody diarrhea in children, rare in the United States
	  ○ Enterotoxigenic: Transmitted by contaminated food and H_2O; secretes heat labile and heat stable A-B exotoxins; similar to *Vibrio cholerae* toxin, it catalyzes adenosine diphosphate (ADP) ribosylation, increasing adenylate cyclase activity and cAMP, causing watery diarrhea

Vibrio cholerae	• Illness results from prototypic A-B exotoxin (choleragen) • Infection is secondary to ingestion of food or H_2O contaminated by this gram-negative, comma-shaped rod • Abrupt-onset intense vomiting and diarrhea are key findings; copious fluid loss via rice-water stools leads to rapid metabolic acidosis and hypovolemic shock; prompt replacement of fluids and electrolytes negates symptoms
Clostridium botulinum	• Gram-positive, spore-forming, anaerobic rod; produces a potent exotoxin that causes flaccid paralysis via suppression of acetylcholine (ACh) release from peripheral nerve axon terminals; toxin can be detected by injection of the food sample into mice • Food poisoning results from ingestion of preformed toxin • Clinical findings include nausea, vomiting, dizziness, cranial nerve palsies, double vision, swallowing and speech problems, muscle weakness, respiratory paralysis, and death in 20% of cases. Antitoxin given early is protective; antibiotics are ineffective. Heat inactivates the toxin, but spores are resistant.

- Intestinal (infant) botulism occurs after spore ingestion and germination in the GI tract; exotoxin disseminates, causing constipation, generalized weakness, loss of head and limb control; only supportive measures are needed; honey is the classic source

Clostridium difficile	• Gram-positive, spore-forming anaerobic rod; often normal GI flora • Many strains are resistant to antibiotics; antibiotics when used for other infections kill gut organisms that normally restrict *C. difficile* growth, resulting in its overgrowth • Produces enterotoxin that causes pseudomembranous colitis and a cytotoxin that kills mucosal cells
Campylobacter jejuni	• A microaerophilic, flagellated, curved rod with a "seagull's wings" appearance; causes an acute, bloody enteritis • Transmitted by poultry products, milk, and via dogs • Can be isolated on special Campy agar at 42°C
Helicobacter pylori	• A microaerophilic, gram-negative, curved rod that invades tissues and causes ulcers, gastritis, and gastric carcinoma • Transmission primarily by fecal–oral route • Produces urease to neutralize stomach HCl; adheres to fucose-containing blood group receptors on gut epithelium
Bacteroides fragilis	• Encapsulated, gram-positive, pleomorphic, anaerobic rod; involved in polymicrobic infections. It is a foul-smelling, frequent cause of GI abscesses after damage to mucosal barriers, possesses a β lactamase.

VIRUSES INVOLVED

Rotavirus	• dsRNA naked viruses; the most common cause of a nosocomial-induced gastroenteritis in children
Norwalk virus	• (+) sense ssRNA virus with an icosahedral nucleocapsid; causes epidemic gastroenteritis; transmission is via food, it cannot be grown in tissue culture
Echoviruses	• (+) sense ssRNA viruses that infect the small intestine; can also cause common colds, fevers, aseptic meningitis, and conjunctivitis
Hepatitis B virus	• Circular dsDNA hepadnavirus that causes liver disease; serum hepatitis is implicated in hepatocellular carcinoma • It requires a viral-coded reverse transcriptase in order to replicate as the virion DNA (the DANE particle) is synthesized from an RNA template • Diagnosis and prognosis are aided by enzyme-linked immunosorbent assay (ELISA) testing for hepatitis B surface antigen (HBsAg) and core-associated antigens (hepatitis E antigen [HBeAg], hepatitis C antigen [HBcAg])

Topic **5**

Urogenital Tract Infections

Must **Knows**

- Organisms involved
- Pathogenic mechanisms

ORGANISMS INVOLVED

Escherichia coli	• The most common causative organism, the main source being one's own fecal flora; it adheres to the urethral mucosa via pili, with inflammation being induced by lipopolysaccharide (LPS) • Cystitis: Characterized by painful, frequent urination; hematuria; and urgency • Pyelonephritis: Ascending infection of the kidneys; symptoms include fever and flank pain and tenderness that may lead to shock • Infection is more common in women because of a shorter urethra and its proximity to the anus • Most strains are susceptible to penicillin and ciprofloxacin
Staphylococcus saprophyticus	• Infection commonly occurs in sexually active young women ("honeymoon cystitis"); differentiated from *Escherichia coli* because *Staphylococci* are gram positive and catalase positive
Proteus mirabilis	• Gram-negative rod typified by swarming growth on blood agar; transmission by catheters and other instruments • Produces a powerful urease that hydrolyzes urea to ammonia and CO_2; causes stones and urinary tract obstruction
Enterococcus faecalis	• Normally non-invasive, opportunist; found in the normal flora; a leading cause of nosocomial infections; including urinary tract infections (UTIs); resistant to many antibiotics
Neisseria gonorrhoeae	• Gram-negative, intracellular-dwelling diplococcus with a "kidney bean" appearance; a frequent pathogen of sexually active young people • Attach to mucosal epithelium by pili and cause damage via LPS

- Urethritis in men and endocervicitis in women result; complications include ependymitis and prostatitis in men and pelvic inflammatory disease (PID), sterility, and arthritis in women
- Resistant to penicillin via a plasmid encoded penicillinase; secretes immunoglobulin A (IgA) protease that destroys early protective antibody
- Conjunctivitis is contracted by newborns during passage through the birth canal of infected women; treatment is topical silver nitrate

Treponema pallidum	• Motile spirochete that causes syphilis
	• Infection initially occurs as a localized, painless chancre with erythema, ulceration, and induration; disseminated infection to almost all tissues and tertiary central nervous system involvement follow
	• Dark-field microscopy of lesion exudates reveals the spirochetes
	• Long-acting penicillin is effective
Chlamydia trachomatis	• Subtypes D to K are important causes of urethritis in men and urethritis, cervicitis, salpingitis, and PID in women; damage results from granuloma formation blocking fallopian tubes, causing infertility; infection is frequently asymptomatic
	• An inclusion conjunctivitis can occur in neonates. It has two forms, an infectious, extracellular form (elementary body), which develops into the second form, an obligate intracellular reticulate body.
Herpes simplex virus	• dsDNA enveloped virus with an icosahedral nucleocapsid, causes latent and acute infections of genitals and lips, often a sexually transmitted disease
	• Neonatal herpes results during passage of newborns through an infected birth canal; delivery by C section is indicated
Human papilloma virus	• Human–human transmission causes genital warts; has been associated with cervical, vulvar, and penile cancers (specifically types 16 and 18)
	• It synthesizes an E6 protein that binds to the protooncogene p53 and an E7 protein that binds to cellular retinoblastoma tumor suppressor (pRb)

Topic **6**

Central Nervous System, Cardiovascular, Ear, and Eye Infections

Must Knows

- Major organisms involved
- Mechanisms of disease

CENTRAL NERVOUS SYSTEM INFECTIONS

***Streptococcus agalactiae* (group B)**	• β hemolytic, gram-positive coccus; can be normal vaginal flora; infections occur in newborns during delivery, meningitis. Sepsis characterizes infection.
	• Polysaccharide capsules are responsible for the five serotypes, which are the major virulence factor; anticapsular antibodies are protective; also secrete a peptidase that inactivates C5a, thus negating a protective polymorphonuclear (PMN) cell influx
	• Clinical disease has two entities:
	○ A highly fatal, early-onset (birth to 7 days) neonatal infection associated with premature birth and obstetric complications
	○ A late-onset (7 days to 4 months) sepsis characterized by meningitis leading to permanent neurologic damage
	• Vaccines are not indicated because infants are poorly responsive to polysaccharide antigens; penicillin G is generally given
Neisseria meningitidis	• Gram-negative, oxidase-positive diplococcus; initially colonizes upper respiratory membranes; can cause an often fatal meningococcemia, mainly in children ages 6 months to 2 years
	• Possesses a capsular polysaccharide that inhibits phagocytosis; also an endotoxin causing disseminated intravascular coagulation (DIC), hemorrhagic purpura, adrenal insufficiency, and shock (Waterhouse-Friderichsen syndrome)
	• Secretes an IgA protease that aids colonization
	• Cranial nerve (CN) VIII deafness may be a complication after recovery
	• A capsular vaccine is available for military and close contacts

Haemophilus influenzae	• Gram-negative, fastidious rod requiring X (hemin) and V (nicotinamide-adenine nucleotide [NAD]) factors for growth (components of chocolate agar); strains causing meningitis have a type B polyribitol capsule
	• Vaccination with the capsule conjugated to a carrier protein is effective in preventing meningitis; the disease in unvaccinated children 3 months to 2 years of age is rapidly progressive, resulting in mental retardation, hearing problems, and other deficits
Streptococcus pneumoniae	• A common cause of meningitis in elderly individuals after pneumonia
Listeria monocytogenes	• Causes meningitis and septicemia in infants and immunocompromised patients
Aseptic viral meningitis	• When bacterial causes are excluded, a diagnosis of aseptic viral meningitis is entertained
	• The coxsackie viruses (enteroviruses), group B and many strains of group A are frequently responsible. Recovery is common in contrast to meningitis caused by the polio viruses.

CARDIOVASCULAR INFECTIONS

Viridans *Streptococci*	• Often a non-invasive opportunist; on access to the blood stream by dental or oral manipulation, it becomes the most frequent cause of subacute bacterial endocarditis (SBE); damage is secondary to inflammation from deposition of the organism on previously damaged heart valves (i.e., congenital defects)
	• α-Hemolytic; uninhibited by Optochin; not bile soluble; the latter two properties distinguish it from *S. pneumoniae*
Enterococci	• Also a common nosocomial cause of SBE in a manner similar to viridans Streptococci
Staphylococcus aureus	• β-Hemolytic, catalase-positive, gram-positive coccus that adheres to native and prosthetic valves causing acute endocarditis
	• Coagulase allows formation of platelet and fibrin clots; these reduce access of phagocytic cells to *S. aureus;* cytolytic toxins damage heart cells; common in intravenous drug abusers
Staphylococcus epidermidis	• Adheres readily to artificial materials in the body (prosthetic heart valves, catheters); causes chronic endocarditis; normal skin flora
Coxsackievirus, type B	• The most common cause of viral heart disease

EAR AND EYE INFECTIONS

C. trachomatis, *N. gonorrhoeae,* *H. influenzae*	• These are suspect organisms in eye infections, in particular neonatal and postnatal purulent conjunctivitis

Streptococcus pneumoniae	• The most common cause of otitis media in infants older than 2 months • Treatment is with penicillin, although resistant strains are now evident
Haemophilus influenzae	• The second most common causative agent of otitis media in children; it recurs often probably because of drug resistance
Pseudomonas aeruginosa	• Causes otitis externa ("swimmer's ear"); also infects multiple other systems (e.g., burns, cellulitis, septicemia, pneumonia) • Possesses an endotoxin, exotoxin A, slime layer capsule, and secretes the enzymes catalase and elastase

Topic **7**

Definition of the Immune System

Must **Knows**

- Role of Th_1 and Th_2 cells
- T- and B-cell antigen receptors
- Function of clusters of differentiation
- Structure and function of antibody classes
- Genetic basis of antibody diversity
- Genetic control of human leukocyte antigen (HLA)

DEVELOPMENT OF THE IMMUNE SYSTEM

T cells

- Multipotent stem cells originate in fetal liver and bone marrow; stem cells migrate to the thymus and acquire phenotypic T-cell characteristics under the influence of thymic hormones
- Clusters of differentiation (CD) appear on the T-cell membrane as proteins at different stages of differentiation in the thymus
  - CD2 and CD3: Major markers retained on all peripheral T cells; labeled anti-CD3 antibodies aid in determining T-cell numbers in circulation
  - CD4: Defines T-helper (T_h) subset, which differentiates in the thymus into Th_1 and Th_2 cells based on differences in cytokine secretion

  ○ CD8: Defines T cytotoxic-suppressor (T_C or T_S) subset that is active in cell-mediated immunity (CMI)
- Th_1 cells secrete interleukin-2 (IL-2), interferon-γ, and tumor necrosis factor-α (TNF-α), which are involved in antibody synthesis and inflammation
- Th_2 cells secrete IL-4, IL-5, IL-6, IL-10, and IL-13, which are involved in antibody synthesis
- T-cell receptor (TCR): Specific for an antigen epitope; exists as one of two types, α:β and γ:δ
  ○ α:β T cells are activated by peptide fragments bound to the major histocompatibility complex (MHC) on antigen-presenting cells (APCs); γ:δ cells are activated by nonpeptide antigens
- A T-cell–dependent homing area exists periarteriolarly in the spleen, the paracortical and deep cortical regions in the lymph nodes, and in the gastrointestinal and bronchus associated tissues
- 1% to 2% leave the thymus for the tissues; others undergo apoptosis

B cells	• Stem cells in bone marrow acquire phenotypic CD markers characteristic of various stages of B cell differentiation: Pro-B, pre-B, immature B, and mature B cells • A membrane-bound, epitope-specific antigenic receptor that is a monomeric immunoglobulin M (IgM) antibody, distinguishes the B cell antigenic receptor from the T-cell receptor; also in contrast to T cells, the B cell receptor links directly to peptide antigen; MHC is not required • Partial maturation of T cells in the thymus and B cells in the bone marrow in utero is followed by migration to and seeding of peripheral lymphoid tissues; after birth, T and B cells differentiate further and gain immunocompetence under antigenic stimuli
Antigens	• Epitope: Short sequence of amino acids or sugars in a molecule that combines with the hypervariable reactive site on an antibody • Hapten: Portion of an antigen that contains the epitope, reacts specifically with antibody, and is incapable of inducing antibody synthesis without a carrier molecule • Superantigens (certain retroviral proteins, Staphylococcal and Streptococcal enterotoxins; toxic shock syndrome toxin 1): Can link the MHC II APC to a T_h site at the Vβ region, which is independent of the specific peptide-binding site; this linkage is not restricted by specificity. So many T cells and APCs are activated, secreting toxic amounts of cytokines. • Thymus-independent antigens activate B cells without T helper involvement; most possess multiple branched polysaccharide repeating units (e.g., LPS from gram-negative bacteria) and activate B cells polyclonally, without regard to B-cell specificity

ANTIBODY

Antibodies	• All five classes have a similar structure: a four-chain protein with two heavy (H) and two light (L) chains linked by disulphide bonds
	• The specific amino acid sequence in H chains is different for the five classes, permitting separate classification; the H chain differences are called isotypes, designated as γ, α, μ, ϵ and δ; L chain isotypes, κ and λ, exist for all five classes
	• Isotypes: Genetic variations all humans possess
	• Allotypes: Alleles with slight amino acid differences (in IgG and IgA) that only some members of a species possess
	• All five classes also are classified together as immunoglobins; they all have an amino acid sequence in common in the L chains
	• H and L chains are divided into constant (CH and CL) and variable region domains (VH and VL)
	◦ The amino acid sequences in constant regions of H and L chains are similar for all antibody molecules within a class
	◦ The amino acid sequences in variable regions of H and L chains show marked differences between antibodies of different specificities
	◦ A hypervariable region exists in each variable region; these regions of H and L chains associate together to form two alike epitope binding regions known as an idiotype
	• Most antigenic preparations give rise to a mixture of antibodies
	• However, antibodies of a single specificity (monoclonal) have many purposes: e.g. specific diagnostic tests and immunotherapy
IgG	• The structure of immunoglobulins has been determined by enzymatic cleavage of IgG
	◦ Papain cleavage: Three fragments; two are similar, termed Fab, each containing only one antigen-binding site; a third fragment (Fc) activates complement, controls catabolism of IgG, fixes IgG to tissues or cells, and mediates placental transfer
	◦ Pepsin: Splits behind a double bond joining the two H chains, permitting the two Fab fragments to remain joined (Fab′2), while the Fc portion is destroyed
	• Has the highest serum concentration of all immunoglobulins (700 to 1500 mg %), and a serum half-life of 18 to 25 days
IgM	• Exists in two forms: A monomer that is an antigen receptor on the B cell membrane and differs for each clone; secreted IgM exists as a pentamer joined together by a J chain, it is the first antibody to appear after antigenic stimuli, an avid fixer of complement
	• Average serum concentration of 150 mg %; a half-life of about 5 days

IgA	• Exists in three forms: A monomer, a dimer, a dimer plus a secretory piece
	○ The dimer is transported across mucosal barriers into the lumen by the secretory piece, which is a receptor for the IgA Fc region
	○ The secretory piece protects IgA from proteolysis
	○ Occurs at high concentrations in secretions; in serum, exists mainly as a dimer with a half-life of 5 days and an average concentration of about 300 mg %
	• Located in and protects mucosal tissues, saliva, tears, and colostrum by blocking bacteria, viruses, and toxins from binding to host cells; does not usually fix complement
IgE	• Occurs at a very low serum concentration because its Fc region binds avidly to FcE receptors on mast cells and basophils
	• Binding of antigen to these IgE-sensitized cells triggers the release of vasoactive amines (e.g., histamine), resulting in atopic disease characterized by hives (local) and anaphylaxis (systemic)
	• Does not cross the placenta or fix complement by the conventional pathway; when bound to Helminths together with IL-5 activated eosinophils, it eradicates these parasites
IgD	• Like IgM, a membrane-bound antigen receptor on mature B cells

IMMUNE SYSTEM GENETICS

Genetic control of immunoglobulin chain synthesis	• Human antibodies exhibit an enormous range (approximately 10^8) of specificities; the genetic basis for diversity involves several factors:
	○ Different genes code for variable and constant regions
	○ Random rearrangement of variable and constant region genes occurs during differentiation. Any one of many different variable region genes can be linked to a single constant region gene, thus conserving DNA.
	○ The joining segment (J) sequence joins the VL region gene to the CL region gene
	○ The diversity segment (D) sequence is also required for H chain formation. This links the VH gene to the J gene; these genes then fuse with the CH gene.
	○ H chain class switching from μ and δ to γ, α, and ε is dictated by a later rearrangement of the class genes in the CH region and is mediated by T-cell cytokines, IL-4, IL-13, interferon-γ, and TGFβ
	○ Random selection by B cells from the variety of V, D, and J germ line genes results in a large number of structural possibilities for VL and VH epitope binding regions; this is primarily responsible for antibody diversity

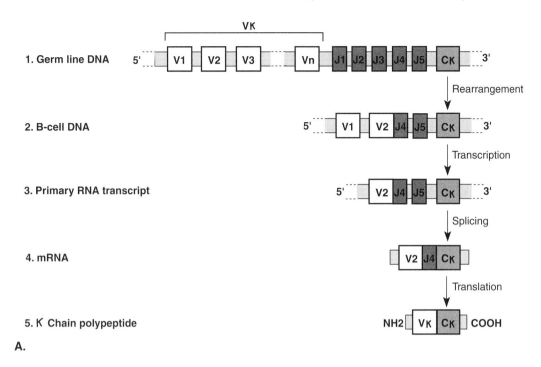

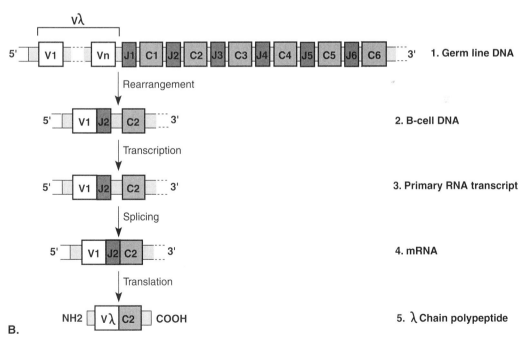

● **Figure V-2** (**A**) Kappa (κ) light (L)-chain synthesis. From the pool of multiple variable (V) region genes on chromosome 2 in the germ line DNA (1), one V region gene is joined to a joining (J) region gene, resulting in B-cell DNA (2). After removal of introns by recombinases, the primary RNA is transcribed (3), resulting in mRNA (4) composed of one V region gene, one J gene, and the constant (Cκ) region gene. Translation of the mRNA results in the κ L-chain polypeptide (5). (**B**) Lambda (λ) L-chain synthesis. Rearrangement and synthesis of the λ L-chain genes occurs in an identical manner on chromosome 22, except for the availability of up to six Cλ exons for union to the VJ combined exon. This availability results in several subtypes. (Part A redrawn with permission from Benjamin E: *Immunology: A Short Course,* 3rd ed. New York, Wiley-Liss, Inc., a subsidiary of John Wiley & Sons, Inc., 1996, p. 98.)

○ Allelic exclusion: Only one of the two parental alleles is expressed by a B cell, resulting in a single H chain isotype and L chain subtype receptor capable of reacting with only one antigenic epitope (Fig. V-2)

Genetic control of human leukocyte antigens (HLAs)	• HLAs are organized into three MHC classes • Class I molecules: Encoded by three gene regions, A, B, and C; they are linked to the cytotoxic T cell via the CD8 molecule and present peptidic epitopes to specific T_C receptors (class I restriction); found on most nucleated cells • Class II molecules: Encoded by three gene regions, DP, DQ, and DR; they are linked to the T_h cell via CD4 and present peptidic epitopes to specific T_h cell receptors (class II restriction); found on dendritic cells, macrophages, and activated T and B cells • Class III molecules control complement • Many alleles of class I and II molecules are present at each locus on chromosome 6; these are major obstacles to organ transplantation • Haplotypes inherited from both parents, expressed codominantly • Binding of CD4 to a class II HLA molecule on the APC triggers humoral immunity; binding of CD8 to class I triggers CMI

Topic **8**

Innate and Humoral Immunity

Must **Knows**

● Components of innate immunity

● Mechanisms of T-cell activation

● Mechanisms of B-cell activation

● Complement activation

INNATE IMMUNITY

Basics	• The initial, rapid recognition system for detection of pathogens; generally leads to humoral immunity (HI), cell-mediated immunity (CMI), or both

- Is nonspecific without previous host adaptation; sentinel cells identify pathogens and recruit other cells via release of cytokines
- Phagocytic cells and physical barriers act to block infection, polymorphonuclear (PMNs) cells are the earliest and most abundant respondent cell

Macrophages	• Phagocytic; use complement receptor to capture complement associated pathogens by the alternate pathway • Alternative pathway: Activated by bacterial cell wall, yeast, and aggregated IgA before antibody synthesis, it does not require $C'1$, $C'4$, or $C'2$; the cell walls bind $C'3b$, which exists in normal serum. This complex binds with serum factors (B, D, and properdin), creating $C'3$ convertase. $C'3bBb$ generates additional $C'3b$. A $C'3bBbC'3b$ complex forms and becomes a $C'5$ convertase leading to reactions that create the membrane attack complex (MAC) (Fig. V-3).

Dendritic cells	• Antigen-presenting cells (APCs); are present in two forms:
	  ○ Immature: Highly phagocytic, itinerant cells expressing low major histocompatability complex (MHC) levels; capture and process pathogens into antigenic fragments; exposure to pathogen molecules activates toll-like receptors (TLR) and triggers maturation
	  ○ Mature: Nonphagocytic, sessile, express abundant MHC in secondary lymphoid organs, resulting in a display of antigenic peptides to naïve T cells and subsequent HI, CMI, or both

Natural killer (NK) cells	• Detect cells expressing decreased levels of MHC I (e.g., virus-infected or transformed cells); capable of initiating cell killing by means of a killer activating receptor (KAR) • Apoptosis is triggered in target cells via perforins and granzymes • NK cells can dock on host cells with a higher concentration of MHC. Inadvertent host cell death is stopped by activating a killing inhibitory receptor (KIR). • Genetically predetermined recognition receptors for pathogens exist on host cells, called pattern recognition receptors (e.g., TLR and endocytosis receptors); these recognize a few highly conserved structures expressed in a large group of microorganisms but not humans; these structures are referred to as pathogen-associated molecular patterns (PAMPS) (e.g., lipopolysaccharide, peptidoglycan, lipoteichoic acid, mannans, bacterial DNA, double-stranded RNA and glucans) • Activation of TLR signals the presence of a pathogen and determines if a CMI response is required

HUMORAL IMMUNITY

Antigen processing	• Viral and intracellular parasite antigens are synthesized endogenously within the APC cytoplasm and endoplasmic reticulum and then processed to peptides by the proteasome.

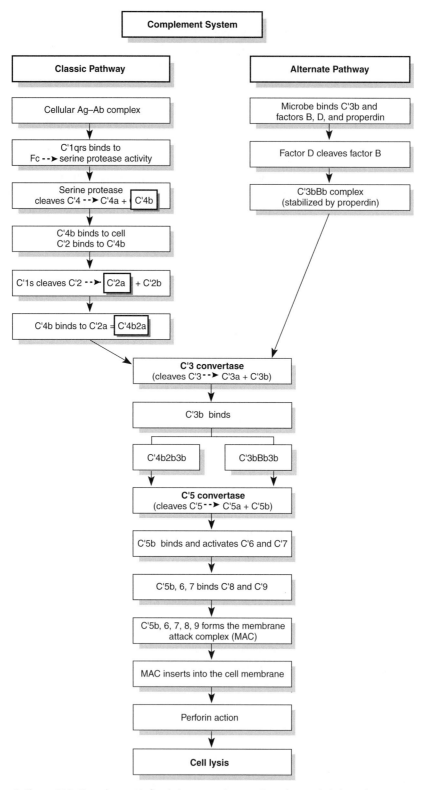

● **Figure V-3** Complement is fixed via two pathways. Complement is lytic and promotes inflammation via its side products, C'3a and C'5a. A receptor for C'3 on phagocytic cells promotes the phagocytosis of Ag–Ab–C' complexes. Ab = antibody; Ag = antigen; C' = complement.

The peptides bind to the H chains of MHC I molecules and migrate to the APC membrane, where they are presented to and activate CD8+ T cells; CMI results.

- Exogenous protein antigens enter an APC by pinocytosis and are processed in endosomal vacuoles; the resulting peptides bind to the cleft in MHC II molecules and are transported to the membrane, where they are presented to and activate CD4+ T cells; HI results

T-cell activation	<ul><li>Activation of CD4+ T cells is initiated by binding of the specific T-cell antigenic receptor to the peptide class II MHC. The CD4 molecule links to the MHC, and an activation signal is transduced by the TCR-CD3 complex, which is composed of three polypeptides (α, δ, and ϵ) and two ζ chains.</li><li>Mandatory accessory T-cell adhesion molecules (CD2, leukocyte function-associated antigen [LFA 1] and CD 28) facilitate adherence of the T_h cell to the APC by binding to LFA 3, ICAM (intracellular adhesion molecule) 1, and B7, respectively; this triggers IL-2 secretion (Fig. V-4)</li></ul>
CD8+ T_h cell activation	<ul><li>Follows the same pathway except CD8 binds to the class I MHC and CD 45R links to CD22, replacing the CD28-B7 linkage</li></ul>
Th$_1$ response	<ul><li>After activation, the Th$_1$ cell clone differentiates, divides logarithmically, and secretes IL-2, interferon γ and TNFα; IL-2 is necessary for T- and B-cell activation</li><li>Interferon γ is a macrophage and NK cell activator; it can trigger HLA antigen presentation by endothelial cells, downregulate IL-4 synthesis by Th$_2$ cells, and thus suppress antibody formation</li><li>TNFα activates macrophages and stimulates the acute phase response by synergizing with IL-1</li></ul>
Th$_2$ response	<ul><li>After antigen activation and stimulation by IL-2, the CD4+ Th$_2$ cell differentiates and divides logarithmically while secreting IL-4, IL-5, IL-10, and IL-13</li><li>IL-4 favors antibody synthesis by stimulating B-cell differentiation. It downregulates interferon-γ by Th$_1$ cells and thus suppresses CMI. It is necessary for a switch to IgE production.</li><li>IL-5 functions synergistically with IL-4 and IL-2 to aid B-cell differentiation. It facilitates IgA synthesis and stimulates growth and differentiation of eosinophils.</li><li>IL-10, similar to IL-4, inhibits Th$_1$ cell release of interferon γ and IL-2, thus negating macrophage activation by interferon γ</li><li>IL-13 mimics IL-4 actions, inhibiting Th$_1$ cytokine release</li></ul>
B-cell response	<ul><li>The B-cell clone with membrane-bound IgM receptor specific for an antigen epitope is selected. Binding of antigen along with stimuli from T-cell cytokines IL-2 and IL-4 triggers differentiation of the clone into large blast cells, and logarithmic division occurs.</li></ul>

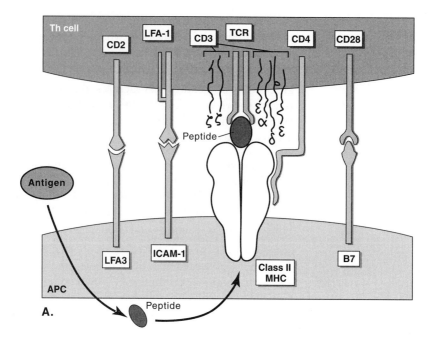

A.

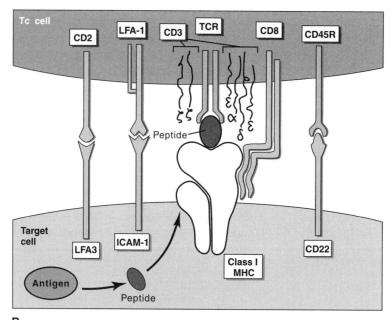

B.

● **Figure V-4** (**A**) Activation of CD4+ helper T (Th) cells. The specific T-cell antigen receptor (αβ: TCR or γδ: TCR) binds to the peptide–class II major histocompatibility complex (MHC) complex by the antigen-presenting cell (APC). The CD4 molecule links to the MHC complex. An activation signal is transduced by the TCR–CD3 complex, which is composed of three polypeptides (α, δ, ε) and two ζ chains. Accessory T-cell adhesion molecules (e.g., CD2, leukocyte function–associated antigen-1 [LFA-1] and CD28) facilitate adherence of the Th cell to the APC and influence interleukin-2 (IL-2) synthesis. (**B**) Activation of CD8+ cytotoxic T (Tc) cells. (From Kuby J: *Immunology*, 3rd ed. ©1992, 1994, and 1997 by W. H. Freeman and Company. Used with permission.)

- IL-5 continues this process, during which the B cell acquires the machinery necessary for antibody synthesis; H and L chains are synthesized, assembled, and under IL-6 influence terminal differentiation to plasma cells and secretion of IgM occurs

- Subsequent gene rearrangements result in a switch to IgG, IgA, IgE synthesis and secretion; IL-4 and interferon-γ influence the switch to IgG. TGFβ influences the switch to IgA, and IL-4 influences the switch to IgE.

- Binding of CD40 on B cells to its ligand on the T_h cell (CD40L) is necessary for switching to occur

- B memory cells are generated independently of the plasma cell lineage; these cells migrate to lymphoid tissues

Topic **9**
Cell-Mediated Immunity

Must Knows

- Dynamics of inflammation
- Mediators of inflammation
- Cell involved in cell-mediated immunity (CMI)
- Types of CMI

INFLAMMATION

Dynamics

- Inflammation is necessary for alleviating and repairing injury; when excessive as occurs in certain T_C reactions or auto-immune disorders, it can be damaging

- It is initiated by injury-induced release of inflammatory mediators, including interleukin-1 (IL-1) and tumor necrosis factor-α (TNFα), as well as alternate pathway complement activation; this changes the resting state of endothelium by the appearance of selectins on the cell surface

- Selectins bind to the counterreceptor on circulating neutrophils, slowing the polymorphonuclear (PMN) cells to "rolling adhesion"

- Release of IL-8, macrophage inflammatory protein (MIP) and monocyte chemotactic protein (MCP) results in activation of integrins on the neutrophil surface, which bind to intracellular adhesion molecules (ICAM) on the endothelial cell surface

- Diapedesis: Facilitated by platelet-endothelial cell adhesion molecules (PECAM-1); migration to injury occurs via chemotaxis
- Antagonism at any point can reduce the inflammatory process

Removal of the inciting condition	• Occurs via phagocytic cells activated by IL-8, MIP, and interferon-γ; phagocytized, membrane-enclosed organisms are destroyed by O_2-dependent killing by lysosomal enzymes and H_2O_2, NO, and O_2^-
Repair	• Requires down regulation by IL-4, IL-10, and TGFβ of IL-8 and cytokines IL-1 and TNFα, which induced the response
	• Platelet-derived growth factor (PDGF), TGFβ, and other factors produce extracellular matrix after increased proliferation and activation of fibroblasts

MEDIATORS OF INFLAMMATION

Chemokines	• Small molecular weight peptides that are released by injury and are active at very low concentrations (10^{-8}–10^{-11} M); they activate and attract leukocytes to tissue damage
	• C-X-C chemokines: have their first two cysteines separated by one amino acid; include IL-8, platelet factor 4, and the interferon-γ–induced proteins (macrophage activation factors and inducible protein 10) that attract neutrophils
	• C-C chemokines: have two adjacent cysteines; they include MCP, MIP, and RANTES; attract monocytes and T cells; some attract eosinophils, basophils, NKs
Cytokines	• Intracellular signaling proteins that act in a paracrine or autocrine manner by binding to high-affinity receptors. The latter can have circulating forms consisting of only the extracytoplasmic portion of the receptor that blocks the cytokine before it reaches its target.
	• IL-1, IL-6, and TNFα induce MCP and IL-8 and the acute phase response; they are endogenous pyrogens
	• TGFβ: a potent wound healing and immunosuppressive agent, inhibiting IL-2 and proliferation of many cell types

CMI EFFECTOR CELLS

Macrophages	• Activated to increased phagocytosis and microbicidal action, primarily by interferon γ released by Th_1 cells after antigenic stimulation; microbial products also induce interferon γ and TNFα release; killing occurs via reactive oxygen species (ROS)
	• Macrophage secretion of IL-12 acts synergistically with IL-2 to induce differentiation of Th_1 and NK cells to CD8+ cytotoxic T cells

- Unlike IgM B cell receptor, TCR is not secreted; immunity is effected by contact with the MHC I on target cells
- After cell–cell contact, T_C lysis occurs by exocytosis of perforins, which cause membrane channels to form in infected cells permitting granzymes, cytolysins, lymphotoxins, and serine esterases to cause osmotic imbalance and rupture

NK cells	• Large granular lymphocytes that kill tumor cells and those infected by virus; prominent in graft-versus-host reactions; contain antagonists similar to cytotoxic T cells • Do not exhibit T- or B-cell phenotypes; lack CD3 and antigen-specific receptors; they do not require prior sensitization to exhibit cytolysis but can be activated by IL-2, IL-12, and interferon-γ

TYPES OF CMI

Basics	• Directed against intracellular-dwelling microorganisms and aberrant endogenous cells (e.g., cancers); antibody is rarely involved
Tuberculin test	• Exemplifies CMI reaction to infectious agents • Although a skin test, it reveals CMI reactions in internal organs; a contained lesion (> 15 mm) of induration and erythema, peaking in 1 to 2 days results from the inflammatory response induced by sensitized T-cell action at the site of antigen (purified protein derivative [PPD]) deposition • Initiated by Langerhans cell presentation of antigen to sensitized delayed-type hypersensitivity T_h cells that have been recruited to the site of antigen deposition by chemokines • PMNs; CD4+ T cells; and the dominant, nonspecific, perivascular accumulation of monocytic or macrophage cells contribute to the destruction of the organisms, tissue, or both
Granulomatous reactions	• Occur if antigen persists in tissues and continues to cause release of chemotactic agents (IL-1, IL-8), causing inflammatory cell influx • IL-4 and interferon-γ promote retention of macrophages and cause fusion of monocytes at the site, leading to a granuloma composed of macrophages, histiocytes, and epithelioid cells
Contact dermatitis	• Result from haptens or irritants deposited in the skin; the combination with a host carrier molecule causes a CMI reaction in sensitized cells. Common eliciting agents include nickel, rubber, poison ivy, poison sumac, and dinitrochlorobenzene. • Reexposure to the agent results in chemokine and cytokine release, monocytic or macrophage infiltration, and a vesiculating lesion with erythema and induration

Topic **10**

Disorders of the Immune System

Must
Knows

- Hypersensitivity reactions
- Immunodeficiency
- Autoimmune disease

HYPERSENSITIVITY REACTIONS

Type I (anaphylaxis)	• The basis for atopic disease (urticaria, asthma, allergic rhinitis) is the adherence of the Fc fragment of IgE to mast cells and basophils; the F(ab)2 remains free to bind an allergen when reintroduced; the resulting membrane perturbation causes degranulation of cells (releasing of histamine, leukotrienes, serotonin, bradykinin); these contract smooth muscle and increase vessel permeability and secretions
	• Mucus secretions and mediator-induced constriction of smooth muscle surrounding the bronchioles cause airway obstruction
	• Anaphylactic shock: Mediators are released systemically, resulting in hypotension and shock caused by arteriolar vasodilation, increased vascular permeability, and upper airway edema, leading to organ failure
	• Repeated injection of certain allergens can achieve a hyposensitive state by favoring the synthesis of IgG. It combines avidly with the allergen in the circulation, blocking union with cell-associated IgE.
Type II (cell surface antigen–antibody cytotoxicity)	• Cytotoxicity results from antibody binding to epitopes on surface membranes of host cells; damage results from osmotic lytic action of complement, opsonization by phagocytic cells or killing by antibody-dependent cell-mediated cytotoxicity (ADCC), T_C lymphocytes, or natural killer (NK) cells
	• Transfusion reactions occur after transfusion of blood containing antigens foreign to the recipient; anemia results from increased phagocytosis and opsonization induced by anti-erythrocyte antibodies; ABO incompatibility reactions are most common; Rh reactions are most severe in utero
	• Erythroblastosis fetalis is caused by the placental transfer of a non-saline agglutinating, maternal anti-Rh IgG (usually anti-D)

that binds to fetal erythrocytes; complement-mediated lysis or rapid phagocytosis causes hemolysis and indirect hyperbilirubinemia, which can cause respiratory and central nervous system (CNS) damage. RhoGAM (anti-D antibody) given within 1 to 2 days of delivery neutralizes the fetal Rh+ antigens and prevents maternal sensitization.

Type III (antigen–antibody complex reactions)	• Circulating antigen–antibody complexes escape phagocytosis and deposit in tissues or on the surface of blood vessels. They cause damage by activating complement and releasing chemotactic factors, which attract neutrophils to the area of deposition, where they release lysosomal enzymes to damage tissue. • Glomerulonephritis (GLN): Antigen-antibody complexes deposit on and behind the renal glomerular basement membrane (GBM) causing inflammation. The release of enzymes by neutrophils results in glomerular destruction and loss of filtration capacity. Implicated antigens are DNA, insulin, thyroglobulin, and group A nephritogenic streptococci. Deposition of these non-kidney complexes is random. Fluorescent antibody testing for antigen, antibody, or complement reveals a "lumpy-bumpy" pattern; this differentiates the cause of GLN from that of type II in which the antibody is directed against renal antigens per se. • Systemic lupus erythematosus (SLE): Can be classified as a type III reaction or an autoimmune disorder. It is characterized by autoantibody complexes against many host antigens. dsDNA is the dominant antigen. dsDNA-anti-dsDNA complexes and other antigen–antibody complexes lodge in the kidney, giving rise to neutrophil enzymatic damage and glomerulonephritis.

IMMUNODEFICIENCY

Developmental immunodeficiency disorders	• Manifest during the prenatal period or early childhood
	• Clinical signs include:
	  ○ History of recurrent infections
	  ○ Low enzyme-linked immunoabsorbent assay (ELISA) values for IgG, IgM, or IgA (normal values in mg% are IgG = 800 to 1400; IgM = 60 to 200; IgA = 100 to 300)
	  ○ Abnormal T/B cell ratios, CD4/CD8 ratios, or both (normal T/B = 2; normal CD4/CD8, approximately 2:1)
	  ○ Diminished in vivo humoral immunity or cell-mediated immunity against standard vaccines

Bruton' agammaglobulinemia	• Affects primarily 5- to 6-month-old boys. The defect may occur in the transition from pre-B to B cells and involves loss of a tyrosine kinase gene. Pre-B cells, the thymus, and CMI are normal.
DiGeorge syndrome	• Congenital thymic aplasia; characterized by hypocalcemia, tetany, and absence of T cells

- Caused by an unknown intrauterine injury to the third and fourth pharyngeal pouches that occurs between the fifth and sixth weeks of gestation. The thymus and parathyroid glands are not developed, but germinal centers, plasma cells, and serum Ig appear normal; CMI is depressed.
- Recent evidence implicates a mutation in the *TBX5* gene as responsible

Wiskott-Aldrich syndrome	<ul><li>X-linked male disorder with three main features: thrombocytopenia, eczema, and recurrent infections</li><li>Respond poorly to bacteria with polysaccharide capsules and possess low serum IgM levels with depressed CMI</li><li>The primary defect is on the short arm of the X chromosome; may result in absence of specific glycoprotein receptors on T cells and platelets</li></ul>
Chronic granulomatous disease	<ul><li>Results from a genetic defect in the nicotinamide adenosine dinucleotide phosphate (NADPH) oxidase system in neutrophils; consequently, their oxidase, superoxidase dismutase activity, and hydrogen peroxide levels are depressed</li><li>Treatment with interferon-γ has been successful</li></ul>
Severe combined immunodeficiency disease	<ul><li>Characterized by a genetic defect in stem cells that results in the absence of the thymus and T and B cells</li><li>An autosomal recessive deficiency in the enzyme adenosine deaminase occurs in 50% of patients. This results in the accumulation of toxic deoxyadenosine triphosphate that inhibits ribonucleotide reductase and prevents DNA synthesis; a sex-linked mutation in the γ chain of the IL-2 receptor gene is found in other patients.</li></ul>
Acquired immunodeficiency disease	<ul><li>Caused by an RNA retrovirus, HIV, that is a member of the Lentivirus family; its major target is the CD4+ T_h cell, which is eventually lysed by the virus; other cells (e.g., macrophages) with much lower membrane levels of CD4 can be infected by low numbers of HIV and may serve as reservoirs of latent virus (Fig. V-5)</li><li>HIV enters cells by binding the CD4 receptor and an obligate chemokine co-receptor (CXCR4) via gp120. Fusion and entry through the cell membrane are mediated by gp41.</li><li>Transcription of viral RNA into DNA is accomplished by a viral reverse transcriptase. Integration of viral DNA into the cell genome is conducted by an integrase, leading to the formation of a provirus that may lie latent for years.</li><li>After activation of the infected T cell by other viruses or antigens, host cell lysis occurs. Depletion of the T_h cells results in a loss of their cytokines and diminished capacity to offset normally non-invasive, infectious agents.<ul><li>At CD4+ T_h levels = 200 to 400 cells/μl, *Candida* sp., *Mycobacteri* sp., and Varicella-zoster infections dominate</li></ul></li></ul>

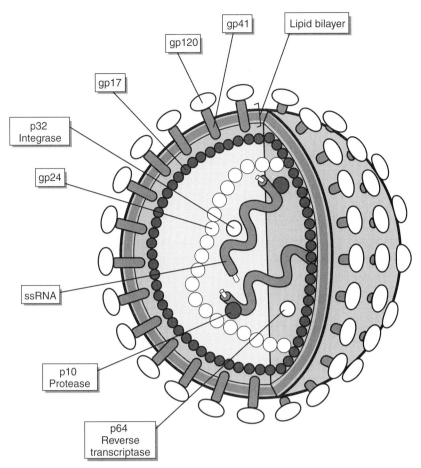

● **Figure V-5** Components of the human immunodeficiency virus (HIV). The virus consists of an envelope formed from glycoproteins (i.e., gp120 and gp41) that houses several core proteins (e.g., p17, p24). The virus has several genes that code for enzymes (e.g., integrase, reverse transcriptase, protease) that play a role in integrating viral DNA into the host genome and degrading polyprotein precursors into smaller proteins and peptides.

- ○ At CD 4 levels < 200 cells/μl, *Pneumocystis carinii*, cytomegalovirus, and *Cryptococcus* sp. are common; Kaposi's sarcoma and B cell lymphomas are also seen

AUTOIMMUNE DISEASE

Basics

- Humans are normally immunologically unresponsive to endogenous molecules secondary to self-tolerance; however, in normal humans, B-cell clones do exist with receptors reacting with endogenous molecules (self-antigens)
- Tolerance to self-antigens is achieved by clonal deletion, clonal anergy, or peripheral suppression. Breakdown in any of these results in aberrant immunologic regulation and autoimmunity.

Clonal deletion	• A loss in self-reactive T and B cells that appear during maturation in the fetal thymus and bone marrow. These are eliminated after contact with self antigens in the thymus or bone marrow.
Clonal anergy	• Follows the loss of T- and B-cell function after exposure to antigens in the absence of mandatory co-stimulatory signals or after exposure to cells lacking major HLA class II molecules
Peripheral suppression	• Occurs if CD8+ T cells or macrophages secrete cytokines (e.g., TGFβ) that downregulate the immune response or if tolerogenic doses of antigen are administered • Tolerance is specific, more readily induced, and lasts longer in T than in B cells
Systemic lupus erythematosus	• Exemplary of the systemic autoimmune disorders • Characterized by multiple autoreactive antibodies against diverse cellular constituents. The patient's signs and symptoms reflect the cells and organs targeted.
Rheumatoid arthritis	• Chronic, systemic inflammatory disease with a genetic predisposition (HLA-Dw4, HLA-DR4+ individuals) • Autoantibodies, usually IgM (rheumatoid factors), appear that react with the Fc domain of altered IgG molecules, thus forming IgM-IgG complexes in the synovial fluid. Complement and cytokines are activated, attracting neutrophils that release lysosomal enzymes destroying articular cartilage.
Multiple sclerosis	• An organ-specific, chronic, relapsing disease characterized by mononuclear cell infiltrates and CNS white matter demyelination • Patients usually have increased IgG in the cerebrospinal fluid and exhibit a decrease in T suppressor cell function, suggesting an immunoregulatory disorder
Myasthenia gravis	• Results from a defect in neuromuscular transmission • Patients exhibit muscle weakness and fatigue as well as thymic hyperplasia or thymoma; anti-acetylcholine (anti-Ach) receptor antibodies are present, which bind to the receptor at the postsynaptic membrane, resulting in receptor endocytosis • An inability to transmit the ACh-induced signal to muscle fibers causes clinical signs
Hashimoto's thyroiditis	• Characterized by autoantibodies and CMI to thyroglobulin or thyroid peroxidase, resulting in destruction of the thyroid gland and hypothyroidism. Antibody-dependent cell-mediated cytotoxicity may be responsible for the tissue damage
Graves' disease	• Characterized by T- and B-cell infiltration of the thyroid gland leading to the formation of autoantibodies to thyroid-stimulating hormone (TSH) receptors and hyperthyroidism. Autoantibodies compete with TSH and induce uncontrolled TSH-like activity. • Clinical features include a diffuse goiter and thyrotoxicosis

Pernicious anemia

- Caused by impaired gastrointestinal (GI) absorption of vitamin B_{12}, resulting in weakness and chronic fatigue. Occurs secondary to T-cell damage to gastric parietal cells that produce intrinsic factor, the agent responsible for the transport of vitamin B_{12} into the blood.

- Antiparietal cell and anti-intrinsic factor antibodies are found in most patients. These block the transport function of intrinsic factor and contribute to disease; injection of vitamin B_{12} bypasses the need for GI absorption and corrects deficiency.

Section **VI**

Biochemistry

10 Top Tips

Biochemistry

Topic	Main Focus	USMLE Example
1 Proteins	Composition of proteins with respect to structure, function, and pathophysiology	• A 15-year-old girl with diabetes mellitus type 1 states that she maintains tight control of her blood sugar. Laboratory testing shows that her HbA_{1c} is well above normal limits, which suggests that her blood sugar level is not nearly as well controlled as she believes.
2 Enzymes	Clinical uses of enzymes for diagnostic purposes	• A 65-year-old man has a sudden onset of severe chest pain and shortness of breath. Laboratory testing reveals elevated plasma levels of troponin-I, which is used to aid in the diagnosis of myocardial infarction.
3 Energetics	Role of uncouplers	• A 16-year-old girl is hyperthermic after taking an aspirin overdose in a suicide attempt. The hyperthermia is a result of uncoupling of the electron transport chain from oxidative phosphorylation.
4 Carbohydrate Metabolism	Inborn errors of metabolism	• A 30-year-old Asian man starts prophylactic chloroquine before embarking on a trip to Africa. He subsequently develops hemolytic anemia caused by a glucose-6-phosphate dehydrogenase deficiency.
5 Lipid Metabolism	Ketone synthesis during diabetes mellitus	• A 40-year-old man is brought to the emergency department unconscious and smelling of fruity alcohol. Laboratory testing reveals severe hyperglycemia, an anion gap acidosis, and ketones in the urine. The

(Continued)

10 Top Tips

Biochemistry   *(Continued)*

Topic	Main Focus	USMLE Example
		man is immediately given insulin for diabetic ketoacidosis.
6 Nitrogen Metabolism	Metabolic defects in amino acid metabolism	• A newborn girl is positive for phenylketonuria (PKU). This metabolic disorder is caused by a deficiency of phenylalanine hydroxylase and, if untreated, may result in mental retardation, failure to walk or talk, seizures, hyperactivity, tremor, microcephaly, and failure to grow.
7 Control of Metabolism	The fasting state	• While running a marathon, a 24-year-old man enters into a catabolic state. In this state, the runner's blood glucose level is maintained by glycogenolysis, gluconeogenesis, and lipolysis.
8 Nutrition	Vitamins	• A 40-year-old purified protein derivative–positive patient has undergone a course of isoniazid. Months later, she complains to her physician that she has tingling and numbness in her extremities. She is immediately started on supplemental pyridoxine.
9 Molecular Biology	Diseases involving trinucleotide repeat expansion	• A 45-year-old man develops severe depression, choreiform movements, and confusion. He is later diagnosed with Huntington's disease.
10 Applications of Biotechnology	Polymerase chain reaction (PCR)	• A 32-year-old pregnant woman with a family history of cystic fibrosis seeks genetic counseling. Her physician recommends an amniotic PCR test to determine if her fetus is affected with this disorder.

Topic **1**

Proteins

Must **Knows**

- The different amino acids and the side chains associated with each
- Significance of the Henderson-Hasselbalch equation
- Examples of important proteins and their role in physiology and pathophysiology

AMINO ACIDS

Carboxyl groups and amino groups	• Every amino acid has a carboxyl group • Every amino acid except proline has an amino group (proline has an imino group) attached to the α-carbon • Both groups are charged at physiologic pH ($-COO^-$ and $-NH_3^+$)
Aliphatic side chains	• Alanine, glycine, isoleucine, leucine, methionine, phenylalanine, proline, tryptophan, valine
Polar side chains	• Asparagine, cysteine, glutamine, serine, threonine, tyrosine
Acidic side chains	• Aspartate, glutamate
Basic side chains	• Arginine, histidine, lysine
Henderson–Hasselbalch equation	• Can be used to calculate the quantitative relationship between the concentration of a weak acid and its conjugate base for amino acids with acidic or basic side chains

PROTEIN STRUCTURE AND FUNCTION

Peptide bonds	• Amino acids are attached to each other by peptide bonds • All α-amino and α-carboxyl groups except the terminal groups on the protein participate in these bonds. These are charged at physiologic pH. • Sequences of amino acids in a peptide are read from the amino-terminal end to the carboxy-terminal end
Forces affecting protein structure	• Hydrophobic interactions: Important for nonpolar amino acids • Hydrogen bonds: Important for polar amino acids

- Disulfide bonds: Formed by two cysteine residues, producing cystine
- Ionic bonds: Formed by acidic and basic side chains; acidic side chains are negatively charged, and basic side chains are positively charged at physiologic pH

Primary structure	• Defined as the linear sequence of its amino acids
Secondary structure	• Defined as regular arrangements of amino acids that are located near to each other in the linear sequence. Examples are the α helix, β sheet, and β bend.
Tertiary structure	• Defined as the fundamental functional and three-dimensional structural units of a polypeptide • It is formed from combinations of motifs. Tertiary structure refers to the folding of the domains and their final arrangement in the polypeptide. • Tertiary structure is stabilized by disulfide bonds, hydrophobic interactions, hydrogen bonds, and ionic bonds
Quaternary structure	• Proteins consisting of more than one polypeptide chain have quaternary structure. The polypeptides are held together by noncovalent bonds.
Denaturation	• Process of unfolding a protein resulting in a nonfunctional unit • Denaturing agents include heat, organic solvents, mechanical mixing, strong acids or bases, detergents, and ions of heavy metals such as lead and mercury
Misfolding and prions	• Protein misfolding is most commonly caused by a gene mutation, which produces an altered protein. An example of this is the amyloid protein that spontaneously aggregates in degenerative diseases such as Alzheimer disease. • The prion protein (PrP) is an infectious protein that converts noninfectious PrP into the infectious form, resulting in diseases such as Creutzfeldt-Jakob disease

PROTEINS AND PHYSIOLOGY

Heme proteins	• Proteins that contain heme as a tightly bound prosthetic group • Examples: Cytochromes, catalase, hemoglobin, and myoglobin
Myoglobin	• Structure: One heme group bound to a single polypeptide • Function: Oxygen carrier within the muscle cell
Hemoglobin (Hb)	• Structure: Four polypeptides, each of which binds a heme group • Function: Oxygen transport within erythrocytes from the lungs to the capillaries of the tissues. Hemoglobin (Hb) exists in two forms: the deoxy form of Hb is called the taut (T) form, and the oxygenated form of Hb is called the relaxed (R) form. The R form is the high oxygen affinity form of Hb.

Factors affecting oxygen tension in hemoglobin	• pO$_2$: Partial pressure of oxygen
	• pH: O$_2$ release increased by decreased pH (Bohr effect). Important for short-term changes such as exercising muscle.
	• pCO$_2$: Partial pressure of CO$_2$
	• 2,3-BPG: Binds to Hb and decreases its oxygen affinity. This allows O$_2$ to be released more easily in peripheral tissues. Important for long-term changes such as of chronic hypoxia or anemia.
Carbon monoxide	• Binds tightly to the Hb iron. It stabilizes the R form of Hb and prevents release of O$_2$ to the tissues. CO toxicity is a result of tissue hypoxia.
	• Treated with 100% O$_2$
Collagen	• Three polypeptides (referred to as α-chains, each 1000 amino acids in length) wound around one another in a triple helix
	• The chains are held together by hydrogen bonds
	• In some collagens (e.g., type 1), the collagen molecules self-assemble into fibrils in which the adjacent triple helices are arranged in a staggered pattern, each overlapping its neighbor by a length approximately three quarters of a molecule
	• The triple helices are cross-linked, giving the fibrillar array great tensile strength
Elastin	• A connective tissue protein with rubber-like properties
	• Composed of elastin and glycoprotein microfibrils, such as fibrillin
	• Found in the lungs, the walls of large arteries, and elastic ligaments

PROTEINS AND PATHOPHYSIOLOGY

Diabetes and HbA$_{1c}$	• HbA$_{1c}$ is formed through nonenzymic glycosylation of hemoglobin and glucose. Increased amounts of HbA$_{1c}$ are found in the erythrocytes of patients with diabetes mellitus because their HbA has contact with higher glucose concentrations in the blood during the 120-day life span of the erythrocyte.
Sickle cell disease (HbS disease)	• Caused by a point mutation in both genes coding for the chain that results in a valine rather than a glutamate at position six. This leads to a polymerization (and therefore decreased solubility) of the deoxy form of Hb, which causes distortion of the erythrocyte membrane. The erythrocytes occlude capillaries, leading to a shortened erythrocyte life span, anemia, tissue anoxia, and painful "crises." Thus, anything that favors the deoxygenated form of Hb (e.g., low pO$_2$, increased pCO$_2$, decreased pH, or an increased concentration of 2,3-BPG) can precipitate a crisis.

Thalassemias	• Hereditary hemolytic diseases in which an imbalance occurs in the synthesis of either α- or β-globin chains

α-Thalassemia	• Due to deletions of the α globin gene. There are four types:
	   ○ Hydrops fetalis: Absence of α chains: results in in utero death of the fetus
	   ○ Hb H = Missing three genes: β tetramers form resulting in severe anemia requiring transfusions
	   ○ α-Thalassemia minor trait: Results in microcytic anemia
	   ○ Missing one & chain gene: Asymptomatic carrier

β-Thalassemia	• There are two types:
	   ○ β^0/β^0 from defective transcription: Results in serious anemia requiring transfusions may see elevated HbF
	   ○ β^+/β^+ from defective translation: Low HbA and some HbF
	   ○ If there is one normal β gene, the anemia will be mild

Ehlers-Danlos syndrome	• A heterogeneous group of generalized tissue disorders that result from inheritable defects in the metabolism of fibrillar collagen molecules. Clinical findings include stretchy skin, loose joints, and vascular problems.
Osteogenesis imperfecta	• Also known as brittle bone syndrome. This is a heterogeneous group of inherited disorders involving mutations in the collagen genes. • Clinical findings: Bones that easily bend and fracture; retarded wound healing and a rotated and twisted spine, leading to a humped-back appearance
Marfan syndrome	• Caused by mutations in the fibrillin gene, which results in defective elastin • Clinical findings: Marfanoid habitus (arm span is longer than height), lens subluxation, high-arched hard palate, mitral regurgitation, and development of aortic aneurism
α_1-Antitrypsin (α_1-AT)	• An enzyme produced in the liver and found in blood and other body fluids that inhibits proteolytic enzymes such as elastase. In the normal lung, activated and degenerating neutrophils release elastase, which is inactivated by α_1-AT. If this inhibitor is absent, lung tissue is destroyed and cannot regenerate, leading to emphysema. • Treatment: Weekly intravenous administration of α_1-AT
Duchenne muscular dystrophy	• A lethal X-linked recessive muscular disease caused by a deletion in the gene coding for the muscle protein dystrophin. This results in progressive muscular weakness starting in early childhood.

Topic **2**

Enzymes

Must **Knows**

- Mechanism of action of enzymes
- Types of inhibition

Enzyme	• Protein catalysts that increase the velocity of a chemical reaction and are not consumed during the reaction they catalyze. Each enzyme has an active site where the substrate binds and is converted to product.
Cofactor	• Some enzymes require cofactors for activity. These can be metal ions or organic molecules that are often derivatives of vitamins. Tightly bound coenzymes are called prosthetic groups.
Mechanism of action of enzymes	• Provides an alternate reaction pathway with a lower free energy of activation. They do not change the free energies of the re-actants or products and, therefore, do not change the equilibrium of the reaction.
Factors affecting reaction velocity	• Substrate concentrations • Temperature • pH
Competitive inhibition	• Reversible • Binds to active site • Increases the apparent K_m (decreases affinity) but does not affect the V_{max} • May be overcome by adding additional substrate
Noncompetitive inhibition	• Reversible • Binds to enzyme at location other than the active site • Decreases the V_{max} but does not affect the K_m of the enzyme • Cannot be overcome by adding additional substrate

| Clinical uses of enzymes for diagnosis | • Enzymes can be found in the plasma either because they were specifically secreted to fulfill a function in the blood or because they were released by dead or damaged cells. Many diseases that cause tissue damage result in an increased release of intracellular enzymes into the plasma. The activities of many of these enzymes (e.g., creatine kinase, lactate dehydrogenase, alanine aminotransferase) are routinely determined for diagnostic purposes in diseases of the heart, liver, skeletal muscle, and other tissues. |

Topic **3**

Energetics

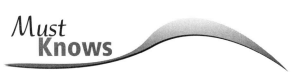

Must Knows

● Definitions of enthalpy, entropy, free energy, and spontaneity

● Purpose of the electron transport chain and its importance to oxidative phosphorylation

Enthalpy	• A measure of the change in heat content of the reactants and products
Entropy	• A measure of the change in the randomness or disorder of the reactants and products
Free energy (ΔG)	• Using enthalpy, entropy, and temperature, free energy predicts the direction in which a reaction will spontaneously proceed
Spontaneity	• If the change in free energy is negative (i.e., the product has a lower free energy than the substrate), the reaction goes spontaneously • If ΔG is positive, the reaction does not go spontaneously • If $\Delta G = 0$, the reactants are in equilibrium • The change in free energy of the forward reaction (A $\rightarrow$ B) is equal in magnitude but opposite in sign to that of the reverse reaction (B $\rightarrow$ A)
Coupling	• The standard free energy changes ($\Delta G°$s) are additive in any sequence of consecutive reactions. Therefore, reactions or processes with a large positive $\Delta G°$ are made possible by coupling them with a reaction with a large negative $\Delta G°$. This large negative $\Delta G°$ is commonly provided by the hydrolysis of ATP.

The electron transport chain	• The reduced coenzymes NADH and FADH$_2$ each donate a pair of electrons to a specialized set of electron carriers, consisting of flavin mononucleotide (FMN), coenzyme Q, and a series of cytochromes, collectively called the electron transport chain. This pathway is present in the inner mitochondrial membrane and is the final common pathway by which electrons derived from different fuels of the body flow to oxygen. The terminal cytochrome is called cytochrome a + a$_3$ and is the only cytochrome able to bind oxygen.
Oxidative phosphorylation	• Electron transport is coupled to the transport of protons (H$^+$) across the inner mitochondrial membrane from the matrix to the intermembrane space. This process creates an electrical gradient and a pH gradient across the inner mitochondrial membrane. After protons have been transferred to the intermembrane space, they can reenter the mitochondrial matrix by passing through a channel in the adenosine triphosphate (ATP) synthase complex, resulting in the synthesis of ATP from adenosine diphosphate (ADP) + Pi, and at the same time dissipating the pH and electrical gradients. Electron transport and phosphorylation are thus said to be tightly coupled. The amount of ATP produced depends on the substrate donating electrons: ○ 1 NADH → 3 ATP ○ 1 FADH2 → 2 ATP
Uncouplers	• Compounds that increase the permeability of the inner mitochondrial membrane to protons. The energy produced by the transport of electrons is released as heat, rather than being used to synthesize ATP. Examples include 2,4-dinitrophenol and high doses of aspirin.

Topic **4**

Carbohydrate Metabolism

Must **Knows**

- The irreversible steps of the glycolytic pathway and the intermediates that regulate them
- The irreversible steps of the tricarboxylic acid cycle and the intermediates that regulate them
- The process of gluconeogenesis
- Glycogen metabolism and the glycogen storage diseases
- The function of the pentose phosphate pathway and the role of its products

GLYCOLYSIS

The irreversible steps of glycolysis	Reaction	Inhibitor	Activator
	Glucose → glucose 6-phosphate = Hexokinase/glucokinase	Glucose 6-P	
	Fructose 6-P → Fructose 1,6-BP = Phosphofructokinase I	Adenosine tri-phosphate (ATP) Citrate	Atrial natriuretic peptide (AMP) Fructose 2,6-BP
	Phosphoenolpyruvate → Pyruvate = Pyruvate dehydrogenase	ATP Alanine	Fructose 1,6-BP

The primary allosteric activator of glycolysis	• Fructose 2,6-bisphosphatase
	○ This activator is paramount for the rate-limiting reaction of glycolysis (the conversion of fructose 6-phosphate to fructose 1,6-bisphosphate by phosphofructokinase I)
	○ Phosphofructokinase II is the enzyme that produces fructose 2,6-bisphosphate from fructose 6-phosphate
	○ This intermediate is also an allosteric inhibitor of fructose 1,6-bisphosphatase. This enzyme is necessary for the process of gluconeogenesis.

Net substrates and products	Substrates	Products
	• 1 Glucose	• 2 ATP
	• 2 ADP	• 2 NADH
	• 2 NAD^+	• 2 Pyruvate

Glucokinase vs. hexokinase	• Glucokinase	• Hexokinase
	○ Found in the liver	○ Found in all other tissues
	○ High K_m and high V_{max}	○ Low K_m and low V_{max}
	○ It is fast and more specific	○ It is slower but less specific

Anaerobic glycolysis	• $NADH$ is reoxidized to NAD^+ by the conversion of pyruvate to lactic acid. This occurs in cells such as erythrocytes that have few or no mitochondria and in tissues such as exercising muscle, where production of NADH exceeds the oxidative capacity of the respiratory chain.

Lactic acidosis	• Occurs when there is a collapse of the circulatory system

Pyruvate kinase deficiency	• Accounts for 95% of all inherited defects in glycolytic enzymes
	• It is restricted to erythrocytes and causes mild to severe chronic hemolytic anemia. Altered kinetics (e.g., increased K_m, decreased V_{max}) most often account for the enzyme deficiency.

Pyruvate dehydrogenase	• Pyruvate + NAD$^+$ + CoA → Acetyl-CoA + CO$_2$ + NADH

• Pyruvate is oxidatively decarboxylated by the pyruvate dehydrogenase complex producing acetyl-coenzyme A (CoA), which is the major fuel for the tricarboxylic acid (TCA) cycle

Cofactors	Inhibitors	Activators
• Thiamine pyrophosphate (TPP; B$_1$)	• ATP	• NAD$^+$
• Flavin adenine dinucleotide (FAD; B$_2$)	• Acetyl-CoA	• CoA
• Nicotinamide adenine din (NAD); B$_3$)	• NADH	• Pyruvate
• CoA (pantothenic acid)		
• Lipoic acid		

Congenital lactic acidosis

• Most commonly caused by pyruvate dehydrogenase deficiency. Because the deficiency deprives the brain of acetyl-CoA, the central nervous system is particularly affected, with psycho-motor retardation and death occurring in most patients.

• Treatment includes a ketogenic diet

THE TRICARBOXYLIC ACID CYCLE

Intermediates of TCA

• Citrate → Isocitrate → α-Ketoglutarate → Succinyl CoA → Succinate → Fumarate → Malate → Oxaloacetate → Citrate

The irreversible steps of the TCA cycle

Reaction	Inhibitor	Activator
Oxaloacetate + Acetyl-CoA → Citrate = Citrate synthase	• ATP • NADH • Succinyl-CoA • Fatty acyl CoA	• ADP
Isocitrate → α-Ketoglutarate + CO$_2$ + NADH = Isocitrate dehydrogenase	• ATP • NADH	• ADP • Ca^{2+}
α-Ketoglutarate → succinyl-CoA + CO$_2$ + NADH = α-Ketoglutarate dehydrogenase	• ATP • NADH • Guanosine 5'-triphosphate (GTP) • Succinyl-CoA	• Ca^{2+}

Products per pyruvate

• 3 NADH × 3 ATP → 9 ATP
• 1 FADH$_2$ × 2 ATP → 2 ATP
• 1 GTP
• 1 CO$_2$
• Σ_{ATP} = 12 ATP/Pyruvate

GLUCONEOGENESIS

Substrates of gluconeogenesis	• Intermediates of glycolysis and the TCA cycle • Glycerol from the hydrolysis of triacylglycerols in adipose tissue • Lactate from anaerobic metabolism • α-Ketoacids from the metabolism of glucogenic amino acids
Irreversible steps of glycolysis	• Reactions catalyzed by pyruvate kinase, phosphofructokinase, hexokinase

Enzymes required to reverse the pyruvate kinase reaction

Reaction	Activators	Notes
Pyruvate + CO_2 + 2 ATP $\rightarrow$ Oxaloacetate + 2 ADP = Pyruvate carboxylase	• Acetyl-CoA	• Located in the mitochondria • Requires biotin and ATP
Oxaloacetate + GTP $\rightarrow$ Phosphoenolpyruvate (PEP) + GMP + CO_2 = PEP carboxykinase		• Located in the cytosol • Requires GTP • Rate-limiting step • Transcription of its mRNA is increased by glucagon and decreased by insulin

Enzymes required to reverse the phosphofructokinase kinase reaction

Reaction	Activators	Inhibitors
Fructose 1,6-bisphosphate $\rightarrow$ fructose 6-phosphate = Fructose 1,6-b_1 = phosphatase	• ATP	• AMP • Fructose-2,6-BP

Enzymes required to reverse the hexokinase reaction

Reaction
Glucose 6-phosphate $\rightarrow$ glucose = Glucose 6-phosphatase

Energy investment required for gluconeogenesis	• 4 ATP • 2 GTP • 2 NADH

GLYCOGEN METABOLISM

Locations of glycogen	• In the liver, glycogen is used to maintain the blood glucose concentration during the fasting state. In skeletal muscle, glycogen serves as a fuel reserve for the synthesis of ATP during muscle contraction.
Structure of glycogen	• Glycogen is a highly branched polymer of α-D-glucose. The primary glycosidic bond is an $\alpha(1\rightarrow4)$-linkage. After about eight to ten glucosyl residues, there is a branch containing an $\alpha(1\rightarrow6)$-linkage.

Glycogenesis	• Uridine diphosphate (UDP)-glucose, the building block of glycogen, is synthesized from glucose 1-phosphate and uridine 5′-triphosphate (UTP) by UDP glucose pyrophosphorylase. UDP glucose is then transferred to the non-reducing ends of glycogen chains by glycogen synthase, which makes $\alpha(1\rightarrow4)$-linkages. • Branches are formed by glucosyl-$\alpha(1\rightarrow4)\rightarrow\alpha(1\rightarrow6)$-transferase, which transfers a chain of five to eight glucosyl residues from the non-reducing end of the glycogen chain (breaking an $\alpha(1\rightarrow4)$ linkage), and attaches it with an $\alpha(1\rightarrow6)$ linkage to another residue in the chain
Glycogenolysis	• Glycogen phosphorylase cleaves the $\alpha(1\rightarrow4)$ bond between glucosyl residues at the non-reducing ends of the glycogen chains, producing glucose 1-phosphate. It requires pyridoxol phosphate as a coenzyme. This sequential degradation continues until four glucosyl units remain on each chain before a branch point. The resulting structure is called a limit dextrin. • Glucosyl-$\alpha(1\rightarrow4)$-$\alpha(1\rightarrow4)$-transferase, removes the outer three of the four glucosyl residues attached at a branch and transfers them to the non-reducing end of another chain, where they can be converted to glucose 1-phosphate by glycogen phosphorylase. Next, the remaining single glucose residue attached by an $\alpha(1\rightarrow6)$ linkage is removed hydrolytically by amylo-$\alpha(1\rightarrow6)$-glucosidase activity, releasing free glucose.
Final products to yield glucose	• Glucose 1-phosphate is converted to glucose 6-phosphate by phosphoglucomutase. In the muscle, glucose 6-phosphate enters glycolysis. In the liver, the phosphate is removed by glucose 6-phosphatase, releasing free glucose that can be used to maintain blood glucose levels at the beginning of a fast.

GLYCOGEN STORAGE DISEASES

Type 1a (Von Gierke disease)	• Deficiency of glucose 6-phosphatase • This prohibits the conversion of glucose 6-phosphate back to glucose for release into the plasma • Clinical findings: Severe fasting hypoglycemia and hepatomegaly
Type II (Pompe disease)	• Deficiency of lysosomal $\alpha(1\rightarrow4)$-glucosidase • Clinical findings: Massive cardiomegaly leading to eventual heart failure
Type V (McArdle disease)	• Deficiency of skeletal muscle glycogen phosphorylase • Clinical findings: Inability to break down muscle glycogen leading to cramps, weakness, myoglobinemia, and myoglobinuria

FRUCTOSE METABOLISM

Sources of fructose	• Sucrose: Disaccharide of fructose and glucose
	• Entry of fructose into cells is insulin independent
Metabolic pathway of fructose	• Fructose is first phosphorylated to fructose 1-phosphate by fructokinase and then cleaved by aldolase B to dihydroxyacetone phosphate and glyceraldehyde. These enzymes are found in the liver, kidney, and small intestinal mucosa.
Hereditary fructose intolerance	• Deficiency of aldolase B
	• Fructose 1-phosphate accumulates resulting in decreased available phosphate, which prevents gluconeogenesis and glycogenolysis
	• Clinical findings: Severe hypoglycemia and liver damage
	• Treatment: Dietary restriction of sucrose and fructose
Essential fructosuria	• Deficiency of fructokinase
	• Clinical findings: Fructosuria, which is a benign condition

GALACTOSE METABOLISM

Sources of galactose	• Lactose
	• The entry of galactose into cells is not insulin-dependent
Metabolic pathway of galactose	• Galactose is first phosphorylated by galactokinase, which produces galactose 1-phosphate. This compound is converted to UDP galactose by galactose 1-phosphate uridyltransferase, with the nucleotide supplied by UDP-glucose.
	• In order for UDP-galactose to enter the mainstream of glucose metabolism, it must first be converted to UDP-glucose by UDP-hexose 4-epimerase
Galactosemia	• Classically from deficiency of galactose 1-phosphate uridyltransferase
	• Galactose 1-phosphate accumulates, trapping phosphate. Excess galactose is converted to galactitol by aldose reductase.
	• Clinical findings: Liver damage, severe retardation, cataracts
	• Treatment: Dietary restriction of galactose and lactose from the diet
	• Less commonly, galactosemia may also occur via deficiency of galactokinase

PENTOSE PHOSPHATE PATHWAY

Pathway summary	• Found in all cells
	• Consists of two irreversible oxidative reactions followed by a series of reversible sugar–phosphate interconversions

- No ATP is directly consumed or produced in the cycle
- Two nicotinamide adenosine dinucleotide phosphate (NADPH) are produced for each glucose 6-phosphate entering the oxidative part of the pathway

Irreversible (oxidative) reactions	- Glucose 6-phosphate is irreversibly converted to ribulose 5-phosphate, and two NADPH are produced. The regulated step is glucose 6-phosphate dehydrogenase (G6PD), which is strongly inhibited by NADPH.
Reversible (nonoxidative) reactions	- Reversible nonoxidative reactions interconvert sugar-phosphates. This part of the pathway is the source of ribose 5-phosphate required for nucleotide and nucleic acid synthesis.
NADPH for lipid synthesis	- NADPH is a source of reducing equivalents in reductive biosynthesis, such as the production of fatty acids and steroids
NADPH for the reduction of H_2O_2	- Glutathione (GSH) is used by glutathione peroxidase to reduce peroxide to water. The oxidized glutathione is reduced by glutathione reductase, using NADPH as the source of electrons.
The cytochrome P450 system	- NADPH provides reducing equivalents for the cytochrome P450 monooxygenase system. This is used in hydroxylation of steroids to produce steroid hormones, bile acid synthesis by the liver, and activation of vitamin D. The system also detoxifies foreign compounds such as drugs and varied pollutants, including carcinogens, pesticides, and petroleum products.
NADPH oxidase	- NADPH provides the reducing equivalents for phagocytes in the process of eliminating invading microorganisms. NADPH oxidase uses molecular oxygen and NADPH to produce superoxide radicals. The superoxide radical can be converted to peroxide, hypochlorous acid, or hydroxyl radicals.
Nitric oxide synthetase	- NADPH is required for the synthesis of nitric oxide (NO), an important molecule that causes vasodilation by relaxing vascular smooth muscle, acts as a kind of neurotransmitter, prevents platelet aggregation, and helps mediate macrophage bactericidal activity
Chronic granulomatous disease	- Defect in NADPH oxidase - Clinical findings: severe, persistent, chronic pyogenic infections
G6PD dehydrogenase deficiency	- G6PD deficiency impairs the ability of the cell to form the NADPH that is essential for the maintenance of the reduced glutathione pool. The cells most affected are the erythrocytes. Free radicals and peroxides formed within the cells cannot be neutralized. This results in protein denaturation. Hemoglobin precipitates into Heinz bodies. The cells become rigid, and they are removed by the reticuloendothelial system of the spleen and liver. Splenic macrophages also pluck out the Heinz bodies in erythrocytes, resulting in bite cells.

- Hemolytic anemia due to G6PD deficiency can be caused by the production of free radicals and peroxides after ingestion of oxidant drugs, ingestion of fava beans, or severe infections. Babies with G6PD deficiency may experience neonatal jaundice appearing 1 to 4 days after birth.

Topic **5**

Lipid Metabolism

Must Knows

- ● Fatty acid metabolism of dietary sources and *de novo* synthesis
- ● Process of β-oxidation
- ● Role of ketogenesis
- ● Synthesis of cholesterol and bile acids

DIETARY LIPIDS

Composition of mixed micelles	• The products of lipid digestion (free fatty acids, 2-monoacyl-glycerol, and cholesterol) plus bile salts form mixed micelles that are able to cross the unstirred water layer on the surface of the brush border membrane. Individual lipids enter the intestinal mucosal cell cytosol.
Fatty acid activation and the synthesis of chylomicrons	• The lipids move to the endoplasmic reticulum, where fatty acyl CoA synthetase converts free fatty acids into their activated CoA derivatives. Fatty acyl CoAs are then used to produce triacylglycerols, cholesteryl esters, and phospholipids. These, together with the fat-soluble vitamins (A, D, E, and K) and a single protein (apolipoprotein [apo] B-48), form a chylomicron. The chylomicron is secreted into the lymphatic system and is carried to the blood.
Formation of functional chylomicrons	• Occurs in the blood when they receive apo C-II and apo-E from circulating high-density lipoprotein (HDL)
Function of apo C-II	• Apo C-II activates lipoprotein lipase, which degrades the chylomicron's triacylglycerol to fatty acids and glycerol. The fatty acids that are released are stored (in the adipose) or used for energy (by the muscle).

Diseases caused by deficiency of apo C-II	• Patients with a deficiency of lipoprotein lipase or apo C-II show a dramatic accumulation of chylomicrons in the plasma (type 1 hyperlipoproteinemia, familial lipoprotein lipase deficiency, or hypertriacylglycerolemia)
Fate of the chylomicron remnant	• After most of the triacylglycerol is removed, apo C-II is returned to the HDL, and the chylomicron remnant—carrying most of the dietary cholesterol—binds to a receptor on the liver that recognizes apo E. The particle is endocytosed and its contents degraded by lysosomal enzymes.
Structure and function of very low-density lipoprotein (VLDL)	• VLDLs are produced in the liver and are composed predominantly of triacylglycerol. They contain a single molecule of apo B-100. Similar to chylomicrons, VLDLs receive apo C-II and apo E from HDLs in the plasma. VLDLs carry triacylglycerol from the liver to the peripheral tissues, where lipoprotein lipase degrades the lipid.
Formation of low-density lipoprotein (LDL)	• As triacylglycerol is removed from the VLDL, the particle receives cholesteryl esters from HDL. This process is accomplished by cholesteryl ester transfer proteins. Eventually, VLDL in the plasma is converted to LDL. Apo CII and apo E are returned to HDLs, but the LDL retains apo B-100, which is recognized by receptors on peripheral tissues and the liver. LDLs undergo receptor-mediated endocytosis, and their contents are degraded in the lysosomes.
Disease caused by deficiency of apo B-100 receptors	• Type II hyperlipidemia (familial hypercholesterolemia)
Reverse cholesterol transport	• Cholesterol in peripheral tissues is transferred to HDL and esterified by phosphatidylcholine cholesterol transferase (PCAT) and is transported to the liver

FATTY ACID METABOLISM

Structure of fatty acids	• A linear hydrocarbon chain with a terminal carboxyl group. A fatty acid can be saturated (contains no double bonds) or unsaturated (contains one or more double bonds).
Essential fatty acids	• Linoleic acid (ω-6) and linolenic acid (ω-3)
De novo synthesis	• Carbons used to synthesize fatty acids are provided by acetyl-CoA, energy is provided by adenosine triphosphate (ATP), and reducing equivalents are provided by NADPH
	• Fatty acids are synthesized in the cytosol. Citrate carries two-carbon acetyl units from the mitochondrial matrix to the cytosol.
	• The regulated step in fatty acid synthesis (acetyl-CoA $\rightarrow$ malonyl CoA) is catalyzed by acetyl-CoA carboxylase, which requires biotin. Citrate is the allosteric activator, and long-chain fatty acyl

CoA is the inhibitor. The enzyme can also be activated in the presence of insulin and inactivated in the presence of epinephrine or glucagon.

- The rest of the steps in fatty acid synthesis are catalyzed by the fatty acid synthase complex, which produces palmitoyl CoA from acetyl-CoA and malonyl CoA, with NADPH as the source of reducing equivalents

Fatty acid degradation	• When lipids are required by the body for energy, adipose cell hormone-sensitive lipase (activated by epinephrine, and inhibited by insulin) initiates degradation of stored triacylglycerol. This results in the liberation of free fatty acids and glycerol. The free fatty acids are carried in the plasma by albumin to the liver and peripheral tissues for oxidation. Glycerol returns to the liver, where it serves as a gluconeogenic precursor.
β-Oxidation	• Occurs in mitochondria. The carnitine shuttle is required to transport fatty acids from the cytosol to the mitochondria. Enzymes required are carnitine palmitoyltransferases I (CPT I, cytosolic side of inner mitochondrial membrane) and II (CPT II, an enzyme of the inner mitochondrial membrane). CPT I is inhibited by malonyl CoA. This prevents fatty acids that are being synthesized in the cytosol from malonyl CoA from being transported into the mitochondria, where they would be degraded.
	• Once in the mitochondria, fatty acids are oxidized, producing acetyl-CoA, NADH, and $FADH_2$. The first step in the β-oxidation pathway is catalyzed by one of a family of four acyl CoA dehydrogenases that each has a specificity for either short-, medium-, long-, or very-long-chain fatty acids.
	• Oxidation of fatty acids with an odd number of carbons proceeds two carbons at a time (producing acetyl-CoA) until the last three carbons (propionyl CoA). This compound is converted to methylmalonyl CoA (a reaction requiring biotin), which is then converted to succinyl CoA by methylmalonyl CoA mutase (requiring vitamin B_{12}). A genetic error in the mutase or vitamin B_{12} deficiency causes methylmalonic acidemia and aciduria.
Diseases caused by carnitine palmitoyltransferase (CPT) deficiencies	• Genetic CPT II deficiency in cardiac and skeletal muscle causes cardiomyopathy and myoglobinemia and weakness after exercise
	• Genetic CPT I deficiency affects the liver, where an inability to use long chain fatty acids for energy during a fast can cause severe hypoglycemia

KETONE METABOLISM

Synthesis and utilization	• Liver mitochondria converts acetyl-CoA derived from fatty acid oxidation into the ketone bodies, acetoacetate, and 3-hydroxybutyrate. (Acetone, a nonmetabolizable ketone body, is produced spontaneously from acetoacetate in the blood.)

Peripheral tissues possessing mitochondria can oxidize 3-hydroxybutyrate to acetoacetate, which can be reconverted to acetyl-CoA, thus producing energy for the cell.

| **Tissues that use ketone bodies** | • Unlike fatty acids, ketone bodies can be used by the brain (but not by cells, such as erythrocytes, that lack mitochondria) and, thus, are important fuels during a fast. The liver lacks the ability to degrade ketone bodies. |

SYNTHESIS OF CHOLESTEROL AND BILE ACIDS

Rate-limiting step of cholesterol synthesis	• Cytosolic HMG CoA reductase • Produces mevalonic acid from hydroxymethylglutaryl CoA (HMG CoA)
Control of cholesterol metabolism	• Sterol dependent regulation of gene expression: Expression of the HMG CoA reductase gene is controlled by a transcription factor that is activated when cholesterol levels are low • Sterol-independent phosphorylation/dephosphorylation: Covalent control through the actions of a protein kinase (inactivates the enzyme) and a protein phosphatase (activates the enzyme) • Hormonal regulation: Insulin up-regulates HMG CoA reductase; glucagon down-regulates • Medications: Drugs such as lovastatin and mevastatin are competitive inhibitors of HMG CoA reductase
Degradation of cholesterol	• The ring structure of cholesterol cannot be metabolized by humans. Cholesterol can be eliminated from the body either by conversion to bile salts or by secretion into the bile.
Synthesis of bile	• Bile consists of bile salts and phosphatidylcholine. Bile salts are conjugated bile acids. The primary bile acids, cholic or chenodeoxycholic acids, contain two or three alcohol groups, respectively. These structures are amphipathic and can serve as emulsifying agents. Before the bile acids leave the liver, they are conjugated to a molecule of either glycine or taurine, producing the primary bile salts (glycocholic or taurocholic acids and glycochenodeoxycholic or taurochenodeoxycholic acids). Bile salts are more amphipathic than bile acids and, therefore, are more effective emulsifiers.
Production of secondary bile acids	• In the intestine, bacteria can remove the glycine and taurine and can remove a hydroxyl group, producing the secondary bile acids, deoxycholic and lithocholic acids

Topic **6**

Nitrogen Metabolism

Must Knows

- The urea cycle
- Catabolism of amino acids
- Metabolic defects in amino acid metabolism

DEAMINATION AND THE UREA CYCLE

Deamination	• Amino groups are transferred to glutamate from all amino acids except lysine and threonine by aminotransferases. The two most important of these enzymes are alanine aminotransferase (ALT) and aspartate aminotransferase (AST). Pyridoxal phosphate is a required coenzyme.
	• Glutamate can be oxidatively deaminated in the liver by glutamate dehydrogenase. This liberates free ammonia that can be used to make urea.
Ammonia transport	• Two mechanisms for transport of ammonia from periphery to liver:
	○ Glutamine from glutamate and ammonia (glutamine synthetase)
	○ Alanine by transamination of pyruvate
	• In the liver, the ammonia group is removed from glutamine by glutaminase and from alanine by transamination
Sources of N in urea	• Free NH_3 and aspartate
The urea cycle	• Carbamoyl phosphate synthetase I produces carbamoyl phosphate in mitochondria from CO_2, NH_3 and two adenosine triphosphate (ATP) molecules
	• Carbamoyl phosphate and ornithine combine to form citrulline, which is transported out of the mitochondria
	• Aspartate and citrulline combine to form argininosuccinate, which is converted to arginine and fumarate
	• Arginase cleaves the arginine, releasing urea and ornithine
	• The cycle repeats
The rate-limiting step of the urea cycle	• Carbamoyl phosphate synthetase I: Requires N-acetylglutamate, a positive allosteric activator

METABOLIC DEFECTS IN AMINO ACID METABOLISM

Phenylketonuria (PKU)	• Deficiency of phenylalanine hydroxylase
	• This enzyme converts phenylalanine to tyrosine. Hyperphenylalaninemia may also be caused by deficiencies in the coenzyme tetrahydrobiopterin.
	• Clinical findings: Mental retardation, failure to walk or talk, seizures, hyperactivity, tremor, microcephaly, and failure to grow
	• Treatment: Dietary restriction of phenylalanine, especially for pregnant women because failure to eliminate phenylalanine results in mental retardation of the fetus. Note that tyrosine becomes an essential dietary component for people with PKU.
Maple syrup urine disease (MSUD)	• Deficiency of branched-chain α-ketoacid dehydrogenase
	• This enzyme decarboxylates leucine, isoleucine, and valine. These amino acids and their corresponding α-ketoacids accumulate in the blood, causing a toxic effect that interferes with brain function. This is a recessive disorder.
	• Clinical findings: Feeding problems, vomiting, dehydration, severe metabolic acidosis, and a characteristic maple syrup smell of the urine. If untreated, the disease leads to mental retardation, physical disabilities, and death.
	• Treatment: Dietary limitation of leucine, isoleucine, and valine
Albinism	• Deficiency of tyrosinase
	• This enzyme is required in the synthesis of melanin from tyrosine. This is a recessive disorder.
Alkaptonuria	• Deficiency of homogentisic acid oxidase
	• This prevents the degradation of tyrosine. It is a recessive disorder.
	• Clinical findings: Dark urine, darkened tympanic membrane on otoscopy, and arthralgias secondary to deposits in joints
Homocystinuria or homocystinemia	• Most often caused by a defect of cystathionine synthase, which converts homocysteine to cystathionine. Cofactor is pyridoxine.
	• Clinical findings: Ectopic lens, marfanoid habitus, mental retardation, and accelerated atherosclerosis
	• Homocystinemia is a "soft" risk factor for heart disease
	• Treatment includes restriction of methionine and supplementation of B_6 (pyridoxine), B_{12}, and folate

PORPHYRIN METABOLISM

Structure	• Cyclic compounds that readily bind metal ions, usually Fe^{2+} or Fe^{3+}
	• Includes heme, myoglobin, cytochromes, and the enzyme catalase

Synthesis	• Carbon and nitrogen atoms are provided by glycine and succinyl CoA. The rate limiting step in heme synthesis is the formation of δ-aminolevulinic acid (ALA) by ALA synthase. This reaction occurs in the mitochondria and requires the coenzyme pyridoxal phosphate.
Lead poisoning	• Lead inhibits ferrochelatase and ALA dehydratase • Clinical findings: Anemia and porphyria
The porphyrias	• Porphyrias are caused by defects in heme synthesis, resulting in the accumulation and increased excretion of porphyrins or porphyrin precursors. Porphyrias are classified as erythropoietic or hepatic, depending where the enzyme deficiency occurs. • With the exception of congenital erythropoietic porphyria, which is a genetically recessive disease, all the porphyrias are inherited as autosomal dominant disorders. Porphyria results in decreased synthesis of heme. Because heme acts as an inhibitor of ALA synthase, the lack of heme allows for increased ALA synthase activity, causing the accumulation of toxic intermediates. • Treatment: Injections of hemin to inhibit ALA synthase. Because some porphyrias result in photosensitivity, avoidance of sunlight is helpful.
Degradation of heme	• Heme is degraded by macrophages to biliverdin (green), which is reduced to bilirubin (red-orange). Bilirubin complexed with albumin is carried via the blood to the liver and is conjugated with glucuronate for excretion. • Bilirubin diglucuronide is transported into the bile canaliculi, where it is first hydrolyzed and reduced by bacteria to yield urobilinogen and is then oxidized by intestinal bacteria to stercobilin (brown). A portion of the urobilinogen is transported by the blood to the kidney for elimination in the urine.

Jaundice	• Jaundice (icterus) refers to the yellow color of the skin, nail beds, and sclerae caused by deposition of bilirubin, secondary to increased bilirubin levels in the blood
	• There are four major forms of jaundice:
	  ◦ Hemolytic: Secondary to massive lysis of erythrocytes. This results in more heme than can be handled by the reticulo-endothelial system
	  ◦ Obstructive: Secondary to obstruction of the bile duct
	  ◦ Hepatocellular: Secondary to damaged liver cells. This decreases the ability of the liver to take up and conjugate bilirubin.
	  ◦ Neonatal: Secondary to decreased hepatic conjugation of bilirubin; especially in premature infants

IMPORTANT AMINO ACID DERIVATIVES

Histidine	• Histamine
Glycine	• Heme
Arginine	• Urea
Tryptophan	• Serotonin and melatonin
Tyrosine	• The catecholamines (dopamine, norepinephrine, epinephrine)

NUCLEOTIDE METABOLISM

Role of 5-phosphoribosyl-1-pyrophosphate (PRPP)	• PRPP is an "activated pentose" that participates in the synthesis of purine and pyrimidine nucleotides and in the salvage of purine bases. It donates the ribose–phosphate unit found in nucleotides. PRPP is produced by PRPP synthetase, an enzyme that is activated by inorganic phosphate and inhibited by purine nucleoside diphosphates and triphosphates (purine nucleotides are the end products of this pathway).
Regulated step in purine synthesis	• Synthesis of 5′-phosphoribosylamine from PRPP and glutamine by glutamine:phosphoribosyl pyrophosphate amidotransferase • Inhibitors: Adenosine monophosphate (AMP), guanosine monophosphate (GMP), and inosine 5′-monophosphate (IMP), the end products of the pathway • Activator: PRPP

The salvage pathway	• Purines that result from the normal turnover of cellular nucleic acids can be reconverted into nucleoside triphosphates and used by the body. Thus, they are "salvaged" instead of being degraded to uric acid. PRPP is the source of the ribose–phosphate unit, and the reactions are catalyzed by:
	  ○ Adenine phosphoribosyltransferase
	  ○ Hypoxanthine-guanine phosphoribosyltransferase (HGPRT)

Synthesis of deoxyribonucleotides	• All deoxyribonucleotides (used to synthesize DNA) are synthesized from ribonucleotides by the enzyme ribonucleotide reductase, which requires thioredoxin as a cofactor • Inhibitor: dATP • Activator: Adenosine triphosphate (ATP)
Degradation of purines	• Purine nucleotides are converted to uric acid through xanthine oxidase
Regulated step in pyrimidine synthesis	• The committed step of this pathway is the synthesis of carbamoyl phosphate from glutamine and CO_2, catalyzed by carbamoyl phosphate synthetase II • Inhibitor: Uridine 5′-triphosphate (UTP) • Activators: ATP and PRPP

Lesch-Nyhan syndrome	• An X-linked recessive disorder caused by the deficiency of HGPRT, resulting in failure of the salvage pathway • Clinical findings: Mental retardation, self-mutilation, involuntary movements
Gout	• Related to high levels of uric acid in the blood • Manifests as podagra (inflammation of the joint of the great toe secondary to uric acid deposition) • Increased uric acid levels may be caused by increased turnover of nucleotides as in myeloproliferative disorders, salvage pathway deficiencies, decreased excretion of uric acid as in renal failure, or lifestyle factors such as excessive consumption of alcohol or red meats.
Adenosine deaminase deficiency	• Results in accumulation of adenosine, which is converted to its ribonucleotide or deoxyribonucleotide forms by cellular kinases. As dATP levels increase, they inhibit ribonucleotide reductase, thus preventing the production of deoxyribonucleotides, so that the cell cannot produce DNA and divide. This causes severe combined immunodeficiency disease (SCID), involving a lack of T and B cells.

Topic **7**

Control of Metabolism

Must
Knows

● Effects of insulin and glucagon on metabolism and how they are involved in the fed versus fasting states

● The pathogenesis of diabetes mellitus

INSULIN TO GLUCAGON RATIO

Functions of insulin	• Anabolic metabolism: Glycolysis, glycogenesis, protein synthesis, lipogenesis, cholesterol synthesis
Functions of glucagon	• Catabolic metabolism: Glycogenolysis, gluconeogenesis, ketogenesis, lipolysis

FED STATE VERSUS FASTING STATE

The fed state
- The pancreas senses increased circulating glucose and amino acids and secretes insulin
- The insulin:glucagon ratio increases
- An anabolic period continues for 2 to 4 hours
- Glycolysis
- Glycogenesis
- Triacylglycerol synthesis $\rightarrow$ very low-density lipoprotein (VLDL) $\rightarrow$ peripheral tissues $\rightarrow$ uptake and lipogenesis
- Protein synthesis

The fasting state
- The pancreas senses a decrease in circulating glucose and amino acids; insulin secretion is decreased and glucagon secretion is increased
- The insulin:glucagon ratio decreases
- A catabolic period begins
- Glycogenolysis
- Muscle protein breakdown for utilization of amino acids for gluconeogenesis
- Gluconeogenesis
- Lipolysis
- Ketogenesis

DIABETES MELLITUS

Diabetes type 1
- Caused by an absolute deficiency of insulin, which may have resulted from an autoimmune mechanism against the pancreatic β cells. Metabolic abnormalities may include hyperglycemia, hypertriglyceridemia, and ketoacidosis. Treatment includes exogenous insulin injected subcutaneously.

Diabetes type 2
- Caused by a relative insulin deficiency attributable to a combination of insulin resistance and dysfunctional pancreatic β cells. Metabolic abnormalities include hyperosmotic coma. Treatment includes weight loss, oral hypoglycemics, and medications with postreceptor effects.

Topic **8**

Nutrition

Must
Knows

● The essential amino acids and dietary fats

● The difference between kwashiorkor and marasmus

● The fat-soluble and water-soluble vitamins and diseases associated with their deficiencies

DIET

Essential amino acids	• PVT TIM HALL = phenylalanine, valine, threonine, tryptophan, isoleucine, histidine, leucine, lysine
Essential dietary fats	• Linoleic (ω-6) and linolenic (ω-3)
Kwashiorkor vs. marasmus	• Kwashiorkor: Protein malnutrition • Marasmus: Protein and energy malnutrition

FAT-SOLUBLE VITAMINS

Vitamin A	• Function: Growth, differentiation of epithelium, vision • Deficiency: Retardation of growth, xerophthalmia, night blindness • Excess: Alopecia, fractures, pseudotumor cerebri
Vitamin D	• Function: When activated, stimulates gut absorption of calcium and phosphate • Deficiency: Rickets (children), osteomalacia (adults), hypocalcemic tetany • Excess: Weakness, constipation
Vitamin E	• Function: Antioxidant • Deficiency: Increased erythrocyte fragility
Vitamin K	• Function: Cofactor in production of clotting factors • Deficiency: Increased prothrombin time (PT) and international normalized ratio (INR)

WATER-SOLUBLE VITAMINS

Vitamin B$_1$ (thiamine)	• Function: Cofactor for pyruvate dehydrogenase (entrance to TCA), α-ketoglutarate dehydrogenase (TCA), and trans-ketolase (PPP) • Deficiency: Beri-beri, Wernicke-Korsakoff syndrome
Vitamin B$_2$ (riboflavin)	• Function: Precursor for flavin adenine dinucleotide (FAD) and flavin mononucleotide (FMN; used in the electron transport chain) • Deficiency: Dermatitis and angular stomatitis
Vitamin B$_3$ (niacin)	• Function: Precursor to nicotinamide adenine dinucleotide (NAD$^+$) and nicotinamide adenosine dinucleotide phosphate (NADPH) • Deficiency: Pellagra (diarrhea, dermatitis, dementia, death)
Vitamin B$_5$ (pantothenic acid)	• Function: Part of coenzyme A (CoA; part of fatty acid synthase) • Deficiency: Rare
Vitamin B$_6$ (pyridoxine)	• Function: Cofactor for transamination and decarboxylation of amino acids • Deficiency: Glossitis and neuropathy; this may be induced by isoniazid
Vitamin B$_{12}$ (cobalamin)	• Function: Cofactor for conversion of homocysteine to methionine and methylmalonyl CoA to succinyl CoA • Deficiency: Megaloblastic anemia and spinal degeneration
Folate	• Function: 1-carbon transfers, especially in nucleic acid synthesis • Deficiency: Megaloblastic anemia
Biotin	• Function: Cofactor for carboxylation reactions • Deficiency: Rare
Vitamin C	• Function: Antioxidant and cofactor in collagen synthesis • Deficiency: Scurvy

Topic **9**

Molecular Biology

Must Knows

- Structure of DNA
- Mechanism of replication
- Organization of eukaryotic DNA
- Process of transcription and translation

DNA STRUCTURE

Structure	• Double-stranded double helix arranged antiparallel around an axis of symmetry
Base pairs	• Adenine with thymine • Cytosine with guanine • Base pairs are held together with hydrogen bonds
Function of histones	• There are five classes of histones, which are positively charged small proteins that form ionic bonds with negatively charged DNA. Two each of histones H2A, H2B, H3, and H4 form a structural core around which DNA is wrapped creating a nucleosome. The DNA connecting the nucleosomes is called linker DNA, and it is bound to histone H1.
Organization of DNA	• Nucleosomes can be packed more tightly to form a polynucleosome (also called a nucleofilament), which is organized into loops that are anchored by a nuclear scaffold containing several proteins. Additional levels of organization create a chromosome.

DNA REPLICATION

Origin of replication	• Eukaryotes have multiple origins of replication that form replication forks. Replication forks consist of a leading strand and lagging (discontinuous) strand.
Single-strand binding proteins	• Attaches to ssDNA after separation • Protects against digestion from DNAses • Does not interfere with replication; displaced by DNA polymerase

Topoisomerase	• Involved with supercoiling DNA
	• It cleaves strands, introduces or removes supercoils, and then reseals strands. No adenosine triphosphate (ATP) is needed to remove supercoils but ATP is needed to introduce. The free ends are never released. Some antibiotics work by inhibiting these enzymes.
Telomeres	• Telomeres are stretches of highly repetitive DNA found at the ends of chromosomes. As cells divide and age, these sequences are shortened, contributing to cell death. In cells that do not age (e.g., germline and cancer cells), the enzyme telomerase replaces the telomeres, thus extending the life of the cell.
DNA polymerase	• There are at least five classes of eukaryotic DNA polymerases.
	○ Pol α is a multisubunit enzyme, one subunit of which performs the primase function
	○ Pol α 5′→3′ polymerase activity adds a short piece of DNA to the RNA primer
	○ Pol δ completes DNA synthesis on the leading strand and elongates each lagging strand fragment using 3′→5′ exonuclease activity to proofread the newly synthesized DNA
	○ Pol β and pol ϵ are involved in carrying out DNA repair
	○ Pol γ replicates mitochondrial DNA
Synthesis	• DNA polymerases read 3′ → 5′ and write 5′ → 3′
	• Beginning with one parental double helix, the two newly synthesized stretches of nucleotide chains must grow in opposite directions, one in the 5′→3′ direction toward the replication fork (leading strand), and one in the 5′→3′ direction away from the replication fork (lagging strand). The lagging strand is synthesized discontinuously.
DNA mutations	• Silent: Base change without change of resulting amino acid
	• Missense: Base change leads to a different amino acid
	• Nonsense: Base change results in an early stop codon
	• Frame shift: Base change results in misreading and a truncated protein
DNA repair	• Exposure of a cell to ultraviolet light can cause covalent joining of two adjacent pyrimidines (usually thymines), producing a dimer. These thymine dimers prevent DNA polymerase from replicating the DNA strand beyond the site of dimer formation. These are removed by UV-specific endonuclease and the resulting gap is filled by DNA polymerases.
Xeroderma pigmentosum	• Deficiency of ultraviolet (UV)-specific endonuclease. Cells cannot repair DNA damaged by UV light. This results in a high incidence of skin cancers.

| Trinucleotide repeat expansion | • Tandem repeats of three bases
• Examples include:
  ◦ Huntington disease: CAG repeats
  ◦ Fragile-X syndrome: CGG repeats
  ◦ Myotonic dystrophy: CTG repeats |

RNA SYNTHESIS AND TRANSCRIPTION

RNA polymerases	• RNA pol I: Synthesizes rRNA • RNA pol II: Synthesizes mRNA • RNA pol III: Synthesizes tRNA
Promoters	• Promoters for class II genes contain consensus sequences, such as the TATA or Hogness box, the CAAT box, and the GC box. They serve as binding sites for proteins called general transcription factors, which, in turn, interact with each other and with RNA polymerase II.
Enhancers	• Enhancers are DNA sequences that increase the rate of initiation of transcription by binding to specific transcription factors called activators
Introns and exons	• Introns are noncoding sequences and are spliced out of mRNA after transcription by snRNPs (small ribonucleoprotein particles) • Exons contain information that codes for proteins and are expressed

TRANSLATION

Transfer RNA	• Aminoacyl-tRNA synthetase uses ATP to charge each tRNA with a specific amino acid at the 3′ end of the tRNA • Each tRNA has a three-base nucleotide anticodon sequence that recognizes the appropriate mRNA codon during translation
Initiation	• Begins with the assembly of the ribosomal subunits, mRNA, tRNA for the first codon, guanosine 5′-triphosphate (GTP), and initiation factors. The 5′-cap on eukaryotic mRNA is used to position the mRNA on the ribosome. The initiation codon is 5′–AUG–3′.
Elongation	• The polypeptide chain is elongated in the 5′→3′ direction by the addition of amino acids to the carboxyl end of its growing chain. The process requires elongation factors. The formation of the peptide bond is catalyzed by peptidyltransferase. After peptide bond formation, the ribosome advances to the next codon (translocation; this process requires GTP). Because of the length of most mRNAs, more than one ribosome at a time can translate a message, forming a polysome.

Termination	• Termination begins when one of the three termination codons moves into the A site. These codons are recognized by release factors. The newly synthesized protein is released from the ribosomal complex, and the ribosome dissociates from the mRNA.
The wobble hypothesis	• States that the first (5′) base of the anticodon is not as spatially defined as the other two bases. Movement of that first base allows nontraditional base pairing with the last (3′) base of the codon, thus allowing a single tRNA to recognize more than one codon for a specific amino acid.

Topic **10**

Applications of Biotechnology

Must Knows

- Cloning, libraries, and probes
- Restriction fragment length polymorphism (RFLP)
- Polymerase chain reaction (PCR)
- Northern blots, Southern blots, and Western blots

Process of cloning	• Amplification of a foreign DNA sequence. The sequence is inserted into a plasmid, which serves as the vector, and is introduced into bacteria or other microorganisms such as yeast, where the DNA is autonomously replicated.
DNA libraries	• A DNA library is a collection of cloned restriction fragments of the DNA of an organism
	• Genomic library: A collection of fragments of double-stranded DNA obtained by digestion of the total DNA of the organism with a restriction endonuclease and subsequent ligation to an appropriate vector. It ideally contains a copy of every DNA nucleotide sequence in the genome.
	• cDNA (complementary DNA) library: Contains only DNA sequences that are complementary to mRNA molecules present in a cell and differ from one cell type to another. Because cDNA has no intervening sequences, it can be cloned into an expression vector for the synthesis of eukaryotic proteins by bacteria.

Probing	• A probe is a single-stranded piece of DNA, usually labeled with a radioisotope. It has a nucleotide sequence complementary to the DNA molecule of interest (target DNA). Probes can be used to identify which clone of a library or which band on a gel contains the target DNA.
Restriction fragment length polymorphism (RFLP)	• The human genome contains many thousands of polymorphisms. A polymorphic gene is one in which the variant alleles are common enough to be useful as genetic markers. An RFLP is a genetic variant that can be examined by cleaving the DNA into restriction fragments using a restriction enzyme. The patterns produced may be linked with a specific disease (e.g., sickle cell anemia).
Polymerase chain reaction (PCR)	• The PCR is a test tube method for amplifying a selected DNA sequence and does not rely on the biologic cloning method. PCR permits the synthesis of millions of copies of a specific nucleotide sequence in a few hours. It can amplify the sequence, even when the targeted sequence makes up less than one part per million of the total initial sample. The method can be used to amplify DNA sequences from any source.
Southern Blot	• Southern blotting is a technique that can be used to detect specific genes present in DNA. The DNA is cleaved using a restriction endonuclease. The pieces are then separated by gel electrophoresis and transferred to a nitrocellulose membrane for analysis. The fragment of interest is detected using a probe.
Northern blot	• Same as a Southern blot except that a radioactive DNA probe is used to detect sample mRNA
Western blot	• Proteins within a sample are separated using gel electrophoresis and are transferred to a filter. A labeled antibody is then used to identify the protein of interest.
Enzyme-liked immunosorbent assay (ELISA)	• Used to quantify antibodies in a sample. To assay for antibodies in the serum of a patient, the serum is added to a sample well that is already coated with the antigen. If antibodies are present in the serum, they will bind with the antigen. Antibodies to human immunoglobulin G (IgG) are then added to the sample. The anti-IgG antibodies bind to the sample IgG that is bound to the antigen. These anti-IgG antibodies are linked to an enzyme. A substrate for the enzyme is then added which changes the color of the solution. The color change is measured. This color change is directly proportional to the amount of sample antibodies that were in the serum.

Pharmacology

10 Top Tips

Pharmacology

Topic	Main Focus	USMLE Example
1 Basic Principles of Pharmacology	Inducers and inhibitors of drug metabolism	• A 65-year-old physician with atrial fibrillation who is taking warfarin for anticoagulation is advised not to drink grapefruit juice after taking the medication. Her cardiologist explains that grapefruit juice is a potent inhibitor of the cytochrome system responsible for warfarin metabolism.
2 Autonomic Drugs	Indirect cholinomimetics	• A 35-year-old woman presents to a neurologist for blurry vision and weakness that progressively worsens throughout the day. Because she improves immediately after edrophonium is administered, she receives a diagnosis of myasthenia gravis.
3 Cardiovascular–Renal Drugs	Role of angiotensin-converting enzyme inhibitors	• A 55-year-old obese man with type II diabetes is found to be hypertensive on three consecutive visits to the physician. The patient is started on lisinopril to both treat the hypertension and to prevent diabetic nephropathy.
4 Drugs That Act on Smooth Muscle	Pharmacologic treatment of asthma	• A 12-year-old boy with asthma must use his inhaler daily. His pediatrician adds fluticasone to his regimen as a controller, and he continues to use albuterol occasionally as a reliever for his asthma symptoms.

(Continued)

10 Top Tips

Pharmacology   (Continued)

Topic	Main Focus	USMLE Example
5 **Nonsteroidal Antiinflammatory Drugs; Antirheumatic Drugs; and Drugs to Treat Diseases of the Skin, Blood, Gastrointestinal Disorders, and Gout**	Anticoagulants, antiplatelets, and thrombolytic drugs	• When a 65-year-old man steps off a plane in New York after flying from Los Angeles, he suddenly develops chest pain and shortness of breath. An electrocardiogram shows tachycardia and right heart strain and a plasma d-Dimer level of 20,000. The man is diagnosed with a pulmonary embolism and is started immediately on enoxaparin.
6 **Neuropharmacology**	Antipsychotic drugs	• 30-year-old man with psychotic symptoms who has been prescribed haloperidol suddenly develops mental status changes, rigidity, and hyperthermia. He is diagnosed with neuroleptic malignant syndrome and is given bromocriptine and dantrolene.
7 **Chemotherapeutic Drugs**	β-Lactam antibiotics	• An 8-year-old boy with a fever of 104°F, mental status changes, and neck rigidity is immediately started on cefuroxime for suspected bacterial meningitis.
8 **Endocrine Drugs**	Estrogens, progestins, selective estrogen receptor modulators (SERMs), uterine stimulants, and tocolytics	• A 28-year-old woman who is 37 weeks pregnant presents to the obstetrics clinic with intractable headaches and a blood pressure of 200/120 mm Hg. She is emergently started on intravenous magnesium for preeclampsia.
9 **Herbs and Vitamins**	Fat-soluble vitamins	• A 32-year-old woman from California presents with complaints of chronic headache and orange-tinted skin. A history reveals that she been taking large quantities of vitamin A supplements.
10 **Toxicology**	Environmental toxins	• A 5-year-old boy who is found unconsciousness in a greenhouse presents to the emergency department with pinpoint pupils, diaphoresis, urinary incontinence, vomiting, and muscle fasciculations. He is administered atropine for organophosphate poisoning.

Topic **1**

Basic Principles of Pharmacology

Must Knows

- The Henderson-Hasselbalch equation
- Basic principles of pharmacokinetics and pharmacodynamics
- Important inducers and inhibitors

PHARMACODYNAMICS

Henderson-Hasselbalch	$$pK - pH = \log\left(\frac{A^-}{HA}\right)$$ • Use this to determine the fraction of ionized drug to nonionized drug for a given physiological pH. HA = unionized form and A^- = ionized form.
Median effective dose (ED$_{50}$)	• The minimum dose required to produce effects in 50% of a population
Therapeutic index	• The ratio of the mean effective dose to the mean toxic dose or mean lethal dose
Efficacy	• The ability to produce a desired therapeutic effect; efficacy is independent of potency
Potency (EC$_{50}$)	• The amount of drug needed to produce 50% of maximal effect • Determined by the affinity of the receptor for the drug
K$_d$	• Concentration of the drug needed to fill 50% of receptor sites. • Measure of affinity • Smaller K_d means greater affinity
Spare receptors	• When the affinity (K_d) is greater than the potency (EC$_{50}$), the maximal effect of the drug will be produced before all receptors are filled

PHARMACOKINETICS

Volume of distribution	$$V_d = \frac{\text{Amount of drug in body}}{\text{Plasma drug concentration}}$$

Clearance (CL)	$$CL = \frac{\text{Rate of elimination}}{\text{Plasma concentration}}$$
Half-life ($t_{1/2}$)	$$t_{1/2} = \frac{0.693 \times V_d}{CL}$$ • Affected by age, renal disease, hepatic disease, congestive heart failure
Bioavailability (BA)	• After administration, BA is the amount of the drug that actually enters into systemic circulation. • For IV drugs, this is usually 1 (100% is available) • For po (by mouth) drugs, this is reduced by incomplete absorption and first-pass metabolism
Loading dose	$$\text{Loading dose} = \frac{V_d \times C_p}{BA}$$ C_p = desired plasma concentration • The dose should be lowered in renal failure
Maintenance dose	$$\text{Maintenance dose} = \frac{C_p}{BA}$$ • This is the desired dose for continuing therapy and may need to be decreased in renal failure
Zero-order metabolism	• The rate of elimination is always a constant amount per unit time • Examples: Ethanol, phenytoin, aspirin (at toxic concentrations)
First-order metabolism	• The rate of elimination is proportional to the drug plasma concentration • The concentration will decrease 50% for each $t_{1/2}$

METABOLISM, ELIMINATION, AND DISTRIBUTION

Important inducers and inhibitors	Inducers • Tobacco smoke • Phenobarbital • Phenytoin • Rifampin • Isoniazid	Inhibitors • Grapefruit juice • Cimetidine • Chloramphenicol • Macrolide antibiotics (erythromycin) • Selective serotonin reuptake inhibitors (SSRIs)

Getting drug to site of action	• Drug must get to its receptor or other site of action
	 • Drug may need to penetrate several barriers to get to site:
	   ◦ Gastrointestinal barrier (if given orally)
	   ◦ Blood–brain barrier (BBB: if needs to be in brain); see topic 6
	   ◦ Penetrate cell membrane if intracellular site of action	

- Drugs need to be lipid soluble and nonionized for maximal absorption across barriers; some drugs have active transport systems

How drugs are distributed in body	<ul><li>Some drugs are distributed throughout body water</li><li>Some drugs stay within the vascular system</li><li>Some drugs are bound to plasma proteins, usually albumin</li><li>Some drugs are sequestered in various places in body (calcium and bisphosphonates go to bone; arsenic is retained in hair; fluoride and some antibiotics are taken up into the teeth)</li></ul>

Topic **2**

Autonomic Drugs

Must Knows

- The organization of the autonomic nervous system, including the names and function of major cholinergic and adrenergic receptors (Tables 2-1 and 2-2)
- Properties and actions of acetylcholine, norepinephrine, and epinephrine
- Cholinomimetics and blockers
- Sympathomimetics, α-blockers, and β-blockers

ORGANIZATION OF THE AUTONOMIC NERVOUS SYSTEM (FIG. VII-1)

Sympathetic division	<ul><li>Sympathetic division prepares body for strenuous muscular activity, stress, and emergencies</li><li>Preganglionic neurons are in the thoracic and lumbar regions of the spinal cord</li><li>Preganglionic fibers are short</li><li>Preganglionic fibers release acetylcholine (Ach) at synapse</li><li>Postganglionic fibers are generally long</li><li>Postganglionic neurons release norepinephrine at postganglionic synapses (epinephrine released at adrenal medulla)</li></ul>
Parasympathetic division	<ul><li>Parasympathetic division is involved with the accumulation, storage, and preservation of body resources</li><li>Preganglionic neurons are in the vertebral ganglia</li><li>Preganglionic fibers are long</li></ul>

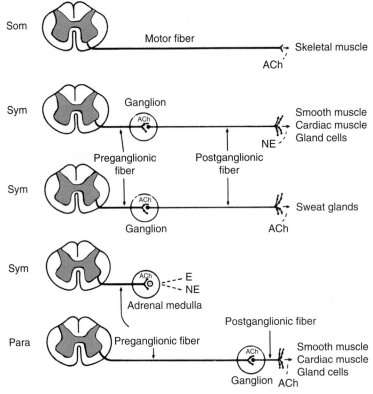

● **Figure VII-1** Anatomical characteristics and neurotransmitters of the somatic (Som), sympathetic (Sym), and parasympathetic (Para) divisions of the peripheral nervous system. Ach = acetylcholine; E = epinephrine; NE = norepinephrine

- Pre- and postganglionic neurons release acetylcholine at synapses

Autonomic receptors	See Tables VII-1 and VII-2

ACETYLCHOLINE, NOREPINEPHRINE, AND EPINEPHRINE

Properties and actions of ACh

- ACh is an ester of choline and acetic acid
- Synthesized by choline acetyltransferase (CAT)
- Binds to muscarinic and nicotinic cholinergic receptors
- Broken down rapidly by acetylcholinesterase (AChE)
- Some agents (i.e., agonists) mimic ACh and are longer lasting than Ach
- Some agents (i.e., antagonists) block ACh
- Muscarinic receptor–blocking drugs decrease secretions, dilate pupils, and are useful in Parkinson's disease, motion sickness, and irritable bowel syndrome
- Nicotinic receptor–blocking drugs have been used to produce paralysis in anesthetic procedures

| TABLE VII-1 | EFFECTS OF AUTONOMIC NERVE ACTIVITY ON ORGAN FUNCTION |

Organ	Sympathetic Nerve Activity	Parasympathetic Nerve Activity
Eye	α—Contracts radial muscle (mydriasis) —	M—Contracts circular muscle (miosis) M—Contracts ciliary muscle
Heart	β_1—Accelerates SA node β_1—Accelerates conduction β_1—increases contractility	M—Decelerates SA node M—Decelerates conduction – –
Vascular smooth muscle	α—Constricts skin, skeletal muscle, and splanchnic vessels β_2—Dilates skeletal muscle vessels M—Dilates skeletal muscle vessels (minor) DA—Dilates renal and mesenteric vessels	M(*)—
Bronchiolar smooth muscle	β_2—Dilates bronchioles	M—Constricts bronchioles
Gastrointestinal tract	β_2—Reduces gut contractility α—Contracts sphincters —	M—Increases gut contractility M—Relaxes sphincters M—Increases secretions
Genitourinary tract	β_2—Reduces bladder motility α—Contracts sphincters α—Contracts the uterus β_2—Relaxes the pregnant uterus α—Ejaculation	M—Increases bladder motility M—Relaxes sphincters – – – – M—Penile erection
Skin	α—Contracts pilomotor smooth muscle M—Induces sweating	– – – –
Metabolic functions	α, β_2—Increases hepatic gluconeogenesis α, β_2—Increases hepatic glycogenolysis β_3—Increases lipolysis	– – – – – –
Glands	α_1—Thick salivary secretions —	M—Thin salivary secretions M—Lacrimal and respiratory secretions
Adrenal gland	N—Secretes EPI and NE	– –
Kidney	β_1—Increases renin release	– –

*Most blood vessels have innervated muscarinic cholinoreceptors. Relaxation involves release of endothelium-derived relaxing factor (EDRF) from the endothelium.
α = α-adrenoceptors; β = β-adrenoceptors; DA = dopamine; EPI = epinephrine; M = muscarinic cholinoceptors; N = nicotinic cholinoceptors; NE = nonepinephrine; SA = sinoatrial; – – = no effect.

| TABLE VII-2 | PROPERTIES OF ACETYLCHOLINE AND ACETYLCHOLINE ANALOGUES |

	Metabolized by Cholinesterases	Nicotinic Activity	GI Activity	CV Activity
ACh	+++	+	++	+++
Methacholine	+	—	+	+++
Carbachol	—	+	+++	+
Bethanechol (*Urecholine*)	—	—	+++	+

ACh = acetylcholine; CV = cardiovascular; GI = gastrointestinal.

- ACh accumulates and may produce serious adverse effects and even death when acetylcholinesterase is inhibited; this is mechanism of nerve gases, such as Sarin

Properties and actions of norepinephrine (NE)	- A catecholamine that is chemically synthesized from tyramine
	- Tyramine → Dopamine → Norepinephrine → Epinephrine
	- Ways to terminate NE's actions:
	- Most important is reuptake into neuron and rerelease
	- Metabolism by monoamine oxidase (MAO)
	- Metabolism by catechol-O-methyl transferase (COMT)
	- Actions of NE:
	- Constricts blood vessels of skin, mucous membranes, and skeletal muscle by effects on α receptor
	- Increase in heart rate and cardiac force by effects at β-receptor effect
	- Therapeutic actions of agonists:
	  ○ Restore or maintain blood pressure
	  ○ Produce mydriasis
	  ○ Treat bronchial asthma
	- Therapeutic actions of antagonists
	  ○ Alpha receptor antagonists: Management of primary hypertension (HTN)
	  ○ β-Receptor antagonists: management of cardiac arrhythmias, angina pectoris, hypertension, glaucoma, "stage fright"

CHOLINOMIMETICS AND BLOCKERS

Direct agonists	- Bethanechol
	  ○ Mechanism: activation of smooth muscle
	  ○ Indications: urinary retention, post-operative ileus
	- Carbachol
	  ○ Mechanism: activation of ciliary muscles in eye
	  ○ Indications: glaucoma (eye drops)

Indirect agonists (inhibit AchE)	- Neostigmine
	  ○ Mechanism: Quaternary amine with low lipid solubility that prevents crossing the BBB
	  ○ Indications: Reversal agent in anesthesia
	- Edrophonium
	  ○ Indication: Diagnosis of myasthenia gravis (administration improves strength temporarily if patient has myasthenia; otherwise, the patient will become weaker)
	- Pyridostigmine
	  ○ Indication: Treatment of myasthenia gravis

Antinicotinic drugs	• Succinylcholine
	  ○ Mechanism: Depolarizing neuromuscular agent
	  ○ Indication: Anesthesia induction
	  ○ Adverse effects: Produces muscle fasciculations and may result in rhabdomyolysis and muscle pain
	• Atracurium, pancuronium, vecuronium
	  ○ Mechanism: Nondepolarizing neuromuscular agent
	  ○ Indications: Anesthesia

Antimuscarinic drugs	• Atropine
	  ○ Mechanism: Nonspecific muscarinic receptor inhibitor
	  ○ Indications: Cardiac resuscitation, organophosphate poisoning
	• Ipratropium
	  ○ Mechanism: Bronchodilation. Limited systemic effects.
	  ○ Indications: Chronic obstructive pulmonary disease and pediatric asthma
	• Scopolamine
	  ○ Mechanism: Inhibits central nervous system (CNS) muscarinic receptors
	  ○ Indication: Motion sickness
	• Benztropine
	  ○ Mechanism: Inhibits CNS muscarinic receptors
	  ○ Indications: Acute dystonias caused by antipsychotic medications, adjunct medication for Parkinson's disease
	• Glycopyrrolate
	  ○ Mechanism: Reduces secretions and gastrointestinal motility
	  ○ Indication: Surgical anesthesia
	• Oxybutynin
	  ○ Indication: Urinary incontinence

Organophosphate poisoning	• Malathion, parathion
	  ○ Mechanism: Inhibits acetylcholinesterase (AChE)
	  ○ Signs related to overstimulation of receptors
	  ○ Miosis, lacrimation, bradycardia, bronchospasm, excessive salivation, diarrhea, urinary incontinence, diaphoresis, tremor
	  ○ Treatment: Large doses of atropine, neostigmine, pralidoxime (regenerates AChE)

Atropine poisoning	• Signs opposite of organophosphate poisoning • Mydriasis; Mental status change; dry mouth; tachycardia; constipation; urinary retention; dry, hot, red skin • Treatment: Physostigmine (an AChE inhibitor that is a tertiary amine allowing for CNS penetration)

SYMPATHOMIMETICS AND ADRENORECEPTOR BLOCKERS

α₁-Selective agonist

- Phenylephrine
  - Mechanism: Direct α-adrenoreceptor agonist
  - Indications: Nasal decongestant, blood pressure (BP) maintenance during spinal anesthesia, termination of paroxysmal atrial tachycardia

α₂-Selective agonists

- Clonidine
  - Mechanism: Central $α_2$ agonist decreases sympathetic outflow
  - Indications: hypertension (HTN), withdrawal from alcohol, heroin
  - Adverse effects: Rebound hypertension, bradycardia, impotence
- Methyldopa
  - Mechanism: Similar to clonidine
  - Indications: HTN of pregnancy
  - Adverse effects: Drug-induced systemic lupus erythematosus (SLE)

β₂-Selective agonists

- Terbutaline, ritodrine, albuterol
  - Indications: premature labor (terbutaline, ritodrine), asthma (albuterol)
  - Adverse effects: Tachycardia, arrhythmias, skeletal muscle tremor
  - Contraindications: Cardiac arrhythmias

α₁-Selective antagonists

- Prazosin, terazosin, doxazosin
  - Indications: HTN and benign prostatic hyperplasia
  - Adverse effects: First dose orthostatic hypotension

α-Nonselective antagonists

- Phenoxybenzamine, phentolamine
  - Mechanism: Irreversible block (phenoxybenzamine), reversible block (phentolamine)
  - Indications: Pheochromocytoma
  - Adverse effects: Orthostatic hypotension, reflex tachycardia

β₁-Selective antagonists

- Atenolol, metoprolol, esmolol
  - Indications: HTN and to block sympathetic cardiac stimulation in patients in whom nonselective β-blockade is contraindicated (asthma, chronic obstructive pulmonary disease [COPD]); Esmolol has very short half-life

β₂-Nonselective antagonists

- Propranolol, nadolol, timolol
  - Indications: HTN, angina, myocardial infarction (MI), congestive heart failure (CHF), arrhythmias, glaucoma (timolol)
  - Contraindications: Asthma, chronic obstructive pulmonary disease (COPD), diabetes, pregnancy, heart block

Drugs that affect release of epinephrine and norepinephrine	• Amphetamine
	○ Indications: Hypotension, resuscitation, narcolepsy
	○ Ephedrine
	○ Indications: Hypotension, bronchodilation, nasal decongestion

Topic **3**

Cardiovascular–Renal Drugs

Must Knows

- Diuretic drugs
- Inhibitors of the renin–angiotensin–aldosterone axis
- Antihypertensive drugs
- Antiarrhythmics
- Cardiac glycosides
- Nitrates
- Intravenous inotropic agents
- Pharmacologic management of congestive heart failure, angina, and myocardial infarction

DIURETICS (FIG. VII-2)

Carbonic anhydrase inhibitors	• Acetazolamide
	○ Mechanism: Inhibits carbonic anhydrase in the proximal convoluted tubule causing loss of $NaCO_3$
	○ Indications: Glaucoma, metabolic alkalosis, altitude sickness
	○ Adverse effects: Hyperchloremic metabolic acidosis
Thiazides	• Hydrochlorothiazide (HCTZ), metolazone
	○ Mechanism: Blocks NaCl resorption in the distal convoluted tubule
	○ Indications: congestive heart failure (CHF), calcium nephrolithiasis, nephrogenic diabetes insipidus, metolazone is effective even if glomerula filtration rate (GFR) < 30
	○ Adverse effects: Hypercalcemia, hyperuricemia, hyperglycemia, hypersensitivity reaction

Major Locations of Ion and Water Exchange in the Nephron

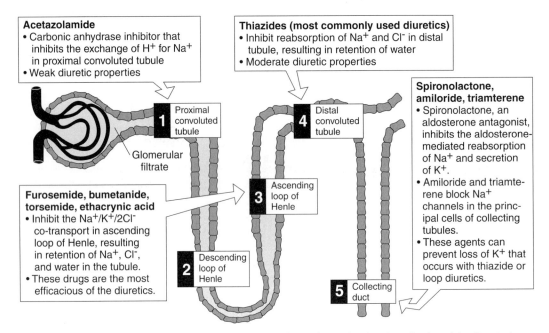

Acetazolamide
- Carbonic anhydrase inhibitor that inhibits the exchange of H^+ for Na^+ in proximal convoluted tubule
- Weak diuretic properties

Thiazides (most commonly used diuretics)
- Inhibit reabsorption of Na^+ and Cl^- in distal tubule, resulting in retention of water
- Moderate diuretic properties

Spironolactone, amiloride, triamterene
- Spironolactone, an aldosterone antagonist, inhibits the aldosterone-mediated reabsorption of Na^+ and secretion of K^+.
- Amiloride and triamterene block Na^+ channels in the principal cells of collecting tubules.
- These agents can prevent loss of K^+ that occurs with thiazide or loop diuretics.

Furosemide, bumetanide, torsemide, ethacrynic acid
- Inhibit the $Na^+/K^+/2Cl^-$ co-transport in ascending loop of Henle, resulting in retention of Na^+, Cl^-, and water in the tubule.
- These drugs are the most efficacious of the diuretics.

1 Proximal convoluted tubule
2 Descending loop of Henle
3 Ascending loop of Henle
4 Distal convoluted tubule
5 Collecting duct

Glomerular filtrate

● **Figure VII-2** Major locations of ion and water exchange in the nephron, showing sites of action of the diuretic drugs. (Redrawn from Mycek MJ, Gertner SB, Perper MM: In Harvey RA, Champe PC, eds, *Lippincott's Illustrated Reviews: Pharmacology, 2nd ed.* Philadelphia, Lippincott-Raven Publishers, 1997, p. 224.)

Potassium-sparing diuretics	• Spironolactone, triamterene, amiloride ○ Mechanism: Spironolactone is an aldosterone antagonist; triamterene and amiloride block sodium resorption in the cortical collecting duct ○ Indications: Hypokalemia, hyperaldosteronism, CHF (first line: spironolactone has anti-remodeling effects on cardiac myocytes) ○ Adverse effects: Hyperkalemia, antiandrogenic effects (spironolactone)
Loop diuretics	• Furosemide, torsemide, bumetanide ○ Mechanism: Inhibit the $Na^+-K^+-2Cl^-$ transporter at the thick ascending loop of Henle ○ Indications: CHF, pulmonary edema, cirrhosis, hypercalcemia ○ Adverse effects: Ototoxicity, hypokalemia, hypovolemia, hypersensitivity reactions

INHIBITORS OF THE RENIN–ANGIOTENSIN–ALDOSTERONE AXIS

The renin–angiotensin–aldosterone system	• This system contributes to routine control of arterial blood pressure

- Inhibition of the renin–angiotensin system with angiotensin-converting enzyme (ACE) inhibitors causes afterload reduction and is considered first line in the treatment of HTN and CHF

ACE inhibitors	• Captopril, enalapril, lisinopril
	  ○ Mechanism: Inhibit ACE
	  ○ Indications: CHF, hypertension, diabetes (protects against the development of diabetic nephropathy)
	  ○ Adverse effects: Chronic dry, hacking cough; hyperkalemia; angioedema
	  ○ Contraindications: Pregnancy (teratogen), renal artery stenosis

Angiotensin receptor blockers (ARBs)	• Losartan, valsartan
	  ○ Mechanism: Angiotensin II receptor antagonist
	  ○ Indications: Usually used when ACE inhibitors are not tolerated
	  ○ Contraindications: Same as ACE inhibitors

OTHER ANTIHYPERTENSIVE MEDICATIONS

Calcium channel blockers (CCBs)	• Dihydopyridines: Nifedipine, amlodipine
	  ○ Mechanism: Peripherally acting Ca^{2+} blockers leading to arteriolar vasodilation
	  ○ Indications: HTN, Raynaud's disease, Prinzmetal's angina
	  ○ Adverse effects: Headache, flushing, peripheral edema; nifedipine is associated with increased risk of myocardial infarction (MI)
	• Centrally acting: Diltiazem, verapamil
	  ○ Mechanism: Block calcium channels in myocytes, thereby causing a negative inotropic and chronotropic response
	  ○ Indications: Arrhythmias, restrictive or hypertrophic cardiomyopathy
	  ○ Adverse effects: Bradycardia, reduced contractility
	  ○ Contraindications: DO NOT USE IN CHF!

Hydralazine	• Mechanism: Arteriolar vasodilation leading to afterload reduction • Indication: HTN, CHF • Adverse effects: Drug induced-systemic lupus erythematosus (SLE), reflex tachycardia
Guanethidine	• Mechanism: Prevents the release of transmitters from peripheral postganglionic sympathetic nerves • Adverse effects: Postural hypotension, sexual impotence

ANTIARRYTHMICS

Class I

- Mechanism: Sodium channel blockers
- Ia: Quinidine, procainamide
  - Indications: Supraventricular tachycardia (SVT), Wolff-Parkinson-White (WPW) syndrome, premature ventricular contraction (PVC), ventricular tachycardia (VT)
  - Adverse effects: ALL MAY INDUCE ARRYTHMIAS! Quinidine: Cinchonism, torsades de pointes (treat with Mg^{2+}); procainamide: drug-induced SLE
- Ib: Lidocaine, mexiletine, phenytoin
  - Indications: VT or ventricular fibrillation (VF), suppression of post-MI arrhythmias (lidocaine is intravenous only, mexiletine is oral and can be used for long-term PVC)

Class II

- Propranolol, atenolol, metoprolol, esmolol
  - Mechanism: Cardiac β-receptors antagonists
  - Indications: Post-MI arrhythmias
  - Contraindications: Bradycardia, asthma

Class III

- Amiodarone, sotalol
  - Mechanism: Potassium channel blockers
  - Indications: Serious life-threatening arrhythmias
  - Adverse effects: Proarrhythmic (may cause torsades de pointes), skin discoloration, amiodarone is notorious for pulmonary fibrosis and hypothyroidism; must do pulmonary function and thyroid function tests!

Class IV

- Diltiazem, verapamil: Block the slow inward Ca^{++} current in heart tissue

CARDIAC GLYCOSIDES

Digitalis

- Digoxin, digitoxin
  - Mechanism: Inhibition of sodium-potassium ATPase leads to increased intracellular sodium; inhibition of the sodium–calcium pump, increased intracellular calcium, increased myocardial contraction; this causes increased inotropy, decreased chronotropy, and increased automaticity
  - Indications: CHF, atrial fibrillation (AF), atrial flutter
  - Adverse effects: PVC, VT, VF, paroxysmal atrial tachycardia (PAT), atrioventricular (AV) block, mental status changes, yellow-green color perception. Adverse cardiac effects are pronounced during hypokalemia
  - Note: The therapeutic index for the cardiac glycosides is narrow, and they do not improve mortality, only morbidity

NITRATES

Nitroglycerin
- Glyceryl trinitrate, isosorbide dinitrate
  - Mechanism: Relaxation of vascular smooth muscle leading to decreased venous tone, increased capacitance, decreased preload, and decreased myocardial O_2 demand; also dilates coronary arteries
  - Indications: Angina, MI
  - Contraindications: Drugs for erectile dysfunction
  - Adverse effects: Flushing, hypotension, dizziness, reflex tachycardia
  - Note: Tolerance will develop. Avoid with intermittent dosing, small doses, and infrequent use

Nitroprusside
- Indications: Hypertensive emergencies
- Adverse effects: Hypotension, tachycardia, cyanide poisoning if used over long period of time

INTRAVENOUS INOTROPIC AGENTS

Phosphodiesterase inhibitors
- Amrinone, milrinone
  - Mechanism: Inhibition of phosphodiesterase leading to decreased cyclic adenosine monophosphate (cAMP), increased intracellular Ca^{2+}, and increased inotropy
  - Indications: Short-term increased cardiac output

Adrenoreceptor agonists
- Dopamine, dobutamine
  - Dopamine acts on α, β_1, and specific dopamine receptors
  - Dobutamine is a direct β_1 agonist
  - Indications: Short-term increased cardiac output; dopamine may also vasodilate renal and splanchnic vasculature at high concentrations, but this is highly debated
  - No serious adverse effects

PHARMACOLOGICAL MANAGEMENT OF CONGESTIVE HEART FAILURE, ANGINA, AND MYOCARDIAL INFARCTION

Congestive heart failure (CHF)
- Mainstay of therapy based on three goals:
  - Decrease salt and water retention (diet: salt and water restriction; diuretics: furosemide, spironolactone, or thiazides)
  - Decrease cardiac work: ACE inhibitor and β-blockers or hydralazine and nitrates
  - Increase contractility: Digoxin

Management of angina pectoris
- Therapy is to terminate or prevent acute attack by:
  - Reducing myocardial O_2 demand: nitrates, β-blockers
  - Prophylaxis of Prinzmetal's: calcium channel blockers (CCBs)

Management of MI

- Mainstay of therapy based on four goals:
  - Reduce pain: Oxygen, morphine
  - Reduce myocardial O_2 demand: β-Blockers, nitrates
  - Improve or restore perfusion: Heparin, aspirin
  - Recognize and treat complications

Topic **4**

Drugs That Act on Smooth Muscle

Must **Knows**

- Histamine antagonists
- Serotonin agonists and antagonists
- Eicosanoids, bradykinin, endothelins, nitric oxide, and asthma drugs

HISTAMINE

Histamine in inflammation

- Histamine is stored in mast cells, basophils, and neurons of the central nervous system (CNS)
- Lewis triple response: Flush, wheal, and flare is the classic picture of histamine release
- Anaphylaxis is the result of rapid release of mast cell histamine

HISTAMINE ANTAGONISTS

Histamine antagonists

- Histamine antagonists cause sedation. This is evidence for histamine being a neurotransmitter in the brain concerned with sleep. The two major histamine receptors are H_1 (involved with allergic reactions) and H_2 (involved with gastric acid secretion)
- Diphenhydramine, chlorpheniramine, loratadine, fexofenadine, cetirizine
  - Mechanism: H_1 antagonists
  - Indications: Rhinitis, urticaria, motion sickness, sleep aids
  - Adverse effects: Sedation (diphenhydramine, chlorpheniramine)
- Cimetidine, ranitidine
  - Mechanism: H_2 antagonists

- Indications: Peptic ulcer, gastroesophageal reflux disease, Zollinger-Ellison syndrome
- Adverse effects: Cimetidine is a potent hepatic inhibitor
- Cromolyn sodium, nedocromil sodium
    - Mechanism: Prevent the release of histamine by mast cells
    - Indications: Asthma

SEROTONIN AGONISTS AND ANTAGONSTS

Agonists
- Sumatriptan, zolmitriptan
    - Indications: Migraine headaches
    - Contraindications: Angina, coronary artery disease

Antagonists
- Odansetron
    - Mechanism: 5-HT$_3$ antagonists at the area postrema
    - Indications: Nausea from surgery, chemotherapy, or hyperemesis gravidum

EICOSANOIDS, BRADYKININ, ENDOTHELINS, NO$_2$, AND ASTHMA DRUGS (FIG. VII-3)

Pathway
- Derived from icosatetraenoic acid (arachidonic acid)
- Arachidonic acid is a precursor for prostaglandins, prostacyclins, and thromboxanes via the cyclooxygenase (COX) pathway or a precursor for leukotrienes via the lipoxygenase pathway

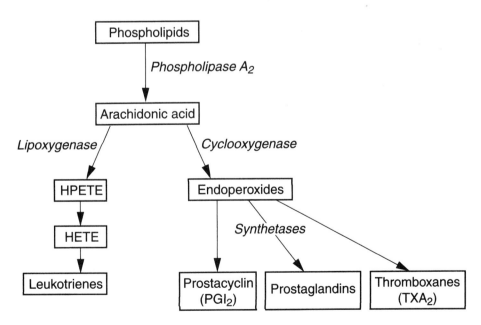

● **Figure VII-3** Synthesis of the eicosanoids. HETE = hydroxyeicosatetraenoic acid; HPETE = hydroperoxyeicosatetraenoic acid.

Prostaglandins	• Alprostadil: Used to maintain patent ductus arteriosus
	• Misoprostol: Used to inhibit ulceration caused by nonsteroidal anti-inflammatory drugs. Also used in combination with mifepristone (RU-486) to induce abortion.
	• Dinoprostone: Causes uterine contraction and is used clinically to induce abortion during the second trimester
Bradykinin, endothelins, and nitric oxide	• Bradykinin is a peptide derived from plasma and tissues and causes vascular smooth muscle relaxation
	• Endothelins are another family of peptides and are the most potent vasoconstrictors known
	• Nitric oxide is a small, unstable free radical that activates guanylate cyclase and leads to an increased production of cyclic guanosine monophosphate (GMP). It serves as a biological messenger in many physiological responses, including vasodilation.
Pharmacological treatment of asthma	• Albuterol, salmeterol
	○ Mechanism: β-Agonist that stimulates β_2 receptors in respiratory smooth muscle, causing relaxation (salmeterol is a long-acting prophylactic β-agonist)
	○ Adverse effects: Skeletal muscle tremor, arrhythmias
	• Ipratropium
	○ Mechanism: Antagonist of muscarinic receptors in respiratory smooth muscle causing relaxation; more effective for pediatric asthma and chronic obstructive pulmonary disease
	• Fluticasone, beclomethasone
	○ Mechanism: Inhaled corticosteroids; effective for control of moderate asthma
	• Prednisone, dexamethasone, methylprednisolone
	○ Mechanism: Oral corticosteroids; effective for control of severe asthma
	○ Adverse effects: Iatrogenic effects include osteoporosis, thin skin, redistribution of fat, adrenal suppression (Cushing's effects)
	• Zileuton
	○ Mechanism: Inhibition of lipoxygenase, preventing synthesis of leukotrienes
	• Zafirlukast, montelukast
	○ Mechanism: Leukotriene receptor antagonist

Topic **5**

Nonsteroidal Anti-Inflammatory Drugs; Antirheumatic Drugs; and Drugs to Treat Diseases of the Skin, Blood, Gastrointestinal Disorders, and Gout

Must Knows

- Nonsteroidal anti-inflammatory drugs (NSAIDs)
- Antirheumatic and gout drugs
- Anticoagulant drugs, antiplatelet and thrombolytic drugs
- Gastrointestinal drugs
- Drugs to treat disorders of the skin

NSAIDs

Aspirin	• Mechanism: Irreversible inhibition of the cyclooxygenase (COX) pathway; inhibition of thromboxane synthesis; inhibition of platelet aggregation • Indications: Analgesia, antipyretic, anti-inflammatory, coronary artery disease, post myocardial infarction • Contraindications: Aspirin-induced asthma, children with viral illness (danger of Reye's syndrome) • Adverse effects: Gastritis, peptic ulcer disease (PUD), uric acid retention
Ibuprofen and naproxen	• Mechanism: Anti-inflammatory action because of their inhibition of prostaglandin synthesis (COX-1 and COX-2) • Indications: Analgesic, antipyretic for dysmenorrhea, arthritis • Adverse effects: Gastritis, PUD
Acetaminophen	• Mechanism: An effective antipyretic but has only weak anti-inflammatory properties • Indications: Analgesic, antipyretic • Adverse effects: Hepatotoxicity

Celecoxib, rofecoxib, and valdecoxib	• Mechanism: COX-2 inhibitors that produce less erosion of the gastrointestinal (GI) mucosa and cause less inhibition of platelet aggregation • Indications: Arthritis, analgesia • Adverse effects: Linked to accelerated cardiovascular disease; life-threatening GI bleeding • Rofecoxib and valdecoxib currently off the U.S. market

ANTIRHEUMATIC AND GOUT DRUGS

Disease-modifying antirheumatic drugs (DMARDs)	• Methotrexate
	  ○ Mechanism: Has a suppressing action on cellular and humoral immunity when used at high doses
	  ○ Adverse effects: Hepatotoxicity, bone marrow suppression
	  ○ Hydroxychloroquine, chloroquine
	  ○ Mechanism: Interference with T lymphocytes
	• Sulfasalazine
	  ○ Mechanism: COX inhibition; it is broken down partially into a salicylate
	• Etanercept
	  ○ Mechanism: Recombinant protein that antagonizes the TNF-α receptor
	• Infliximab
	  ○ Mechanism: Monoclonal antibody that binds TNF-α, inactivating it

Drugs used for gout	• Probenecid
	  ○ Mechanism: Inhibits uric acid reabsorption in the proximal tubules
	  ○ Indication: Chronic gout; DO NOT USE FOR ACUTE ATTACKS!
	• Allopurinol
	  ○ Mechanism: Inhibition of xanthine oxidase that leads to decreased serum urate
	  ○ Indication: Chronic tophaceous gout
	  ○ Adverse effects: Rashes, GI problems, hepatotoxicity
	• Colchicine
	  ○ Mechanism: Impairs leukocyte chemotaxis
	  ○ Indication: Used only for acute attacks
	  ○ Adverse effects: Diarrhea

ANTICOAGULANT, ANTIPLATELET, AND THROMBOLYTIC DRUGS

Anticoagulant drugs	• Anticoagulants are indicated in deep vein thrombosis (DVT), arterial embolism, atrial fibrillation, unstable angina, and disseminated intravascular coagulation
	• Heparin, enoxaparin
	○ Mechanism: There are two types of heparin used clinically. The first is standard (unfractionated) heparin. The second is called low-molecular-weight heparin (LMWH) and is derived from the first type. Heparin inhibits both in vitro and in vivo clotting of blood.
	○ Adverse effects: Hemorrhage, thrombocytopenia
	• Warfarin
	○ Mechanism: inhibits production of clotting factors II, VII, IX, and X
	○ Adverse effects: Hemorrhage, cutaneous necrosis, drug interactions
Antiplatelet drugs	• Aspirin, Clopidogrel, ticlopidine, dipyridamole
	○ Mechanism: Inhibits platelet aggregation and prolongs bleeding time by inhibiting the synthesis of platelet thromboxane A (TxA_2 – aspirin), inhibits adenosine diphosphate (ADP)-induced aggregation (clopidogrel, ticlopidine), or inhibits phosphodiesterase (PDE), causing increased cyclic adenosine monophosphate (cAMP), resulting in inhibition of platelet aggregation (dipyridamole)
	○ Indications: Prophylaxis of arterial thrombosis and therapeutic management of myocardial infarction (MI) and stroke
Thrombolytics	• Streptokinase, urokinase, reteplase
	○ Mechanism: Lysis of a formed thrombus to reestablish tissue perfusion
	○ Indications: MI, pulmonary embolism (PE), DVT, cardiovascular accident (CVA)
	○ Adverse effect: Bleeding

GASTROINTESTINAL DRUGS

Drugs for diarrhea	• Medications for diarrhea
	○ Metoclopramide: Stimulates GI tract motility by acting as dopamine antagonist and stimulates acetylcholine release
	○ Adverse effects: Fatigue and (rare) Parkinson-like effects
	○ Opioids: Have a constipating action and are used to treat diarrhea
	○ Adverse effects: Addiction liability

> ○ Kaolin (Kaopectate) and bismuth subsalicylate (Pepto-Bismol): Absorb intestinal toxins and are useful in diarrhea

Drugs for constipation	• Medications for constipation
	
	  ○ Docusate, Colace: Stool softeners; are not absorbed from GI tract and act by increasing bulk
	
	  ○ Methylcellulose (Citrucel), psyllium seed (Metamucil): Bulk-forming laxatives
	
	  ○ Polyethylene glycol: Osmotic laxative; colorless and tasteless
	
	  ○ Milk of Magnesia: Saline laxatives; do not use with renal failure

Antiemetic drugs	• Antiemetics
	
	  ○ Antihistamines: Useful in preventing vomiting associated with motion sickness and inner ear dysfunction
	
	  ○ Scopolamine: An anticholinergic drug that prevents motion sickness when applied as a patch to the ear
	
	  ○ Marijuana: Useful in preventing vomiting caused by cancer chemotherapeutic drugs

Drugs to decrease or neutralize gastric acid secretion	• Antacids: Buffer gastric acidity and have limited usefulness
	• May interfere with the absorption of certain drugs
	• Cimetidine, ranitidine, famotidine
	
	  ○ Mechanism: Histamine receptor antagonists (H_2-blockers)
	
	  ○ Indications: Gastritis, peptic ulcers
	
	  ○ Reduce dose if renal insufficiency is present
	• Omeprazole, lansoprazole, esomeprazole
	
	  ○ Mechanism: Proton pump inhibitors that inhibit gastric acid secretion by blocking the H^+-K^+ATPase enzymes (proton pumps)
	
	  ○ Indications: Peptic ulcer disease (PUD), esophagitis
	
	  ○ Adverse effects: Diarrhea and headaches

Statins	• Lovastatin, simvastatin, atorvastatin
	
	  ○ Mechanism: HMG-CoA (beta-hydroxy-β-methylglutaryl-coenzyme) reductase inhibitor
	
	  ○ Indication: Hypercholesterolemia
	
	  ○ Adverse effects: Myopathy, drug-induced hepatitis

Drugs to treat inflammatory bowel disease	• Sulfasalazine (5-aminosalicylates)
	
	  ○ The mainstay of treatment for ulcerative colitis. It is a prodrug that is converted to sulfapyridine and 5-aminosalicylic acid.
	
	  ○ Adverse effects: Nausea and vomiting
	• Infliximab: A monoclonal neutralizing antibody to human TNF-α, an inflammatory cytokine that is useful in Crohn's disease

Miscellaneous GI drugs	• Misoprostol: A prostaglandin used for prevention of NSAID-induced ulceration by stimulating gastric mucous production • Sucralfate: Used for prophylaxis of stress-induced gastritis in patients in intensive care units

SKIN DRUGS

Drugs to treat skin disorders	• Isotretinoin, topical tretinoin, acitretin
	    ○ Mechanism: Retinoid analogues of vitamin A
	    ○ Indication: Acne
	    ○ Acitretin is useful in severe psoriasis
	    ○ Adverse effects: Teratogenicity; women should not conceive for at least 1 month after discontinuation of isotretinoin or acitretin

Topic **6**

Neuropharmacology

Must Knows

● Blood–brain barrier

● Agents affecting neuromuscular transmission

● General anesthetics

● Local anesthetics

● Central nervous system stimulants and depressants

● Parkinson's disease

● Antiepileptic drugs

● Drugs for mood disorders

● Antipsychotic drugs

Blood–brain barrier	• Highly ionized drugs, large-molecular-weight agents, and highly water-soluble agents are excluded from entering the brain. • Biologically active substances (e.g., neurotransmitters) pass into the brain very poorly • To penetrate into the brain, drugs must be lipid soluble, nonionized, and relatively low molecular weight

Gas laws	• Henry's law states that the concentration of gas dissolved in a liquid is directly proportional to the partial pressure of the agent. The solubility of an anesthetic agent in blood is inversely proportional to its rate of producing anesthesia. That is, agents with low solubility in blood produce anesthesia rapidly because the blood becomes saturated and releases the agent to the brain. Conversely, agents that are very soluble in blood have a slower onset because the blood must be relatively saturated before the agent enters the brain in significant amounts.

THE ANESTHETICS

Inhalational anesthetics	• Halothane: Has been a widely used agent for many years. Halothane hepatitis is a rare syndrome that resembles viral hepatitis.
• Enflurane: A similar agent that is associated with seizure-like electrocardiographic (EEG) changes in deep anesthesia
• Isoflurane: An isomer of enflurane that is considered particularly safe in patients with ischemic heart disease. It also does not produce seizure-like EEG changes.
• Desflurane: Irritates the respiratory tract and causes a decrease in blood pressure
• Sevoflurane: Is not pungent, a characteristic that permits smooth induction of anesthesia
Nonhalogenated gaseous anesthetics	• Nitrous oxide (N_2O): Deep levels of anesthesia are unattainable even with the highest concentration. It is often combined with another inhalational anesthetic to decrease dosage requirements and toxicity.
Intravenous anesthetics	• Agents that are highly lipid soluble and penetrate rapidly into the brain. As the drug is removed from the brain tissue to other, less richly perfused tissues or by elimination by metabolism or excretion or both, levels in the brain decline rapidly and the anesthetic rapidly decreased.
• Barbiturates (thiopental, thiamylal, and methohexital): Three ultra short-acting barbiturates that are used as intravenous induction agents. All are very lipid soluble.
• Benzodiazepines: Midazolam is the most popular for induction of anesthesia
• Flumazenil: A benzodiazepine antagonist
• Propofol: Rapidly acting, with a short $t_{1/2}$. It possesses antiemetic properties.
• Ketamine: Used some in pediatrics. It can be administered intramuscularly in children who resist inhalational induction. Ketamine causes cardiac stimulation and has a propensity to evoke excitatory and hallucinatory phenomena as the patient emerges from anesthesia.

Local anesthetics	• Esters: Cocaine, benzocaine, procaine, tetracaine
	• Amides: Lidocaine, mepivacaine
	○ Mechanism: Interfere with the generation of the action potential in nerve by binding at or near to sodium channels and interfere with the normal passage of Na^+ through the cell membrane
	○ Adverse effects: They may produce central nervous system (CNS) stimulation characterized by restlessness, disorientation, tremors, and sometimes convulsions. Local anesthetics may induce depression of cardiac conduction that may progress to severe hypotension and cardiac arrest.
Neuromuscular-blocking agents	• Succinylcholine
	• Nondepolarizing blockers
	• Baclofen: Useful for treating spinal spasticity and spasticity associated with multiple sclerosis. It is an agonist at the $GABA_B$ (γaminobutyric acid$_B$) receptors.
	• Dantrolene: Used in the treatment of spasticity caused by stroke, spinal injury, multiple sclerosis, or cerebral palsy. It is also the agent of choice in treatment of malignant hyperthermia.

CENTRAL NERVOUS SYSTEM STIMULANTS AND DEPRESSANTS

CNS stimulants	• Amphetamine, methylphenidate
	○ Indications: Attention deficit hyperactivity disorder, narcolepsy
	• Methylxanthines: Caffeine, theophylline
	○ Indications: Mild CNS stimulation
Benzodiazepines	• Alprazolam, diazepam, lorazepam, triazolam (Fig. VII-4)
	○ Mechanism: Bind to $GABA_A$ receptors, increasing chloride conductance leading to hyperpolarization of the cells and therefore to a diminished synaptic transmission (inhibition)
	○ Indications: Anxiolytic, sleep aids
	○ Pharmacokinetics: Some have active metabolites and long half lives. An exception is alprazolam; it is not metabolized. Use it for elderly patients and those with decreased hepatic function.

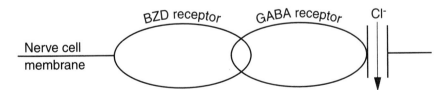

● **Figure VII-4** Relationship of the benzodiazepine (BZD) receptor to the γ-aminobutyric acid (GABA) receptor. Enhanced chloride inflow hyperpolarizes (inhibits) central nervous system neurons, leading to sedative, antianxiety, and hypnotic effects.

Nonbenzodiazepine anxiolytics and sleep aids	• Buspirone: Used for generalized anxiety disorder • Zolpidem: Popular non-addictive, fast-acting sleep aid • Hydroxyzine: H_1 histamine antagonist effective as an anxiolytic and sleep aid

Therapy for Parkinson's disease	• Levodopa/carbidopa
	  ○ Mechanism: Agonist of dopamine receptors in the basal ganglia. If levodopa is given alone, it is extensively metabolized in the liver. This is prevented with the enzyme inhibitor carbidopa.
	  ○ Adverse effects: Unpredictable fluctuations between mobility and immobility (on-off phenomenon). There may also be abnormal movement disorders (dyskinesias).
	• Bromocriptine, pergolide, pramipexole
	  ○ Mechanism: Dopamine receptor agonist
	  ○ Adverse effects: Psychosis, movement disorders
	• Selegiline
	  ○ Mechanism: Inhibitor of monoamine oxidase-B (MAO-B) an enzyme for metabolism of dopamine in the brain
	  ○ Contraindications: Selegiline should not be coadministered with tricyclic antidepressants or selective serotonin uptake inhibitors because of the possibility of severe adverse events (e.g., hyperpyrexia, agitation, delirium, coma).
	• Tolcapone, entacapone
	  ○ Mechanism: Inhibitor of Metabolism by catechol-O-methyl transferase (COMT), another enzyme that metabolizes dopamine
	• Amantadine
	  ○ Mechanism: An antiviral agent that stimulates dopamine release and has moderate effects
	  ○ Indication: Used in early stages of Parkinson's disease
	• Trihexyphenidyl, biperiden
	  ○ Mechanism: Cholinergic agonists
	  ○ Indications: Treatment of drug-induced parkinsonism from the use of antipsychotic drugs

ANTIEPILEPTIC DRUGS

Agents that block sodium channels	• Phenytoin
	  ○ Indications: Effective in partial and generalized seizures
	  ○ Pharmacokinetics: Shows saturation kinetics (zero-order) at high therapeutic doses. If this occurs, a buildup of phenytoin levels may ensue with consequent cerebellar

toxicity, seen as ataxia, vertigo, nystagmus, and diplopia.

- ○ Adverse effects: Cerebellar toxicity, gingival hyperplasia, hirsutism, teratogen, Stevens-Johnson syndrome
- Fosphenytoin
  - ○ Indication: Status epilepticus. This medication is the soluble phosphate salt of phenytoin that can be administered intravenously.
- Carbamazepine
  - ○ Indications: Partial and generalized seizure disorders, bipolar disorder, trigeminal neuralgia
  - ○ Adverse effects: Ataxia, diplopia
- Lamotrigine
  - ○ Indications: Partial and generalized seizures
  - ○ Adverse effects: Rash, Steven-Johnson syndrome (can reduce likelihood of rash by slowly increasing the dose)

Agents that potentiate GABA	• Tiagabine
	  ○ Mechanism: Blocks GABA uptake and prolongs the actions of GABA
	  ○ Indications: Status epilepticus
	• Vigabatrin
	  ○ Mechanism: An irreversible inhibitor of GABA metabolism (inhibits GABA transaminase) and leads to elevated levels of GABA
	  ○ Indications: Status epilepticus

Agents that block Ca²⁺ channels	• Valproic acid (blocks sodium and calcium channels)
	  ○ Indications: Absence, partial, and generalized seizures; impulsivity
	  ○ Adverse effects: Hepatic failure in children, teratogen (spina bifida)
	• Ethosuximide
	  ○ Blocks transient (T) calcium channels
	  ○ Indications: Drug of choice for absence seizures
	  ○ Adverse effects: Nausea, vomiting, abdominal pain

Agents with unknown mechanisms	• Gabapentin
	  ○ Indications: Seizure adjunct, neuropathic pain
	• Zonisamide
	  ○ Mechanism: May have multiple actions; there is evidence that it blocks sodium channels and has carbonic anhydrase inhibitor activity. It is a long-acting compound with a half-life of about 60 hours.

DRUGS FOR MOOD DISORDERS

Selective serotonin reuptake inhibitors (SSRIs)	• Fluoxetine, sertraline, fluvoxamine, paroxetine, citalopram, escitalopram
	  ○ Mechanism: SSRIs have little or no affinity for cholinergic, β-adrenergic, or histaminergic receptors and do not interfere with cardiac conduction
	  ○ Indications: Depression, obsessive-compulsive disorder (OCD), anxiety disorders
	  ○ Side effects: Insomnia, nausea, loose stools, and sexual dysfunction such as decreased libido, delayed ejaculation, or anorgasmia

Miscellaneous agents	• Trazodone
	  ○ Mechanism: Inhibits reuptake of serotonin
	  ○ Indications: Depression with features of anxiety
	  ○ Adverse effects: Sedation, priapism
	• Venlafaxine
	  ○ Mechanism: Inhibits the reuptake of both norepinephrine and serotonin
	  ○ Indication: Depression
	  ○ Side effects: Anxiety, agitation, insomnia
	• Bupropion
	  ○ Mechanism: Has weak effects on the reuptake of norepinephrine, dopamine, and serotonin
	  ○ Indications: Depression, smoking cessation
	  ○ Adverse effects: Agitation, hypertension, seizures
	  ○ Contraindication: Seizure disorders
	• Mirtazapine
	  ○ Mechanism: α_2-Antagonist, 5-HT receptor antagonist
	  ○ Adverse effects: Agranulocytosis, sedation, increased appetite

Tricyclic antidepressants (TCAs)	• Imipramine, desipramine, amitriptyline, nortriptyline, clomipramine, desipramine
	  ○ Mechanism: Inhibit reuptake of norepinephrine or serotonin or both
	  ○ Adverse effects: Anticholinergic effects causing symptoms such as dry mouth, constipation, tachycardia, blurred vision, urinary retention, lower seizure threshold, ventricular arrhythmias
	  ○ Indications: Major depression, pain syndromes and fibromyalgia (amitriptyline), OCD (clomipramine)
	• Maprotiline and amoxapine
	  ○ Mechanism: Different chemically but otherwise have the same clinical profile as the tricyclics

Monoamine oxidase inhibitors (MAOIs)	• Phenelzine, tranylcypromine ◦ Adverse effects: Serotonin syndrome (when used with SSRIs), hypertensive crisis (when tyramine is consumed—wines, cheese)

Treatment of bipolar disorder	• Lithium
	  ◦ Mechanism: Not well understood
	  ◦ Indication: Bipolar disorder. It is effective in up to 80% of patients within 5 to 21 days of treatment.
	  ◦ Adverse effects: Plasma levels should be maintained below 1.5 mEq/L. At concentrations above 2.5 mEq/L, effects include mental confusion, hyperreflexia, gross tremor, seizures, coma, and death. Adverse effects that may be seen at lower blood levels include hypothyroidism and nephrogenic diabetes insipidus.

Mood stabilizers	• Antiepileptic drugs: Valproic acid and carbamazepine • The atypical antipsychotic agent olanzapine is approved for acute mania and mixed episodes associated with bipolar disorder

ANTIPSYCHOTIC DRUGS

Typical antipsychotics	• Haloperidol, chlorpromazine, thioridazine
	  ◦ Mechanism: antagonist of dopamine D_2 receptors
	  ◦ Adverse effects: Extrapyramidal symptoms
	    ▪ Hours: Acute dystonia and akathisia
	    ▪ Weeks: Parkinson-like side effects; usually responds favorably to central antimuscarinic agents
	    ▪ Years: Tardive dyskinesia: It is the most serious adverse effect of antipsychotics and can occur in 20% to 40% of chronically treated patients. There is no established therapy, and reversibility upon removing the drug may be limited.

Atypical antipsychotics	• Clozapine, risperidone, olanzapine, quetiapine, ziprasidone, aripiprazole
	  ◦ Mechanism: These agents have activity at other sites, such as D_1 receptors, H_1, α_1, and serotonergic receptor sites
	  ◦ Indications: All can be used for schizophrenia; they are also used as adjuncts for mood disorders
	  ◦ Adverse effect: Fewer extrapyramidal side effects than typical, prolongation of QT interval (ziprasidone), agranulocytosis (clozapine)

Neuroleptic malignant syndrome	• A rare medical emergency involving extrapyramidal symptoms that occurs in about 1% of patients taking antipsychotics. It is fatal in about 10% of patients affected. • Treatment: Short-term therapy with dantrolene in combination with dopamine agonists such as bromocriptine

Topic **7**

Chemotherapeutic Drugs

Must Knows

- Synthetic organic antimicrobials
- β-Lactam antibiotics and other cell wall inhibitors
- Inhibitors of protein synthesis antibiotics
- Drugs used against mycobacterium
- Antiviral drugs
- Antifungal drugs
- Antiparasitic drugs
- Anticancer drugs

SYNTHETIC ORGANIC ANTIMICROBIALS

Principles of antibiotic therapy	• Drugs can kill organisms (cidal effect) or inhibit growth (static effect)
	• Inappropriate use of antibiotics is common and accelerates the development of resistance
	• Resistance is the greatest reason for therapeutic failure
	• Treatment must often be continued for several days after signs and symptoms of infection have disappeared
Sulfonamides	• Sulfisoxazole, sulfamethoxazole, sulfadiazine
	○ Mechanism: Structural analogues of *p*-aminobenzoic acid (PABA). PABA is required for the bacteria to synthesize folic acid and sulfonamides competitively block PABA incorporation. Because this is reversible, these are bacteriostatic drugs.
	○ Effective against many bacterial strains, including gram-positive and some gram-negative organisms, but resistance is common
	○ Indications:
	▪ Urinary tract and ear infections. Sulfonamides, such as sulfadiazine, in combination with pyrimethamine, are

considered the treatment of choice for symptomatic toxoplasmosis.

- Burns: Topical sulfadiazine or mafenide
- Inflammatory bowel disease: Sulfasalazine
  - Adverse effects: Hypersensitivity reactions, rarely Stevens-Johnson syndrome
  - Contraindications: Newborns or women during the last 2 months of pregnancy because of risk of kernicterus in newborn

Trimethoprim	• Mechanism: Competitively inhibits dihydrofolate reductase; because trimethoprim and sulfonamides have their effects at different sites in the folic acid synthetic pathway, a synergistic effect results when the two are used together • Indications: Combination of trimethoprim and sulfamethoxazole is used in the treatment of genitourinary, gastrointestinal (GI), and respiratory tract infections caused by susceptible bacteria. It is also used in treatment of shigellosis, pneumocystic carinii pneumonia, and traveler's diarrhea in adults. • Adverse effects: Stevens-Johnson syndrome, agranulocytosis, aplastic anemia, and fulminant hepatic necrosis

Fluoroquinolones	• Mechanism of action: Inhibits DNA synthesis through inhibition of DNA gyrase
	
	• Examples:
	  ○ First generation (nalidixic acid); Have limited gram-negative activity
	  ○ Second generation (norfloxacin, ciprofloxacin, enoxacin): More active against gram-negative organisms
	  ○ Third (levofloxacin, gatifloxacin) and fourth (trovafloxacin, moxifloxacin) generations: Show greater activity against gram-positive organisms
	
	• Indications: Urinary and respiratory tract infections; GI and abdominal infections; sexually transmitted diseases; and bone, joint, and soft tissue infections
	
	• Adverse effects: Damage to developing ligaments and joints in children; some fluoroquinolones prolong the QT interval; convulsions have occurred
	
	• Interactions: Poor absorption when taken with antacids

β-LACTAM ANTIBIOTICS AND OTHER CELL WALL INHIBITORS (FIG. VII-5)

- Mechanism of action: Blocks transpeptidases, inhibiting cell wall growth
- Resistance has developed by hydrolysis of the β-lactam ring by β-lactamases. Inhibitors of β-lactamases include clavulanic acid, sulbactam, and tazobactam.

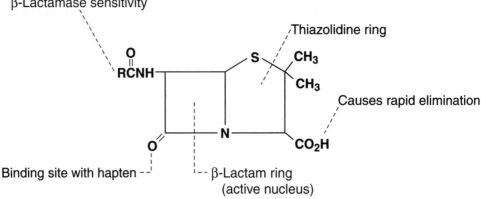

R group determines:
  Spectrum
  Kinetics
  Acid sensitivity
  β-Lactamase sensitivity

Thiazolidine ring

Causes rapid elimination

Binding site with hapten

β-Lactam ring
(active nucleus)

● **Figure VII-5** The general structure of the penicillins.

Penicillins	• Classified into four groups:
	○ Natural penicillins (G and V): Penicillin G is poorly absorbed orally and is rapidly excreted into the urine
	○ Antistaphylococcal (penicillinase-resistant) penicillins: Nafcillin, oxacillin, cloxacillin, dicloxacillin
	○ Aminopenicillins: Ampicillin and amoxicillin
	○ Antipseudomonal penicillins: Ticarcillin, piperacillin
Cephalosporins	• Classified into four generations:
	○ First generation (cefazolin, cephalexin): Active against gram-positive organisms; used for skin infections and commonly as antimicrobial prophylaxis before surgery
	○ Second generation (cefuroxime, cefoxitin, cefotetan): Gram-positive coverage with increased activity against gram-negative organisms; intra-abdominal infections (cefoxitin)
	○ Third generation (ceftriaxone, ceftazidime): Increased activity against gram-negative organisms, penetrate the central nervous system (CNS); bacterial meningitis, antipseudomonas (ceftazidime)
	○ Fourth generation (cefepime): Extended spectrum for high-power empiric coverage
Carbapenems and carbacephem	• Imipenem, meropenem
	○ Mechanism of action: Same as the β-lactams. It is β-lactamase resistant.
	○ Indications: Empirical treatment of polymicrobial pulmonary, intraabdominal and soft tissue infections; drug of choice for *Enterobacter* sp. infections

	○ Pharmacokinetics: Imipenem is combined with cilastatin to prevent renal inactivation
	○ Adverse effects: Seizures affect about 1% of patients (imipenem)
Monobactams	• Aztreonam
	○ Indication: Active against gram-negative organisms; can be used with patients with penicillin allergies
Vancomycin	• Mechanism: Inhibits cell wall synthesis. Bactericidal.
	• Indication: Methicillin-resistant *S. aureus* (MRSA) infection
	• Adverse effects: Nephrotoxicity, ototoxicity, flushing
Bacitracin	• Mechanism: Inhibits cell wall synthesis
	• Indication: Topical
	• Adverse effects: Nephrotoxicity
Polymyxins	• Mechanism: Disrupt cell membranes
	• Indications: Topical therapy in external otitis caused by *P. aeruginosa* infection
	• Adverse effects: Nephrotoxicity, neurotoxicity

INHIBITORS OF PROTEIN SYNTHESIS

Aminoglycoside antibiotics	• Amikacin, gentamicin, kanamycin, tobramycin
	○ Mechanism: Bind to 30S ribosome, disrupting formation of the initiation complex. Also induces translation errors.
	○ Indications: Gram-negative infections. They are synergistic with β-lactams.
	○ Toxicity: Nephrotoxicity, ototoxicity; can also cause neuromuscular blockade by displacing Ca^{++} from the neuromuscular junction; this is important when considering anesthesia
Tetracyclines	• Tetracycline, doxycycline, demeclocycline
	○ Mechanism: Bind to the 30S ribosome and prevents the binding of tRNA to the acceptor site on the 50S ribosomal unit
	○ Indications: Drugs of choice for *Vibrio, Rickettsia, Chlamydia,* and *Coxiella* sp.; granuloma inguinale; syndrome of inappropriate antidiuretic hormone (demeclocycline causes diabetes insipidus)
	○ Adverse effects: Staining of teeth in children younger than age 8 years, photosensitivity
Macrolide antibiotics	• Erythromycin, clarithromycin, azithromycin
	○ Mechanism: Bind to the 50S subunit; bacteriostatic
	○ Indications: *Mycoplasma pneumoniae* infection, Legionnaires' disease, prevention of secondary pneumonia in neonates
	○ Adverse effects: GI upset

Chloramphenicol	• Mechanism: Inhibits 50S peptidyl transferase • Indications: Typhoid and paratyphoid fever • Toxicity: Potentially fatal bone marrow suppression, gray baby syndrome

Lincosamides	• Lincomycin, clindamycin
	  ○ Mechanism: Block peptide bond formation by binding to the 50S ribosomal subunit
	  ○ Adverse effects: Hypersensitivity rashes, diarrhea

DRUGS USED AGAINST MYCOBACTERIUM

Principles of tuberculosis (TB) treatment	• Treatment must consist of multiple drugs to prevent resistance • The drugs must be taken regularly • Drug treatment must continue for a sufficient time

First-line drugs used in TB	• Isoniazid, rifampin, pyrazinamide, ethambutol, and streptomycin
	• Isoniazid: Most active drug for the treatment of TB
	  ○ Mechanism: Inhibits cell wall synthesis
	  ○ Adverse effects: Hepatitis and neurotoxicity. Should be administered with pyridoxine to help prevent neurotoxicity.
	• Rifampin
	  ○ Mechanism: Inhibits RNA synthesis
	  ○ Adverse effect: Hepatotoxicity
	• Pyrazinamide
	  ○ Adverse effect: Hepatotoxicity
	  ○ Mechanism: Unknown
	• Ethambutol
	  ○ Used with isoniazid, pyrazinamide, and rifampin in patients infected with resistant strains. It is bacteriostatic.
	• Streptomycin:
	  ○ Final first-line drug; binds to 30S ribosomal subunit
	  ○ Adverse effects: Ototoxicity, nephrotoxicity

Drugs used in leprosy	• Dapsone: Mechanism of action similar to the sulfonamides • Clofazimine: Used in combination with dapsone or for dapsone intolerance; adverse effect is skin discoloration • Rifampin: Inhibits DNA dependent RNA polymerase, a potent inducer

ANTIVIRAL DRUGS (FIG. VII-6)

Herpes virus drugs	• Acyclovir, valacyclovir ○ Mechanism: Activated by viral thymidine kinase and inhibits herpes DNA polymerase. Valacyclovir is the prodrug of acyclovir.

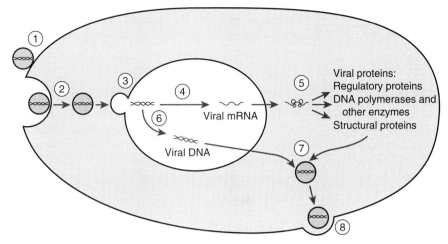

● **Figure VII-6** Replicative cycle of a herpesvirus, an example of a DNA virus showing possible sites for antiviral drug action. **(1)** Attachment. **(2)** Membrane fusion. **(3)** Release of viral DNA through nuclear pores. **(4)** Transcription of viral mRNA. **(5)** Synthesis of viral proteins by host cell's ribosomes. **(6)** Replication of viral DNA by viral polymerases. **(7)** Assembly of virus particles. **(8)** Budding and release of progeny virus.

- Indication: herpes simplex virus (HSV), varicella zoster virus (VZV)
- Ganciclovir, valganciclovir (prodrug)
    - Mechanism: Inhibits cytomegalovirus (CMV) DNA polymerase
- Cidofovir
    - Mechanism: Inhibits DNA polymerase
    - Indications: CMV retinitis, musculocutaneous HSV, human papilloma virus
- Foscarnet
    - Mechanism: Directly inhibits HSV DNA polymerase
    - Indications: CMV retinitis in AIDS patients, acyclovir-resistant HSV, ganciclovir-resistant CMV
    - The enhanced production of the cytokines called interferons is one of the body's earliest responses to a viral infection. Several interferons have been approved and are used for the treatment of several viral infections in humans.

Amantadine, rimantadine	• Mechanism: Interfere with the unseating of virus • Indications: Influenza prophylaxis; amantadine used some in Parkinson's Disease • Adverse effects: Ataxia, dizziness, slurring of speech, and insomnia
Immune globulin (γ-globulin)	• Mechanism: Blocks viral adsorption and penetration, providing the patient with passive immunity
Interferons (IFN-α, IFN-β, IFN-γ)	• Mechanism: Inhibit peptide chain initiation, stimulate degradation of mRNA, inhibit elongation • Indications: Hepatitis B virus (HBV), hepatitis C virus (HCV), posttransplant CMV activation

Therapy of human immunodeficiency virus (HIV)	• Nucleoside reverse transcriptase inhibitors (NRTIs): Zidovudine, stavudine, didanosine, lamivudine
	○ Resistance occurs rapidly
	○ Adverse effects: Hepatotoxicity, pancreatitis (didanosine)
	• Non-nucleoside reverse transcriptase inhibitors (NNRTIs): Efavirenz, nevirapine, delavirdine, tenofovir
	○ When combined with NRTIs or protease inhibitors, the NNRTIs produce additive and possibly synergistic effects against HIV
	• Protease inhibitors: Saquinavir, indinavir, ritonavir, nelfinavir
	○ Adverse effects: Vomiting, diarrhea, paresthesia
	○ Interact with a large number of drugs because they are metabolized by and inhibit the cytochrome P450 enzyme system (especially ritonavir)
	○ Nelfinavir is probably the most commonly used protease inhibitor because of its low incidence of serious adverse effects
Highly active antiretroviral therapy (HAART)	• A protocol that increases the effectiveness of HIV treatment
	• Consists of combining 2 NRTIs with a protease inhibitor

ANTIFUNGAL DRUGS

Amphotericin	• Mechanism: Disrupts fungi cell membrane
	• Indications: Drug of choice for serious disseminated yeast and dimorphic fungal infections in immunocompromised hospitalized patients
	• Adverse effects: Nephrotoxicity, fever, chills, nausea, vomiting, thrombophlebitis at intravenous sites
Azoles	• Mechanism: Inhibits ergosterol synthesis
	○ Ketoconazole: Drug of choice for candida; inhibits steroid synthesis, resulting in gynecomastia and loss of libido and increased liver transaminases
	○ Fluconazole: Effective in the treatment of infections with *Candida* sp., especially esophageal and vaginal candidiasis
	○ Itraconazole: Most useful in the long-term suppressive treatment of disseminated histoplasmosis in AIDS
	○ Clotrimazole: A broad-spectrum agent used in the topical treatment of oral, skin, and vaginal infections with *C. albicans*
Flucytosine	• Mechanism: Converted to 5-fluorouracil and incorporated into RNA, causing dysfunction
	• Indications: Administered with amphotericin for cryptococcus meningitis and deep candida infections
Nystatin	• Mechanism: Similar to amphotericin B
	• Indications: Mucocutaneous candidiasis, thrush (swish and swallow)

Griseofulvin	• Indications: Oral fungistatic agent used in the long-term treatment of dermatophyte infections caused by *Epidermophyton*, *Microsporum*, and *Trichophyton* sp.

ANTIPARASITE DRUGS

Antiprotozoal drugs	• Metronidazole: Exerts activity against most anaerobic bacteria and several protozoa; is the most effective agent available for the treatment of all forms of amebiasis and giardiasis • Suramin: Drug of choice to treat African trypanosomiasis (sleeping sickness)
Antimalarial drugs	• Chloroquine is an older drug that may still be the drug of choice for prophylaxis in most areas where chloroquine resistance is not a problem • Mefloquine may be used as prophylaxis in chloroquine-resistant areas • Primaquine is effective against the liver forms of the disease • Pyrimethamine and trimethoprim inhibit the conversion of dihydrofolic acid to tetrahydrofolic acid and inhibit the ability of the malarial parasite to synthesize folic acid
Anti-nematode (roundworms)	• Mebendazole and thiabendazole: Active against *Trichuris trichiura*, *Enterobius*, *Ascaris*, and hookworms (*Necator and ancylostoma* sp.) • Piperazine: Active against *Ascaris* and *Enterobius* sp. • Diethylcarbamazine: Drug of choice for lymphatic filariasis (*Wuchereria bancrofti*) • Ivermectin: Drug of choice for onchocerciasis (*Onchocerca volvulus*)
Anti-cestode (tapeworms) drugs	• Praziquantel: Active against *Schistosomes, Paragonimus westermani, Opisthorchis sinensis, Fasciola hepatica*
Anti-trematode (flukes) drugs	• Niclosamide: Active against *Taenia solium* and *Diphyllobothrium latum* • Albendazole: Active against *Echinococcus granulosus* and neurocysticercosis

ANTICANCER DRUGS (FIG. VII-7)

Principles of cancer chemotherapy	• One classification scheme for cancer chemotherapy drugs divides the drugs into three categories: ○ Class 1 agents exert their cytotoxicity in a nonspecific manner and kill both normal and malignant cells to the same extent

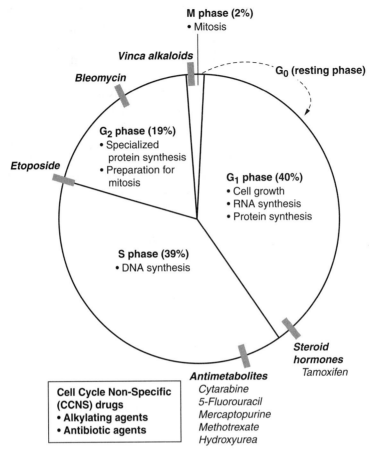

M phase (2%)
• Mitosis

Vinca alkaloids

Bleomycin

G$_0$ **(resting phase)**

G$_2$ phase (19%)
• Specialized
protein synthesis
• Preparation for
mitosis

Etoposide

G$_1$ phase (40%)
• Cell growth
• RNA synthesis
• Protein synthesis

S phase (39%)
• DNA synthesis

*Steroid
hormones*
Tamoxifen

Antimetabolites
Cytarabine
5-Fluorouracil
Mercaptopurine
Methotrexate
Hydroxyurea

**Cell Cycle Non-Specific
(CCNS) drugs**
• **Alkylating agents**
• **Antibiotic agents**

● **Figure VII-7** Cell cycle–specific antineoplastic drugs. The percentages indicate the approximate percentage of time spent in each phase by a typical malignant cell. The duration of the G$_1$ phase, however, can vary markedly.

- ○ Class 2 agents are phase specific and reach a plateau in cell kill with increasing dosages
- ○ Class 3 agents kill proliferating cells in preference to resting cells
- Cytotoxic drugs act by first-order kinetics; that is, at a given dose, they kill a constant fraction of the tumor cells rather than a fixed number of cells. Many cancers are resistant to therapy, some early in the course of treatment and some later as cancer cells become resistant. Many kinds of biochemical resistance to anticancer drugs have been described. Tumor cells may become generally resistant to a variety of cytotoxic drugs on the basis of decreased uptake or retention of the drugs. This form of resistance is termed *pleiotropic,* or *multidrug,* resistance, and it is the major form of resistance to anthracyclines, vinca alkaloids, etoposide, paclitaxel, and dactinomycin. The gene that confers multidrug resistance (termed *mdr I*) encodes a high-molecular-weight membrane

protein called P glycoprotein, which acts as a drug efflux pump in many tumors and normal tissues. Most of the drugs used in cancer treatment exert toxic effects on both normal and tumor tissues even at optimal doses. Most anticancer drugs damage hair follicles and produce partial or complete alopecia. The value of combination chemotherapy has been proved in humans. The combined use of two or more drugs is often superior to single-agent treatment of many cancers. Adjuvant chemotherapy involves the use of antineoplastic drugs when surgery or radiation therapy has eradicated the primary tumor but historical experience with similar patients indicates a high risk of relapse because of micrometastases.

Antineoplastic agents	• Classification of the anticancer drugs: Classification of each type is listed in the left column; drugs are listed in the right column
	• Indication of where in cell cycle the drug is most effective
	• G_1 phase; G_2 phase; G_o phase; m = mitosis; ns = nonspecific; s = s phase
Alkylating agents	• Cyclophosphamide (ns)
	○ Indications: Non-Hodgkin's lymphoma (NHL), breast and ovarian cancer
	○ Adverse effects: Bone marrow toxicity, hemorrhagic cystitis (prevent with hydration and mercaptoethane sulfonate [MESNA])
	• Cisplatin, carboplatin (ns)
	○ Indications: Ovarian and testicular cancer
	○ Adverse effects: Neurotoxicity, nephrotoxicity
Antimetabolites	• Methotrexate (s): Used for choriocarcinoma, leukemia, lymphoma
	• 5-Fluorouracil (s): Used for basal cell carcinoma, solid tumors
	• Cytarabine (s): Used for myelogenous leukemia
	• 6-mercaptopurine (s): Used for acute lymphoblastic leukemia (ALL), chronic myelogenous leukemia (CML)
Antibiotics	• Doxorubicin (s)
	○ Mechanism: Intercalating agent and generates free radicals, causing strand breakage
	○ Indications: Breast, ovary, endometrium, bladder, and thyroid cancers and small cell carcinoma
	○ Adverse effects: Cardiotoxic, myelosuppression
Vinca alkaloids	• Vincristine, vinblastine, paclitaxel (s and m)
	○ Mechanism: Inhibit tubulin, causing cellular arrest in metaphase during mitosis, preventing cell division
	○ Indications: Leukemia, breast cancer, ovarian cancer

Enzymes	• L-asparaginase catalyzes the hydrolysis of L-asparagine to aspartic acid and ammonia. Depletion of exogenous asparagine and glutamine inhibits protein synthesis in sensitive cells, leading to inhibition of nucleic acid synthesis and cell death. L-asparaginase differs from most cytotoxic drugs in its lack of toxicity to bone marrow, the gastrointestinal tract, and hair follicles.
Hormonal agents	• Tamoxifen (G_2): Synthetic antiestrogen used in the treatment of breast cancer • Flutamide (ns): Antiandrogen that competes with testosterone for binding to androgen receptors • Estramustine (G_2, m) phosphate: A hybrid structure that combines estradiol and a nitrogen mustard in a single molecule and is used in prostatic carcinomas
Miscellaneous	• Hydroxyurea (s): Inhibits the enzyme *ribonucleotide reductase* and causes a specific impairment of DNA synthesis • Procarbazine (G_2): Autoxidizes spontaneously and releases reactive products that may degrade DNA • Mitotane (ns): Produces adrenocortical necrosis and has been used in the palliative care of inoperable adrenocortical adenocarcinomas • Bleomycin (G_2): Causes DNA strand breaks; used in testicular cancer, Hodgkin's lymphoma (HL), NHL, bladder cancer • Etoposide (G_2): Inhibits topoisomerase II; used in testicular cancer
Immunomodulating agents	• Levamisole (ns): Enhances T-cell function and cellular immunity • Interferons (ns); α-2b and aldesleukin enhance T-lymphocyte cytotoxicity, induction of natural killer cell activity, and induction of interferon-γ production
Cellular growth factors	• Filgrastim: A human recombinant granulocyte colony-stimulating factor (rG-CSF) • Sargramostim: A human recombinant granulocyte and macrophage colony-stimulating factor
New drugs	• Imatinib mesylate: Inhibitor of the tumor-specific bcr-abl kinase • Herceptin: A monoclonal antibody directed against the HER-2 antigen that is overexpressed on the tumor cell surface in about 25% of breast cancer patients • Iressa: Orally active tyrosine kinase inhibitor selective for the epidermal growth factor receptor tyrosine kinase

Topic **8**

Endocrine Drugs

Must **Knows**

- Pituitary hormone analogs
- Immunomodulating drugs
- Corticosteroids, antagonists, and inhibitors
- Estrogens, progestins, selective estrogen receptor modulators (SERMs), uterine stimulants, and tocolytics
- Androgens, steroids and drugs for erectile dysfunction
- Thyroid drugs
- Drugs affecting calcium homeostasis
- Diabetes drugs

PITUITARY HORMONE ANALOGS

Gonadotropin-releasing hormone (GnRH) agonists	• Leuprolide, goserelin, nafarelin
	   ○ Mechanism: During pulse dosing, stimulates gonadotropin release; during continuous dosing, inhibits gonadotropin release
	   ○ Indications: Prostate cancer, endometriosis

Dopamine agonists	• Bromocriptine, pergolide, cabergoline ○ Indications: Galactorrhea, neuroleptic malignant syndrome
Antidiuretic hormone (ADH; vasopressin) analogue	• DDAVP (desmopressin) ○ Indications: Pituitary diabetes insipidus, enuresis (children)

IMMUNOMUDULATING DRUGS

Introduction to use of immunomodulating drugs	• Three major indications for immunotherapy are in the treatment of autoimmune diseases, primary immunodeficiency diseases, and organ transplantation
Organ transplantation	• Cyclosporine: Inhibits T cells without significantly impairing B cells

- Tacrolimus and sirolimus: Inhibit transcription of specific lymphokine genes in T lymphocytes
- Corticosteroids: Used as an adjunct with cyclosporine and other agents
- Mycophenolate mofetil: Impairs the proliferation of both T and B lymphocytes and may be used in conjunction with cyclosporine and corticosteroids to prevent the acute rejection of transplanted organs

Immunostimulating agents	• Bacillus Calmette-Guérin (BCG): Stimulates natural killer cells and is used in the treatment of bladder cancers • Levamisole: Potentiates the stimulatory effects of antigens, mitogens, lymphokines, and chemotactic factors on lympho- cytes, granulocytes, and macrophages and has been shown to increase T-cell–mediated immunity • Interleukin-2 (IL-2): Promotes the proliferation, differentia- tion, and recruitment of T and B lymphocytes, natural killer cells, and thymocytes

CORTICOSTEROIDS, ANTAGONISTS, AND INHIBITORS

Glucocorticoids	• Prednisone, hydrocortisone, dexamethasone
	   ◦ Mechanism: Inhibits phospholipase A_2, resulting in decreased leukotrienes and prostaglandins
	   ◦ Indications: Inflammatory states such as autoimmune and rheumatologic diseases, asthma, immunosuppression after transplantation
	   ◦ Adverse effects: Osteoporosis, Cushing's syndrome, adrenal crises (if chronic therapy is suddenly stopped)

Mineralocorticoids	• Fludrocortisone
	   ◦ Mechanism: Aldosterone receptor agonist
	   ◦ Indications: Addison's disease, adrenocortical insufficiency

Spironolactone	• Mechanism: Aldosterone receptor antagonists • Indications: Congestive heart failure, hypertension (HTN), hypokalemia

Corticosteroid synthesis inhibitors	• Aminoglutethimide, ketoconazole
	   ◦ Mechanism: Competitive inhibitor of the enzyme that catalyzes the conversion of cholesterol to pregnenolone
	   ◦ Indications: Hirsutism, metastatic breast and prostate cancer because it diminishes the levels of circulating sex hormones

ESTROGENS, PROGESTINS, SERMS, UTERINE STIMULANTS, TOCOLYTICS

Estrogens and progestins	• Indications: Oral contraceptives, hormone replacement therapy, osteoporosis

- Adverse effects:
  - Cardiovascular: Pulmonary embolism, cardiovascular accident, thromboembolism, HTN
  - Gastrointestinal: Hepatoma, gallbladder disease
  - Weight gain, breast tenderness
- Benefits include decreased incidence of:
  - Ectopic pregnancy
  - Pelvic inflammatory disease
  - Benign breast disease

Mifepristone (RU486)	- Mechanism: Progesterone receptor antagonist at the uterus - Indications: Induction of abortion

Selective estrogen receptor modulators (SERMs)	- Tamoxifen, clomiphene, and raloxifene
	  - Mechanism: SERMS are nonhormonal pharmacologic agents that act as an estrogen agonist in one or more tissues and as an estrogen antagonist in one or more other estrogen target organs
	  - Tamoxifen is a partial estrogen agonist in breast and is used to treat and prevent breast cancer
	  - Clomiphene antagonizes estrogen and stimulates secretion of follicle-stimulating hormone and luteinizing hormone and is used for the induction of ovulation
	  - Raloxifene is approved for use in the prevention and treatment of osteoporosis

Uterine stimulants	- Oxytocin: A natural hormone that is generally considered to be the drug of choice for inducing labor at term - Misoprostol: A prostaglandin analogue that stimulates uterine smooth muscle - Ergonovine, methylergonovine: Stimulate uterine smooth muscle. They are capable of shortening the final stage of labor and aid in the reduction of postpartum bleeding.
Tocolytics	- Terbutaline: a β_2-adrenoceptor agonist that relaxes uterine smooth muscle - Mg^{2+}: Relaxes smooth muscle and is also used for preeclampsia

ANDROGENS, STEROIDS, AND DRUGS FOR ERECTILE DYSFUNCTION

Androgens and anabolic steroids	- Testosterone, nandrolone, methandrostenolone, oxandrolone
	  - Indications: Used to stimulate appetite and muscle mass in persons with advanced malignancy or other conditions characterized by advanced malnutrition
	  - Often abused by athletes trying to build muscle mass
	  - Adverse effects: Fluid retention, changes in cholesterol levels that may contribute to increased risk of atherosclerosis and coronary disease

Antiandrogens	• Flutamide
	  ◦ Mechanism: A nonsteroidal androgen receptor antagonist that inhibits androgen binding to its nuclear receptor
	  ◦ Indication: Prostate cancer; induces prostatic regression
	• Finasteride
	  ◦ Mechanism: A 5α-reductase inhibitor that blocks the conversion of testosterone to dihydrotestosterone
	  ◦ Indication: Benign prostatic hyperplasia

Drugs used in the treatment of erectile dysfunction	• Sildenafil, vardenafil, tadalafil
	  ◦ Mechanism: Inhibition of the degradation of cyclic guanosine monophosphate (cGMP)-phosphodiesterase-5. This enzyme facilitates the release of nitric oxide and smooth muscle relaxation of the corpus cavernosa, resulting in erection.
	  ◦ Indication: Erectile dysfunction
	  ◦ Contraindications: Patients with angina who are taking nitrates
	  ◦ Adverse effects: Headache, flushing, priapism

THYROID DRUGS

Thyroid agonists	• Levothyroxine ◦ Indication: Hypothyroidism

Antithyroid drugs	• Thioamides: Propylthiouracil (PTU), methimazole
	  ◦ Mechanism: Inhibit thyroid hormone synthesis
	  ◦ Adverse effects: Dermatitis, vasculitis, agranulocytosis
	• Iodine
	  ◦ Mechanism: Temporary inhibition of thyroid hormone synthesis

Drugs used for thyroid storm	• Iodide • β-blockers (inhibit peripheral conversion and are cardio-protective from tachycardia and arrhythmias) • Ipodate (radiocontrast media; inhibits peripheral conversion) • Corticosteroids • Thioamides

DRUGS THAT AFFECT CALCIUM HOMEOSTASIS

Bisphosphonates	• Alendronate, risedronate, ibandronate
	  ◦ Mechanism: Inhibition of osteoclast bone resorption
	  ◦ Indications: Hypercalcemia, postmenopausal osteoporosis
	  ◦ Adverse effects: Dysphagia, esophagitis, PUD
	  ◦ Contraindication: Hypocalcemia

| **Calcitonin** | • Mechanism: Decreases bone resorption
• Indications: Acute reduction of hypercalcemia; not for long-term use |

DIABETES DRUGS

Insulin	Type	Onset (h)	Peak (h)	Duration (h)
	Lispro	< 0.25	0.5–1.5	< 5
	Insulin	0.5–0.75	2–4	5–7
	Neutral protamine Hagedorn (NPH), Lente	1–4	6–14	18–24
	Ultralente	4–6	18–26	> 24
	Glargine	> 4	None	> 24

| **Sulfonylureas** | • Glyburide, glipizide, glimepiride
   ○ Mechanism: Stimulation of insulin release from the pancreatic β-cells
   ○ Indication: Type 2 diabetes
   ○ Adverse effect: Hypoglycemia |

| **Metformin** | • Mechanism: Inhibits gluconeogenesis and sensitizes peripheral insulin receptors for increased glucose uptake
• Indication: Type 2 diabetes
• Adverse effects: Gastrointestinal (GI) upset, lactic acidosis
• Contraindications: Patients with renal or hepatic disease |

| **Thiazolidinediones** | • Pioglitazone, rosiglitazone
   ○ Mechanism: Increased peripheral insulin sensitivity; will not cause hypoglycemia
   ○ Indications: Type 2 diabetes; can also be used with insulin in type 1 diabetes mellitus
   ○ Adverse effect: Hepatotoxicity |

| **α-Glucosidase inhibitors** | • Acarbose
   ○ Mechanism: Inhibits absorption of glucose
   ○ Indication: Type 2 diabetes
   ○ Adverse effects: Gas, GI upset, diarrhea |

Topic **9**

Herbs and Vitamins

Must **Knows**

● Properties of useful herbal preparations

● Therapeutic use of fat-soluble and water-soluble vitamins

Important herbal preparations	• Echinacea comes from the purple coneflower. It appears to stimulate the number and activity of immune cells in the body. Its major uses have been in the treatment of upper respiratory viral symptoms. Its efficacy has not been established, but it appears to be very safe.
	• Feverfew is a common European composite herb that is used for the treatment of migraine headaches. Its efficacy has also not been established. It should be avoided in pregnancy and lactation.
	• Ginkgo biloba leaf extract is reputed to enhance cognitive function and is used in memory loss, dementia, and cerebrovascular insufficiency; a number of well-designed clinical trials indicate modest benefit in Alzheimer's disease
	• Kava has been used for short-term treatment of anxiety. Prolonged or excessive use may create psychological dependency and health problems.
	• Saw palmetto is used to treat benign prostatic hypertrophy (BPH) and is a well-tolerated alternative to finasteride for long-term treatment of BPH
	• St. John's wort is probably effective for mild to moderate depression. A major concern is its numerous herb–drug interactions mediated by its induction of the cytochrome P450 enzyme system.
Therapeutic use of fat-soluble vitamins	• Vitamin A
	○ Mechanism: Essential for the proper maintenance of the functional and structural integrity of epithelial cells
	○ Deficiency: night-blindness, xerophthalmia, dermatitis, immunosuppression
	○ Toxicity: Drowsiness, headache, vomiting

- Vitamin D
  - Mechanism: Conversion to 1,25-dihydroxycholecalciferol → stimulates gut absorption of calcium and phosphate and bone resorption
  - Deficiency: Rickets, osteomalacia
  - Toxicity: Hypercalcemia, nausea, stupor, nephropathy
  - Indication: Osteoporosis
- Vitamin K
  - Mechanism: Cofactor for synthesis of clotting factors II, VII, IX, X
  - Deficiency: Increased PT
  - Indications: Increased PT attributable to warfarin administration

Therapeutic use of water-soluble vitamins	- B_1 (thiamine): Beriberi, alcoholism - B_3 (niacin): Pellagra; high doses also inhibit lipolysis and may be used as treatment for hyperlipidemia - B_6 (pyridoxine): Supplement during isoniazid therapy - B_{12}: Pernicious anemia - Folate: Megaloblastic anemia; used to prevent neural tube defects by administering during pregnancy

Topic **10**

Toxicology

Must Knows

- Common poisons and their treatment
- Drug over dosage and treatment

ENVIRONMENTAL TOXICOLOGY

Lead poisoning	- Acute effects: Abdominal colic, encephalopathy leading to irritability and seizures - Chronic: Peripheral neuropathy leading to motor dysfunction, and wrist drop and foot drop; anorexia; developmental delay

- Microcytic hypochromic anemia by inhibition of alpha linoleic acid (ALA) dehydratase and ferrochelatase; basophilic stippling is also seen on smear
- Lead lines at the tooth–gum junction
- Lead lines at the epiphysis of long bones (do not confuse with open growth plates of children)
- Treatment: Calcium ethylenediaminetetraacetic acid (Ca EDTA), dimercaprol, succimer, or penicillamine

Carbon monoxide	• Binds to hemoglobin tighter than oxygen
	• Clinical findings: Headache, mental status changes, tachycardia, cherry-red skin
	• Treatment: Removal from exposure plus 100% O_2 (consider hyperbaric therapy)

Solvents (cleaners, glues, benzene, toluene)	• Acute exposure: Central nervous system (CNS) depression, nausea, vertigo, headache
	• Chronic: Hepatotoxicity, nephrotoxicity, CNS atrophy

Organophosphates (malathion, parathion)	• Mechanism: Inhibits acetylcholinesterase (AchE)
	• Clinical findings: Pinpoint pupils, sweating, salivation, lacrimation, bronchospasm, vomiting, diarrhea, fasciculations, paralysis, respiratory failure
	• Treatment: Atropine, pralidoxime
	NOTE: CHEMICAL WARFARE AGENTS (SARIN, VX, TABUN) ACT SIMILARLY AND ARE TREATED SIMILARLY.

Methanol	• Clinical findings: Blindness; acidosis
	• Treatment: Bicarbonate, fomepizole, dialysis

Ethylene glycol	• Clinical findings: Formation of calcium oxalate stones
	• Treatment: Alcohol, fomepizole, dialysis

Nitrite poisoning	• Clinical findings: Headache, dizziness, tachycardia
	• Treatment: Methylene blue

Cyanide	• Mechanism: Inhibits electron transport; can occur as result of excessive sodium nitroprusside
	• Clinical findings: Almond smell, cyanosis, unconsciousness, seizures
	• Treatment:
	◦ Nitrites: Convert hemoglobin to methemoglobin, which has a higher affinity for cyanide
	◦ Sodium thiosulfate: Converts cyanomethemoglobin to methemoglobin and thiocyanate, which is excreted in the kidney
	◦ Methylene blue: Converts methemoglobin back to hemoglobin

OVERDOSES AND TREATMENTS

Acetaminophen	• Mechanism: Hepatic necrosis • Clinical findings: Nausea, vomiting, diarrhea, jaundice • Treatment: Acetylcysteine
Aspirin	• Acute findings: Respiratory alkalosis leading to metabolic acidosis • Chronic findings: Headache, dizziness, tinnitus, nausea, vomiting, diarrhea, gastrointestinal (GI) bleeding • Treatment: Alkalinize urine, dialysis
Iron	• Findings: Nausea, vomiting, GI bleeding, lethargy, vascular collapse • Treatment: Chelation with deferoxamine
Heparin	• Treatment: Protamine sulfate
Warfarin	• Treatment: Vitamin K, fresh frozen plasma
Benzodiazepines	• Treatment: Flumazenil
Opioids	• Clinical triad: Pinpoint pupils, unconsciousness, respiratory depression • Treatment: Naloxone, respiratory support

Abbreviations

1°	primary
2°	secondary
2,3-DPG	diphosphoglycerate
5-HT	5-hydroxytriptamine
α1-AT	α1-antitrypsin
Ab	antibody
ABL	antigen-binding lymphocyte
ACE	angiotensin-converting enzyme
ACh	acetylcholine
AChE	acetylcholinesterase
ACL	anterior cruciate ligament
ACTH	adrenocorticotropic hormone
AD	autosomal dominant
ADCC	antibody-dependent cell-mediated cytotoxicity
ADH	antidiuretic hormone
ADHD	attention deficit hyperactivity disorder
ADP	adenosine diphosphate
AF	atrial fibrillation
AFP	alpha fetoprotein
AIDS	acquired immunodeficiency syndrome
ALA	alpha linoleic acid
ALL	acute lymphoblastic leukemia
ALP	alkaline phosphatase
ALS	amyotrophic lateral sclerosis
ALT	alanine aminotransferase
AML	acute myelogenous leukemia
AMP	adenosine monophosphate
ANP	atrial natriuretic peptide
ANS	autonomic nervous system
APC	antigen-presenting cell
APC	adenomatosis polyposis coli/antigen-presenting cell
apo	apolipoprotein; apoenzyme
AR	autosomal recessive
ARB	angiotensin receptor blocker
ARDS	adult respiratory distress syndrome
AST	aspartate aminotransferase
ATI	angiotensin I
ATII	angiotensin II
ATP	adenosine triphosphate
ATPase	adenosine triphosphate
AV	atrioventricular

AVM	arteriovenous malformation
AZT	azidothymidine
BA	bioavailability
BBB	blood–brain barrier
BCG	Bacillus Calmette-Guérin
BMPR	bone morphogenetic protein receptor
BMR	basal metabolic rate
BP	blood pressure
BPH	benign prostatic hypertrophy
BSE	bovine spongiform encephalopathy
BUN	blood urea nitrogen
CABG	coronary artery bypass graft
CAD	coronary artery disease
CA EDTA	calcium ethylenediaminetetraacetic acid
CAG	calcium gluconate
CALLA	common acute lymphoblastic leukocyte antigen
cAMP	cyclic adenosine monophosphate
CAT	choline acetyltransferase
CCK	cholecystokinin
CD4/8	cluster of differentiation 4/8
cDNA	complementary DNA
CEA	carcinoembryonic antigen
CF	clinical features
CFTR	cystic fibrosis transmembrane conductance regulator
cGMP	cyclic guanosine monophosphate
CH	constant heavy (protein chain)
CHF	congestive heart failure
CIN	cervical intraepithelial neoplasia
CIS	carcinoma in situ
CK	creatine kinase
CK-MB	creatine kinase muscle brain isoenzyme
CL	clearance; constant light
CLL	chronic lymphocytic leukemia
CMI	cell-mediated immunity
CML	chronic myelogenous leukemia
CMV	cytomegalovirus
CN	cranial nerve
CNS	central nervous system
CoA	coenzyme A
COMT	catechol-O-methyl transferase
COPD	chronic obstructive pulmonary disease
COX	cyclooxygenase
Cp	desired plasma concentration
CPT	carnitine palmitoyltransferase
CRH	corticotropin-releasing hormone
c/s	cycles per second
CSF	cerebrospinal fluid
CT	computed tomography
CTG	cardiotocogram
CVA	cardiovascular accident
CVS	cardiovascular system

CXCR	chemokine coreceptor
CXR	chest x-ray
DA	ductus arteriosus
Da	daltons
DAD	diffuse alveolar damage
DCC	deleted in colorectal carcinoma
DDAVP	desmopressin
DHEA-S	dehydroepiandrosterone-sulfate
DHT	dihydrotestosterone
DIC	disseminated intravascular coagulopathy
DIT	diiodotyrosine
DJD	degenerative joint disease
DM	diabetes mellitus
DMARDS	disease-modifying antirheumatic drugs
DNA	deoxyribonucleic acid
DRG	dorsal root ganglion
DS- (ss-) DNA	double-stranded (single-stranded) deoxyribonucleic acid
DST	distal straight tubule
DTaP	diphtheria, tetanus toxoids, and acellular pertussis
DVT	deep vein thrombosis
DX	diagnosis
EBV	Epstein Barr virus
EC	potency
ECF	extracellular fluid
ED	emergency department
ED50	median effective dose
EDV	end-diastolic volume
EEG	electrocardiogram
EGD	esophagogastroduodenoscopy
EKG	electrocardiogram
ELISA	enzyme-linked immunoabsorbent assay
EM	electron microscopy
EMG	electromyogram
EPI	epidemiology
ER	emergency room
ERV	expiratory reserve volume
ESR	erythrocyte sedimentation rate
ESV	end-systolic volume
ETI	endotracheal intubation
EtOH	ethanol/ethyl alcohol
EWS	Ewing sarcoma
EXT	external
FAB	French-American-British
FAD	flavin adenine dinucleotide
FC	constant fragment
FEV	forced expiratory volume
FF	filtration fraction
FFP	fresh frozen plasma
FMN	flavin mononucleotide
FSH	follicle-stimulating hormone
FVC	forced vital capacity

FX	function
G6PD	glucose 6-phosphate dehydrogenase deficiency
GABA	γaminobutyric acid
GALT	Gut-associated lymphoid tissue
GBM	glomerular basement membrane
Gen	general
GERD	gastroesophageal reflux disease
GFR	glomerular filtration rate
GH	growth hormone
GHRH	growth hormone–releasing hormone
GI	gastrointestinal
GIP	gastric inhibitory peptide
glc	glucose
GLN	glomerulonephritis
GM-CSF	granulocyte macrophage colony-stimulating factor
GMP	guanosine monophosphate
GnRH	gonadotropin-releasing hormone
GRP	gastrin-releasing peptide
GSH	glutathione
GTP	guanosine 5′-triphosphate
G/U	genitourinary
HAART	highly active antiretroviral therapy
HACEK	*Haemophilus parainfluenzae, Actinobacillus, Cardiobacterium, Eikenella, Kingella*
HAV	hepatitis A virus
Hb	hemoglobin
HBV	hepatitis B virus
hCG	human chorionic gonadotropin
HCT	hematocrit
HCTZ	hydrochlorothiazide
HCV	hepatitis C virus
HDL	high-density lipoprotein
HER	human c-erb 2
HEV	hepatitis E virus
Hg	Hemoglobin
HGPRT	hypoxanthine-guanine phosphoribosyltransferase
HHV	human herpes virus
HI	humoral immunity
HIV	human immunodeficiency virus
HL	Hodgkin's lymphoma
HLA	histocompatibility locus antigen
HMG-CoA	beta-hydroxy-β-methylglutaryl-coenzyme A
HMP	hexose monophosphate
HNPCC	hereditary non-polyposis colon cancer
HPV	human papilloma virus
HR	heart rate
HSV	herpes simplex virus
HTLV	human lymphotropic virus
HTN	hypertension
HUS	hemolytic uremic syndrome
Hx	history
ICAM	intracellular adhesion molecules

ICP	intracranial pressure
ICF	intracellular fluid
IF	immunofluorescence
IGF	insulin-like growth factor
IFN	interferon
Ig	immunoglobulin
IL	interleukin
IMA	inferior mesenteric artery
IMP	inosine 5'-monophosphate
INR	international normalized ratio
IP3	inositol triphosphate
IRV	inspiratory reserve volume
ITP	idiopathic thrombocytopenic purpura
IVC	inferior vena cava
IVDA	intravenous drug administration
JG	juxtaglomerular
JVD	jugular venous distension
KAR	killer-activating receptor
KD	concentration
KIR	killing inhibitory receptor
L	liter
Labs	laboratory tests
LAD	left anterior descending artery
LCT	lateral corticospinal tract
LDL	low-density lipoprotein
LFA	leukocyte function associated
LH	luteinizing hormone
LLQ	left lower quadrant
LMCA	left main coronary artery
LMN	lower motor neuron
LMWH	low-molecular-weight heparin
LP	lumbar puncture
LPS	lipopolysaccharide
LR	lateral rectus muscle
LRI	lower respiratory tract infection
LV	left ventricle
m	mitosis
MAC	membrane attack complex
MAO	monoamine oxidase
MAP	mean arterial pressure
MCP	monocyte chemotactic protein
MCV	mean cell volume
MD	macula densa
mdrI	multidrug resistance
MEN	multiple endocrine neoplasia
MESNA	mercaptoethane sulfonate
MHC	major histocompatability complex
MI	myocardial infarction
MIF	Müllerian inhibitory factor
MIP	macrophage inflammatory protein
MIT	monoiodotyrosine

MLCK	myosin light-chain kinase
MMR	measles, mumps, rubella
MRI	magnetic resonance imaging
MRSA	methicillin resistant *S. aureus*
MS	multiple sclerosis
M/S	musculoskeletal
MSUD	maple syrup urine disease
MTP	metatarsophalangeal
MV	mitral valve
MYC	oncogen called MYC
MYCN	MYC oncogene of N variant
NAD	nicotinamide adenine dinucleotide
NADPH	nicotinamide adenosine dinucleotide phosphate
NE	norepinephrine
NHL	non-Hodgkin's lymphoma
NK	natural killer
NMJ	neuromuscular junction
NOS	nitric oxide synthase
NPH	neutral protamine Hagedorn
NRTI	nucleoside reverse transcriptase inhibitors
Ns	nonspecific
NSAID	nonsteroidal anti-inflammatory drug
NSGCT	nonseminomatous germ cell tumor
OCD	obsessive-compulsive disorder
PABA	p-aminobenzoic acid
PAF	platelet activating factor
PAH	para-aminohippuric acid
PALS	periarteriolar lymphatic sheaths
PAMP	pathogen-associated molecular patterns
p-ANCA	perinuclear anticytoplasmic antibody
PAP	pulmonary artery pressure
PAS	periodic acid Schiff reagent
PAT	paroxysmal atrial tachycardia
PCAT	phosphatidylcholine cholesterol transferase
PCN	penicillin
PCR	polymerase chain reaction
PDA	patent ductus arteriosus
PDE	phosphodiesterase
PDGF	platelet-derived growth factor
PE	physical examination; pulmonary embolism
PECAM	platelet-endothelial cell adhesion molecules
PFT	pulmonary function test
PG	pathology
PGE	prostaglandin E
PID	pelvic inflammatory disease
PIPS	proximal interphalangeal joint
PKD	polycystic kidney disease
PKU	phenylketonuria
PMN	polymorphonuclear
PND	paroxysmal nocturnal dyspnea
PNET	primitive neuroectodermal tumor

PNS	peripheral nervous system
Pol	polymerase
POMC	proopiomelanocortin
PPD	purified protein derivative
PrP	prion protein
PRPP	5-phosphoribosyl-1-pyrophosphate
PSA	Prostate-specific antigen
PT	physical therapy; prothrombin time
PTEN	phosphatase and tensin homolog
PTH	parathyroid hormone
PTHrP	parathyroid hormone–related peptide
PTT	partial thromboplastin time
PTU	propylthiouracil
PUD	peptic ulcer disease
PVC	premature ventricular contraction
RA	rheumatoid arthritis
RANTES	regulated on activation, normal T-cell expressed and secreted
RAS	rat-associated sarcoma
RB1	retinoblastoma 1
RBF	renal blood flow
RCA	right coronary artery
RDS	respiratory distress syndrome
rER	rough endoplasmic reticulum
RFLP	restriction fragment length polymorphism
rG-CSF	recombinant granulocyte colony-stimulating factor
RNA	ribonucleic acid
ROS	reactive oxygen species
RPF	renal plasma flow
R/S	respiratory system
RSV	respiratory syncytial virus
RU-486	mifepristone
RUQ	right upper quadrant
RV	residual volume; right ventricle
RVH	right ventricular hypertrophy
Rx	treatment
s	s phase
S1 (S2,S3)	first (second, third) heart sounds
S&S	signs and symptoms
SA	sinoatrial
SBE	subacute bacterial endocarditis
SCFE	slipped capital femoral epiphysis
SCID	severe combined immunodeficiency disease
sER	smooth endoplasmic reticulum
SERMS	selective estrogen receptor modulators
SGLT	sodium glucose cotransporter
SIADH	syndrome of inappropriate antidiuretic hormone
SLE	systemic lupus erythematosus
SR	sarcoplasmic reticulum
SS-A	Sjögren syndrome (antigen) A
SSRI	selective serotonin reuptake inhibitor
ss-RNA	single-stranded ribonucleic acid

STD	sexually transmitted disease
SV	stroke volume
SVC	superior vena cava
SVT	supraventricular tachycardia
$t_{1/2}$	half-life
T3	triiodothyronine
T4	thyroxine
TB	tuberculosis
TBG	thyroid-binding globulin
TBW	total body water
TCA	tricyclic antidepressants
TCP	thrombocytopenia
TCR	T-cell receptor
TdT	terminal deoxynucleotidyl transferase
TE	tracheoesophageal
TF/P	tubule fluid-to-plasma ratio
TFT	thyroid function test
TIBC	total iron-binding capacity
TLC	total lung capacity
TLR	toll-like receptor
TNF	tumor necrosis factor
TNM	tumor, node, metastasis
TP53	tumor protein 53
TPR	total peripheral resistance
tRNA	transfer ribonucleic acid
TRH	thyroid-releasing hormone
TSH	thyroid-stimulating hormone
TSI	Thyroid-stimulating immunoglobulin
TRAP	tartrate resistant acid phosphatase
TTP	thrombotic thrombocytopenic purpura
TTX	tetrodotoxin
TV	tidal volume
UDP	uridine diphosphate
UMN	upper motor neuron
URI	upper respiratory infection
URTI	upper respiratory tract infection
UTI	urinary tract infection
UTP	uridine 5′-triphosphate
VD	volume of distribution
VF	ventricular failure
VH	variable heavy
VHL	von Hippel-Lindau
VIP	vasoactive intestinal peptide
VL	ventrolateral; variable light (protein chain)
VLDL	very low-density lipoprotein
VMA	vanillylmandelic acid
VPL	ventroposterolateral
V/Q	ratio of alveolar ventilation to pulmonary blood flow
VDRL	venereal disease research laboratory (test)
VSD	ventricular septal defect
VT	ventricular tachycardia

VuIN	vulvar intraepithelial neoplasia
vWF	von Willebrand factor
VX	U.S. Army code for deadly nerve poison
VZV	varicella zoster virus
WAIHA	warm autoimmune hemolytic anemia
WPW	Wolff-Parkinson-White syndrome
WT (1,2)	Wilms tumor
XLR	X-linked recessive
XR	X-ray

Index

Page numbers in *italics* denote figures; those followed by a *t* denote tables.